Coercion in Community Mental Health Care

International Perspectives

Edited by

Andrew Molodyns
Consultant Psychiatrist,
Oxford Health NHS Foundation Trust, UK;
Honorary Clinical Senior Lecturer,
Oxford University, UK

Jorun Rugkåsa
Senior Researcher,
Health Services Research Unit,
Akershus University Hospital, Lørenskog, Norway;
Senior Researcher,
Social Psychiatry Group, Department of Psychiatry,
University of Oxford, Warneford Hospital, UK

Tom Burns
Professor Emeritus of Social Psychiatry,
University of Oxford, Department of Psychiatry,
Warneford Hospital, UK;
Fellow Emeritus of Kellogg College,
University of Oxford, UK

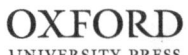

OXFORD
UNIVERSITY PRESS

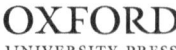

OXFORD

UNIVERSITY PRESS

Great Clarendon Street, Oxford, OX2 6DP,
United Kingdom

Oxford University Press is a department of the University of Oxford.
It furthers the University's objective of excellence in research, scholarship,
and education by publishing worldwide. Oxford is a registered trade mark of
Oxford University Press in the UK and in certain other countries

Published in the United States of America by Oxford University Press
198 Madison Avenue, New York, NY 10016, United States of America

British Library Cataloguing in Publication Data

Data available

Library of Congress Control Number: 2016932535

ISBN 978-0-19-878806-5

Printed in Great Britain by
Ashford Colour Press Ltd, Gosport, Hampshire

Coercion in Community Mental Health Care

International Perspectives

For Cyd, Poppy, and Helen
—A.M.

For Danny
—J.R.

Acknowledgements

We are grateful to many people for their assistance in this endeavour. First, Lauren Dunn and Peter Stevenson at OUP have at all times been unstinting in their help and support and have helped to make the process pleasant and fun. The book would have been longer in coming and much less polished without them.

We are grateful to all the chapter authors who met different kinds of challenges to bring together such a wide-ranging and rich body of information and insights. We had heard 'horror stories' regarding the process of editing books but our contributors made our lives easy—we are grateful!

The volume has been a long time in preparation and many people have supported us. A.M. would like to thank his clinical team in Didcot for their hard work, clinical excellence, and ongoing support and humanity during the process and Anneliese Guerin-LeTendre for her wisdom and insights. Most of all he would like to thank Helen for putting up with him during the last few months of preparation.

Special thanks must go to Jane Wood, who has diligently read through this whole volume to ensure its grammatical quality, while at the same time being endlessly helpful and supportive.

Contents

Contributors

Atalay Alem
Professor, Department of Psychiatry, School of Medicine, College of Health Sciences; Consultant Psychiatrist, Amanuel Specialized Mental Hospital, Addis Ababa, Ethiopia

Mariam Ali
Imperial College London, UK

Beth Angell
Associate Professor, School of Social Work, Rutgers, State University of New Jersey, USA

Tom Burns
Professor Emeritus of Social Psychiatry, University of Oxford, Department of Psychiatry, Warneford Hospital, UK; Fellow Emeritus of Kellogg College, University of Oxford, UK

Krysia Canvin
Honorary Research Fellow, Department of Psychiatry, University of Oxford, Oxford Health NHS Foundation Trust, UK

Frank Huang-Chih Chou
President, Taiwanese Society of Psychiatry, Taiwan; Professor, Graduate Institute of Health Care, Meiho University, Taiwan; Medical Advisor, Superintendent Office, Kaohsiung Municipal Kai-Syuan Psychiatric Hospital, Kaohsiung, Taiwan

John Dawson
Professor, Faculty of Law, University of Otago, New Zealand

John Gray
Adjunct Professor, Department of Psychiatry, Western University, Ontario, Canada

Angelo Fioritti
Medical Director, Azienda USL Bologna, Italy

Tania Gergel
Visiting Research Fellow in Philosophy and Psychiatry, Department of Psychological Medicine, Institute of Psychiatry, Psychology and Neuroscience, King's College London, UK; Visiting Research Fellow in Ancient Philosophy, Department of Classics, King's College London, UK

Steve Kisely
Professor, Discipline of Psychiatry, School of Medicine, The University of Queensland, Princess Alexandra Hospital, Queensland, Australia; Professor, Departments of Psychiatry, Community Health and Epidemiology, Dalhousie University, Nova Scotia, Canada; Professor, Population and Social Health Research Programme, Griffith University, Queensland, Australia

Catherine Manning
Psychiatric Registrar, South London and Maudsley NHS Foundation Trust, UK

Thomas Marcacci
Psychologist, Department of Mental Health, Azienda USL Bologna, Italy

Andrew Molodynski
Consultant Psychiatrist, Oxford Health
NHS Foundation Trust, UK;
Honorary Clinical Senior Lecturer,
Oxford University, UK

Stéphane Morandi
Service of Community Psychiatry,
Department of Psychiatry, University
Hospital of Lausanne, Switzerland

Anthony J. O'Brien
Senior Lecturer, School of Nursing,
Faculty of Medical and Health Sciences,
The University of Auckland, New
Zealand; Nurse Specialist (Liaison
Psychiatry), Auckland District Health
Board, Auckland, New Zealand

Richard O'Reilly
Professor, Department of Psychiatry,
Western University, London, Ontario,
Canada; Professor of Psychiatry,
Northern Ontario School of Medicine,
Ontario, Canada; Director of Psychiatric
Research, Parkwood Institute, St Joseph's
Health Care, London, Ontario, Canada

Soumitra Pathare
Coordinator, Centre for Mental Health
Law and Policy, Indian Law Society,
Pune, India; Consultant Psychiatrist,
Ruby Hall Clinic, Pune, India

David Pilgrim
Honorary Professor of Health and Social
Policy, University of Liverpool UK and
Visiting Professor of Clinical Psychology,
University of Southampton, UK

B. N. Raveesh
Director, Dharwad Institute of Mental
Health and Neurosciences (DIMHANS),
Dharwad, India

Genevra Richardson
Professor of Law, Dickson Poon School
of Law, King's College London, UK

Diana Rose
Service User Research Enterprise
(SURE), PO34 Institute of Psychiatry,
Psychology & Neuroscience, King's
College London, de Crespigny Park,
London SE5 8AF, UK

Jorun Rugkåsa
Senior Researcher, Health Services
Research Unit, Akershus University
Hospital, Lørenskog, Norway; Senior
Researcher, Department of Psychiatry,
University of Oxford, Warneford
Hospital, UK

Swaran P. Singh
Head of Division, Mental Health and
Wellbeing, Warwick Medical School,
University of Warwick, UK; Honorary
Consultant Psychiatrist, Birmingham
and Solihull Mental Health Foundation
Trust, UK

Stefan Sjöström
Associate Professor in Social Work,
Department of Social Work, Umeå
University, Sweden

George Szmukler
Emeritus Professor of Psychiatry
and Society, Institute of Psychiatry,
Psychology and Neuroscience, King's
College London, UK

Ksenija Yeeles
Research Fellow, Department of
Psychiatry, University of Oxford, UK

Hui Ching Wu
Professor at Department of Social
Work, National Taiwan University,
Taipei, Taiwan

Chapter 1

Introduction

Jorun Rugkåsa, Andrew Molodynski,
and Tom Burns

Why this book?

Coercion in psychiatry is often associated with the large, impersonal, and sometimes inhumane asylums of the late nineteenth and early twentieth centuries. However, the vast majority of people with severe and enduring mental illness are now cared for in the community. This is either because mental health hospitals are few or nonexistent where people live, or because current policy in their country directs these services to take place in a community setting. As a result, most of the coercive practices used with people with mental illness occur outside hospitals.

Power imbalances in mental health care have always been a cause of controversy. There is a difficult balance to strike between respecting autonomy and ensuring that those in need of treatment and support are provided for. While mental health professionals believe coercive practices are necessary to help patients or ensure safety, others may perceive this as surveillance and social control. Both the World Health Organization and the United Nations suggest that some coercive practices within psychiatry may violate people's fundamental human rights. The growing service-user movements in many parts of the world argue in a similar vein, advocating for individuals' rights to retain control over their own lives, even when unwell. Such criticisms have been particularly prominent in those parts of the world where compulsion is exercised on behalf of the state and regulated by mental health legislation. In the research literature this is often called *formal coercion*. While this has traditionally taken place in hospitals, it is now progressively being moved to community settings.

Debates on legal compulsion notwithstanding, many of the coercive practices in the community are not regulated by law. Such practices, often referred to as *informal coercion*, may be imposed on patients by health-care professionals, family members, traditional healers, community leaders, housing providers, and financial management systems. They can also stem from social norms and cultural expectations more widely and are usually linked with how mental illness is understood in different cultural traditions and what are considered to be the best methods for treating it and for helping the patient and those around him or her.

Despite the often vigorous debate about the benefits or otherwise of coercion, there has been relatively little research into the extent, effect, and experience of coercive practices in community care. The evidence that does exist is patchy. In the era of evidence-based medicine, this is both remarkable and concerning. Despite mental ill-health being increasingly recognized as a global issue, almost no research exists on either formal or informal community coercion outside Western societies. What we hope to achieve with this book is to bring together what is currently known internationally, to identify what is not known, and to highlight some of the clinical, sociological, ethical, and legal issues raised.

What is coercion?

Conceptualization of coercion

The *Oxford English Dictionary* defines coercion as 'constraint, restraint, compulsion; the application of force to control the action of a voluntary agent'. We readily accept coercion in many aspects of life (mandatory education, taxation, or restricted liberty for those who break the law, for example) when it is considered beneficial for individuals or society in that it represents an improvement on the 'baseline' (Wertheimer 1987). Coercion is rare in health-care settings. It is justified by its benefits for health and safety, but this is complicated because the fundamental principle of patient autonomy is breached. In order to test whether coercion can be justified by the benefits it accrues for psychiatric patients it has been conceptualized and operationalized in different ways.

As already mentioned, coercion may be considered either as formal compulsion, which includes measures sanctioned by mental health law, or as informal coercion, including all other pressures applied to encourage adherence to treatment or to change the patient's behaviour in other ways. While compulsion is defined by law and is thus relatively easy to measure, informal coercion has proved harder to operationalize in research efforts. Monahan et al. (2005) applied the notion of 'leverage' to measure some aspects of informal coercion. Leverage involves making, or proposing to make, the provision of services conditional on the patient's adherence to treatment. Monahan's study found that half of public mental health patients in the USA had experienced at least one of the measured forms of leverage. This study brought the prevalence of informal coercive practices in mental health services to the consciousness of the research community.

To gain a better understanding of the complex social dimensions of coercive practices, researchers often distinguish between its subjective and objective elements. Coercion can be perceived both as what is *done to someone* and what is *experienced by someone*: 'it is thus both an objective set of actions and a subjectively experienced result of particular actions' (Hoge et al. 1993, p. 282). The notion of *perceived coercion* has increasingly been applied in efforts to conceptualize coercion and it represents what the patient[1] experiences to be coercive. It is an important perspective because it

---

[1] The term for those receiving mental health care is contested and 'patient', 'client', 'service user', and, indeed, 'consumer' are all used. Terminology is particularly problematic when referring to people who are receiving treatment against their own will. We use 'patient' in this Introduction, but in the subsequent chapters several of the authors have chosen different terms.

has been found that even when treated voluntarily patients may feel that they are being coerced or that their freedom to make decisions is constrained (Hoge et al. 1997). Voluntary patients who have been subjected to compulsion in the past may interpret statements that they 'should' do something as more pressurizing than patients who have never been compelled. Perceived coercion may therefore reduce patients' sense of autonomy (Stensrud et al. 2015) and shape their treatment decisions and pathways through care systems by acting as a barrier to help-seeking (Van Dorn et al. 2006). As a result, it could potentially delay presentation and increase the likelihood of involuntary hospitalization.

In the literature, a wide range of terminology is used to describe coercion in the community. Formal coercion is usually referred to by the name of local legislation such as 'community treatment orders' (CTOs; this is the most common term and the one applied in this volume), 'mandated outpatient commitment', 'involuntary outpatient commitment', and more recently the perhaps misleading 'assisted outpatient treatment'. Informal coercion is variously described as 'treatment pressures', 'therapeutic limit setting', 'influencing behaviours', or 'leverage'. Many of these terms are used interchangeably and there is no consensus on what the different terms signify or which ones best reflect the phenomenon under study. A further difficulty in researching 'coercion' is that it is simultaneously an analytical term applied by researchers *and* an emotive notion with clear intuitive meanings to those at the giving and at the receiving ends. These meanings may differ: what is considered an acceptable form of influence by one person may be understood as coercive by another. While there often is a cultural dimension to what is seen as coercive, there will always be different opinions within a cultural tradition. Coercion is thus a moralized concept that is sensitive to context (Hoge et al. 1993). It touches on a wide range of discourses and has been investigated from medical, social, cultural, personal, legal, and ethical perspectives. While this book will present all these perspectives, a common aim of the chapters that follow is to illuminate coercive practices imposed on people with mental illness living in the community, with a particular focus on the services delivered to them (or not).

Community services and informal coercion

The deinstitutionalization of mental health services in many Western countries has led to a huge reduction of beds in psychiatric hospitals and an increase in community services. This process is driven by a number of factors. These include developments in drug therapies making it feasible to treat people while they live in the community, major changes in social attitudes towards the socially disadvantaged, and the financial savings in closing large hospitals and replacing them with the delivery of mixed-economy care with involvement of the state, private, and voluntary sectors. More recently there has been an increasing focus on family caregiving as well as growing pressure from service-user advocates and organizations who challenge the interpretations of needs inherent in professional models of care (Williams 2009).

New models for community services focus on helping patients to manage their symptoms and live fulfilling lives in their own homes despite their mental illness. This presents new challenges for health professionals with regard to patients who do not wish to receive treatment. Non-adherence can result in repeated involuntary readmission to hospital, and this 'revolving door syndrome' can be dramatic and damaging for patients and their families and expensive for services and for the wider community. More assertive forms of service delivery have therefore developed, and these are often delivered via case-management approaches by multidisciplinary teams consisting of psychiatrists, nurses, psychologists, social workers, and support workers (Burns 2004). Many of these services place emphasis on outreach, and professionals become involved in a wide range of patients' daily activities. They also interact with family members and other services with remits for housing, social care, and social security benefits (Szmukler and Appelbaum 2008). In attempts to assist reluctant patients, professionals in these services apply different types (and degrees) of influence or pressure. These have been described as a continuum of increasing restrictiveness spanning from

> ... encouragement or admonition ('That behaviour keeps getting you into trouble'), contingent support or contracting ('Once you manage your medication reliably, we'll see about getting you that job'), involvement of others ('You seem to need help managing your money'), informal coercion ('You can enter the hospital voluntarily, or we will have to commit you') ...

> Neale and Rosenheck (2000, p. 499)

to the use of formal coercion. These new service models have generally been found to improve patients' engagement and clinical outcomes. Assertive community treatment (ACT) is the most intensively researched of these approaches (Marshall and Lockwood 2000).

Formal coercion in the community

Compulsion outside hospitals has been made possible in around 75 jurisdictions (see Box 1.1) over the last four decades with the introduction of various legal regimes for CTOs. In brief, CTOs make adherence to treatment a legal requirement and facilitate rapid admission to hospital when necessary. They may be applied to provide a 'least restrictive alternative' to hospital detention, or they may be seen as 'preventative' of deterioration and hospitalization. CTOs are the most researched form of coercion in the community. The evidence remains contested, but as we will see in Chapter 4, CTOs do not seem to confer benefits to patients or reduce readmission rates despite significantly limiting personal liberty. Despite this they remain the preferred policy solution to the problem of the 'revolving door' phenomenon.

CTOs are complex social interventions, and continue to be the subject of clinical, legal, and ethical debate. They also provide an interesting example of how implementation of this kind of legislation relies to a large extent on the opinion of the individual psychiatrist or health authority. Huge variation has been observed in the use of this legal power between different psychiatrists and hospitals within the same jurisdiction. In order to fully understand how such laws work in practice, there is a need to understand micro-level interactions.

Community coercion at the micro-level

Building trusting relationships with individual patients is central to the job of a mental health professional: coercive practice, it is reported, often results from a failure to do

Box 1.1 Jurisdictions permitting CTOs or extended conditional discharge

Australian states: New South Wales, Northern Territory, Western Australia, South Australia, Queensland, Victoria, Tasmania

Belgium

Canadian provinces and territories: Alberta, British Columbia, Manitoba, Newfoundland and Labrador, Nova Scotia, Ontario, Prince Edward Island, Saskatchewan, Quebec

Denmark

England and Wales

Fiji

France

Germany

Gibraltar

Hong Kong

Israel

Luxembourg

New Zealand

Norway

Portugal

Samoa

Scotland

Spain

Sweden

Swiss cantons: Aargau, Appenzell Inner Rhodes, Appenzell Outer Rhodes, Basel-Landschaft, Basel-Stadt, Bern, Fribourg, Geneva, Glarus, Graubünden, Jura, Lucerne, Neuchâtel, Nidwalden, Obwalden, Sankt Gallen, Schaffhausen, Schwyz, Solothurn, Thurgau, Ticino, Uri, Valais, Vaud, Zug, Zurich

Taiwan

Tonga

US states/district: Alabama, Arizona, Arkansas, California, Colorado, Florida, Georgia, Hawaii, Idaho, Illinois, Indiana, Iowa, Kansas, Kentucky, Louisiana, Maine, Michigan, Minnesota, Mississippi, Missouri, Montana, Nebraska, New Hampshire, New Jersey, New York, North Carolina, North Dakota, Ohio, Oklahoma, Oregon, Pennsylvania, Rhode Island, South Carolina, South Dakota, Texas, Utah, Vermont, Virginia, Washington, West Virginia, Wisconsin, Wyoming, District of Columbia so. Also, it can be difficult to maintain trust when needs to coerce formally or discuss the need for compulsion (Nath et al. 2012). This is recognized by patients receiving community care (Laugharne et al. 2012).

The distinction between what constitutes formal and informal coercion may be unclear to patients as they experience health professionals' roles simultaneously as empowering and controlling—the same people help them, persuade them, and, at times, compel them (Angell and Mahoney 2007). While this is also true in the hospital setting, the consequences may be more pronounced in outpatient services where professionals often are involved across different spheres of patients' lives (Rugkåsa et al. 2014).What is experienced as coercive might, however, depend on what the individual perceives as constituting a legitimate use of authority. Very limited research has investigated the 'personal experiences' within which perceived coercion exists or the socio-cultural *meanings* attached to coercion in the community setting. While leverage and informal coercion are recognized by patients, pre-defined questionnaire items may not fully account for the multiple forms and sources of pressure that influence them. For example, patients can experience considerable internalized pressure arising from socio-cultural expectations about social roles and obligations, such as being a good parent (Canvin et al. 2013), but this is rarely reflected in research.

Family members are often identified as a source of coercion. This may be unsurprising as they have a vested interest in the patient's adherence to treatment. Mental illness can create unusual relationships between services and the families it affects, as patients can be detained against their will with or without the family's cooperation. Even when this leads to improved care, conflicting views occur. Insight into personal experiences of patients, health professionals, and family members has the potential to enhance our understanding of how community coercion unfolds. In those parts of the world where mental health services or mental health legislation is limited or absent, families, communities, and alternative service providers in particular play a prominent role. As will be highlighted in Part 3 of this volume, many of the same processes of informal coercion exist across different continents.

How this book is organized

The potential territory for a book about community coercion is enormous. We have limited its scope to the treatment of adults with severe mental illness. Where appropriate, however, the authors comment on co-morbidity, substance abuse, and other age groups. While the main setting is the community, it has been impossible to focus exclusively on this, particularly where there is a lack of community services or where the demarcation between inpatient and outpatient services is not clear cut.

The book is written so that readers who are particularly interested in some of the topics can read chapters in isolation from each other. To allow this, the authors of each chapter clarify contextual issues and the terminology they use, which means there is a small degree of overlap. The authors also cross-refer to other chapters where this might be helpful to readers.

The aim of the following chapters is to draw together current knowledge about coercion in the community from around the world. In doing so we address a number of questions. What coercive practices take place in the community setting? What are their purposes? Do they work? How are they experienced by those on the giving and the receiving end? How do these practices vary across populations and continents? What ethical issues are raised by community coercion and how is it regulated by law? Collectively, our contributors address these questions from a variety of perspectives, drawing on diverse disciplines such as law, sociology, medicine, anthropology, history, and psychology.

The book is divided into five parts. In Part 1, *Coercion in the community: origins and extent*, Tom Burns (Chapter 2) provides an overview of the shift from hospitals to the community setting. He focuses in particular on how CTOs have emerged—despite a lack of evidence for their effectiveness—and developed in many parts of the world as a response to public concern about patient welfare and public safety. This is followed up in Chapter 3 where John Dawson gives a comparative overview of legal frameworks that surround community compulsion, showing that despite some variation in detail, different CTO legislations overlap considerably in terms of criteria and legal processes.

Part 2, *The evidence*, presents what we know about the effect of coercive practices. Compared with other areas of medicine, there is a relatively modest amount of research in this field so it is possible to discuss it in some detail. Stéphane Morandi (Chapter 4) provides an overview of descriptive and epidemiological studies of CTOs, focusing on the processes and practical applications involved, the characteristics of the people placed on such orders across different jurisdictions, and the inconsistencies in the outcomes observed in these kinds of studies. Steve Kisely (Chapter 5) reviews experimental studies of the effectiveness of CTOs and discusses methodological issues impacting on research design and generalizability. In Chapter 6, Ksenija Yeeles outlines the research measuring outcomes of informal coercion in community care. She shows that, where they are studied, informal coercive practices are heavily used but there is no strong evidence for what predicts experiences of perceived coercion. In the final chapter of Part 2, Diana Rose (Chapter 7) summarizes service-user-led research on coercion in the community. She sets out the case for how such research can provide a different perspective and she provides an outline of how a user-led research programme could be constructed.

Part 3, *The experiences*, is concerned with coercion as a social phenomenon, covering its objective and subjective manifestations and its impact on people's lives. It sheds light on how formal and informal coercion are often intertwined. Stefan Sjöström (Chapter 8) investigates the micro-level enactment of coercion in community settings, in particular how 'coercion contexts' may be invoked, often inadvertently, and how this may help to explain the interconnectedness of formal and informal coercion. Krysia Canvin (Chapter 9) summarizes current research on patient experiences and perceptions of coercion, with particular attention to qualitative studies. A complex picture emerges of how patients perceive negative and positive dimensions of interventions, including obligations, safety, and the threats they have encountered. The variation in views among patients is also reported by family caregivers, and the literature on the role of the family in community coercion is reviewed by Jorun Rugkåsa (Chapter 10). Family members may exert influence directly or when engaged in the formal or informal coercive practices of professionals but may also experience themselves as being coerced. Finally, Beth Angell (Chapter 11) reviews the literature on the experience of mental health professionals in applying community coercion. This includes both compulsion and the full range of informal practices. From the perspective of health professionals these practices become deployed as tools in tasks that can be difficult and unpredictable and include both clinical and legal responsibilities.

While the chapters in Parts 2 and 3 are primarily empirically oriented, Part 4, *The context*, presents overarching perspectives from different positions. First, David Pilgrim (Chapter 12) presents a sociological perspective on the socio-ethical challenge of detention without trial. Outlining the phenomena from the theoretical positions of social causationism, labelling theory, and social history he calls for more a context-specific understanding of coercion as a social process. Next, Genevra Richardson (Chapter 13) discusses the human rights implications of community compulsion, in particular the implication of the UN Convention on the Rights of People with Disabilities and how community mental health care may need to be reshaped to reflect the principles of this fundamental challenge to both formal and informal coercive practices. In Chapter 14, Tania Gergel and George Szmukler suggest that community compulsion represents a new 'grey area' in the ethical debate and that different levels of coerciveness (spanning from persuasion, interpersonal leverage, inducements and threats to compulsion) require different ethical justifications. They propose a capacity-based approach as a way forward.

The fact that the vast majority of existing research on coercion has been conducted in Western industrialized countries unfortunately means that the first four parts of the book are not truly global in scope. Part 5, *International perspectives*, attempts to outline current practice, law, and policy in all continents. These have been particularly challenging chapters to write. In some continents, such as North America and Europe, there is a wealth of material that is difficult to condense into one chapter, while in others it has been hard, if not impossible, to obtain basic information about legislations or mental health systems. Reliable information on informal coercion has been particularly difficult to obtain. As a result, the authors have needed to make judgements about what information to include, and in how much detail. This means some countries or areas are inevitably described in more depth than others. Together, however, these chapters demonstrate the enormous variations in mental health care between continents and between countries within them. The chapters are as follows: Richard O'Reilly on the Americas (Chapter 15), B. N. Raveesh, Swaran P. Singh, and Soumitra Pathare on Asia (Chapter 16), Hui Ching Wu, Frank Huang-Chih Chou, Mariam Ali, and Andrew Molodynski on Southeast Asia (Chapter 17), Angelo Fioritti and Thomas Marcacci on Europe (Chapter 18), Atalay Alem and Catherine Manning on Africa (Chapter 19), and Anthony J. O'Brien on Oceania (Chapter 20). In the penultimate chapter, Andrew Molodynski (Chapter 21) draws together the major themes from the six regional chapters and distils implications for future global mental health. A central theme is the intrinsic coerciveness stemming simply from a lack of available services or treatment in large parts of the world. Finally, in Chapter 22, the editors bring together some ideas for the future of this complex, hard to measure, and important aspect of psychiatry.

References

Angell B, Mahoney C (2007). Reconceptualizing the case management relationship in intensive treatment: a study of staff perceptions and experiences. *Administration and Policy in Mental Health*, 34:172–188.

Burns T (2004). *Community mental health teams: a guide to current practices*. Oxford: Oxford University Press.

Canvin K, Rugkåsa J, Sinclair J, et al. (2013). Leverage and other informal pressures in community psychiatry in England. *International Journal of Law and Psychiatry*, 36:100–106.

Hoge SK, Lidz C, Mulvey E, et al. (1993). Patient, family, and staff perceptions of coercion in mental hospital admission: an exploratory study. *Behavioral Sciences and the Law*, 11:281–293.

Hoge SK, Lidz CW, Eisenberg M, et al. (1997). Perceptions of coercion in the admission of voluntary and involuntary psychiatric patients. *International Journal of Law and Psychiatry*, 20:167–181.

Laugharne R, Priebe S, McCabe R, et al. (2012). Trust, choice and power in mental health care: experiences of patients with psychosis. *International Journal of Social Psychiatry*, 58:496–504.

Marshall M, Lockwood A (2000). Assertive community treatment for people with severe mental disorders. *Cochrane Database of Systematic Reviews*, CD001089.

Monahan J, Redlich AD, Swanson J, et al. (2005). Use of leverage to improve adherence to psychiatric treatment in the community. *Psychiatric Services*, 56:37–44.

Nath SB, Alexander LB, Solomon PL (2012). Case managers' perspectives on the therapeutic alliance: a qualitative study. *Social Psychiatry and Psychiatric Epidemiology*, 47:1815–1826.

Neale MS, Rosenheck RA (2000). Therapeutic limit setting in an assertive community treatment program. *Psychiatric Services*, 51:499–505.

Rugkåsa J, Canvin K, Sinclair J, Sulman A, et al. (2014). Trust, deals and authority: community mental health professionals' experiences of influencing reluctant patients. *Community Mental Health Journal*, 50:886–895.

Stensrud B, Hoyer G, Granerud A, et al. (2015). 'Life on hold': a qualitative study of patient experiences with outpatient commitment in two Norwegian counties. *Issues in Mental Health Nursing*, 36:209–216.

Szmukler G, Appelbaum PS (2008). Treatment pressures, leverage, coercion, and compulsion in mental health care. *Journal of Mental Health*, 17:233–244.

Van Dorn RA, Elbogen EB, Redlich AD, et al. (2006). The relationship between mandated community treatment and perceived barriers to care in persons with severe mental illness. *International Journal of Law and Psychiatry*, 29:495–506.

Wertheimer A (1987). *Coercion*. Princeton, NJ: Princeton University Press.

Williams F (2009). *Claiming and framing in the making of care policies: the recognition and redistribution of care*. Geneva: United Nations Research Institute for Social Development. Retrieved 15 March 2015 from: http://www.unrisd.org/80256B3C005BCCF9/search/F0924 AD817FE8620C125780F004E9BCD?OpenDocument.

Part 1

Coercion in the community: origins and extent

Chapter 2

Compulsion in community mental health care: historical developments and current provisions

Tom Burns

Compulsion in inpatient settings

The origins of modern mental health care can be dated to the end of the eighteenth century. Pinel's iconic striking off of the lunatics' chains in the Paris Salpêtrière in 1793 and the opening of the York Retreat by the Tuke family in 1796 signalled a sea change in the understanding and care of the mentally ill. Madhouses were replaced by asylums and the era of moral therapy was introduced. The removal of shackles and prohibition of punishment did not, however, imply the abandonment of compulsion. All asylum patients were detained against their will and they had to be 'certified' as insane. Initially asylum admissions and discharges were determined not by doctors but by magistrates or similar local authorities (town mayors, watch committees etc.). Apart from some advanced institutions in Switzerland it was not until as late as 1930 that voluntary admissions to public asylums were permitted.

Although compulsion was a ubiquitous feature of asylum care, that did not mean that society was comfortable with it. Public concern about the possibility of unjustified incarceration remained from the era of unregulated madhouses with their tales of families locking away members to avoid embarrassment and scandal or to influence inheritances. Most developed states introduced legislation during the nineteenth century to ensure both the provision and supervision of asylum care. The UK, for example, passed national Asylum Acts in 1808 and 1828, a Lunatics Act in 1845, and finally the 1890 Lunacy Act that surrounded admission with so many bureaucratic hurdles that it hindered early intervention for half a century.

The need for compulsory care for mentally ill individuals who are sufficiently unwell to require 24-hour nursing and supervision has been broadly accepted in most developed countries. Indeed a significant proportion of detained patients themselves acknowledge after discharge that their care was necessary (Katsakou and Priebe 2006). Most mental health legislation has been phrased in terms of the 'need for detention', assuming that compulsory treatment could only be indicated for individuals requiring such 24-hour care.

The 1970s witnessed a sustained international challenge by both civil rights organizations (Gostin et al. 1975) and anti-psychiatrists (Szasz 1972) to the use of compulsory powers. There are currently very profound differences in the thresholds imposed on the use of compulsion and in the extent of its use. Variations within Europe currently exceed a ten-fold difference which cannot be explained by any obvious health-care factors or, indeed, by details of their legislation (Salize and Dressing 2004). The most striking difference, however, is between the USA and Europe. The USA has always had a much stronger emphasis on the importance of individual liberty and, since the Lessard decision (Eastern District of Wisconsin 1972) in 1972, it has restricted compulsory care to patients who demonstrate '. . . an extreme likelihood of . . . immediate harm to self or others'. Most jurisdictions worldwide include terms such as 'risk' or 'harm' in their definitions of liability to compulsory detention. However, European practitioners usually define this as risk to health, widely interpreted to include deterioration in mental health. Some jurisdictions such as the Netherlands, Austria, and Switzerland responded to the civil rights challenges by removing the legal provision for compulsory *treatment* of competent individuals but retained the provision for compulsory *detention* (Zinkler and Priebe 2002).

Deinstitutionalization

The last 50 years has been marked by the shift of care from large institutions to the community. In the aftermath of World War II most developed countries introduced forms of a welfare state which provided at least minimal provision for income support, accommodation, and access to health care for all their citizens. At the same time disillusionment with asylum care set in, fuelled by a recognition of its potentially damaging effects on long-term patients (Barton 1959; Goffman 1960) and emerging stories of abuse and neglect (Department of Health 1969; Talbott 1978). The discovery of the first effective antipsychotic, chlorpromazine, in 1952 and of antidepressants in the late 1950s accelerated this move out of the asylum. The process of deinstitutionalization with the down-sizing and eventual closure of most of these large hospitals came to be the defining feature of mental health care in the Western world in the second half of the twentieth century.

How well deinstitutionalization was managed varied considerably. In much of Europe it was conducted reasonably well (Leff et al. 2000; Priebe et al. 2002) with a systematic re-provision of care and accommodation for disabled patients. Italy took a radically different approach by passing a law in 1978 ('law 180') which effectively abolished mental hospitals and prevented admissions (Mangen 1989). In the USA, however, deinstitutionalization was not matched by the provision of either adequate accommodation or effective community mental health services (Bachrach 1982; Talbott et al. 1987). The US problems were exacerbated by the very rapid closure of beds but also by the Lessard decision, which severely restricted clinicians' ability to provide prolonged rehabilitative care for patients with severe psychosis who rejected treatment. The result was a wave of incarceration of such patients and a growing concern about the criminalization of mental illness.

Informal community coercion

With deinstitutionalization, community services have found themselves faced with caring for a substantial number of patients with severe and complex problems. Many of these patients (particularly 'revolving-door' psychosis patients) remain doubtful of the reality of their illness or the value of the treatment offered. Only recently has attention been paid to the way in which clinicians regularly employ a wide range of techniques to encourage, persuade, and cajole such patients to comply with their prescribed treatment. The extensive literature on assertive community treatment (Mueser et al. 1998; Burns and Firn 2002; Wright et al. 2004) focused essentially on its structure rather than its process. However, the rationale behind such services has always been to engage patients in treatment that they fundamentally do not want.

It has become clear that many voluntary outpatients do not experience their care as fully consensual—they feel coerced to a greater or lesser degree. Appelbaum and Szmukler (2008) have organized these pressures into a hierarchy from encouragement to compulsion (see also Chapter 14). Monahan and colleagues have examined the extent to which the most explicit of these informal pressures (so-called 'leverage' where a clear benefit is made contingent on accepting treatment) is used in public mental health services in five US states (Monahan et al. 2005). Over half of their 1000 patients reported that they had been required to cooperate with treatment in exchange for access to accommodation, finance, or leniency within the criminal justice service. European rates are generally lower, but still substantial—about 30–35% in the UK, although they vary between different clinical groups (Burns et al. 2011). What this research indicates is that (as New Zealand patients have reported; Gibbs et al. 2005) CTOs have to be understood within a context of a continuum of pressures in community mental health care. They are not simply an isolated binary choice between entirely voluntary care or compulsion.

'Least restrictive' CTOs

The criminalization of the mentally ill and the large numbers of patients being held in US jails for want of alternative provision generated considerable disquiet and led to an unlikely alliance between civil rights activists and clinicians. Having campaigned vigorously to restrict compulsory care, civil rights groups now backed legislation for the introduction of CTOs with the aim of providing care in less restrictive environments. Rather than being detained in prisons to receive active treatment the new legislation would allow patients, albeit still obliged to receive treatment, the relatively greater freedom of living their own lives. The conditions for imposing a 'least restrictive CTO' were exactly the same as those for inpatient detention (i.e. the imminent risk of significant danger). The first state to introduce such legislation was North Carolina in 1977. By 1985, 42 US states had some form of CTO on their statute book (Miller 1985).

Least restrictive CTOs appealed to civil rights groups, as they continued to protect patients' rights but ensured that they would have maximum personal liberty and receive treatment. Unfortunately they rapidly ran into trouble clinically, were rarely used, and generated tension and animosity between the courts and clinicians. The problem with them is easy to understand. If an individual poses an imminent and serious risk to their own or others' safety then it is difficult to see how they can be managed in the community. In addition, if the treatment is even marginally effective they are likely to fail to meet this threshold within days or, at most, weeks. Clinicians wanted a CTO that gave them powers to continue to treat and stabilize patients while they were still ill, though no longer an immediate danger.

'Preventative' CTOs

By the mid 1980s most US states had introduced CTO legislation in a form that allowed a lower threshold for compulsion, so-called preventative CTOs. Preventative CTOs were explicitly constructed to authorize continuing treatment in partially recovered patients to forestall deterioration and relapse. Three features are common to most preventative CTO regimes. First, the wording of the legislation for their use distinguishes their threshold from that required for inpatient care and they usually have their own separate process and paperwork. Second, they recognize the right to intervene before there is a clear deterioration in mental state. Third, they usually outline a mechanism for their implementation—specific clinical procedures that must be followed, or reporting structures that must be in place. This requirement to outline what is offered is, in part, an attempt to respond to the ethical principle of 'reciprocity'. Reciprocity requires that when something is forfeited (liberty) something (treatment or care) should be offered in exchange (Eastman 1994). The surprising alliance between clinicians and civil rights groups was now at an end and preventative CTOs have become the dominant model internationally.

The first CTOs to be introduced outside the USA were in Australia and New Zealand. Their orders have some features of both the least restrictive and the preventative approaches. The conditions for inpatient detention and community compulsion are the same; indeed clinicians do not need to specify where compulsion will be exerted. However, the threshold for their imposition allows compulsion based on a longitudinal assessment of risk. Thus, in practice, stable patients can be (and are) maintained on CTOs for months and even years. A mixed approach was also adopted in Wisconsin, USA, in 1998, where a patient could 'waive' their rights in a mental health court and 'voluntarily' comply with treatment. In Israel the 1991 wording is as for a least restrictive CTO but 'clinical discretion' has been allowed which effectively ensures it operates as a preventative CTO.

Public safety or patient benefit?

Apart from the earliest US least restrictive CTOs (whose aim was to provide an alternative to incarceration) the declared aim of CTOs has invariably been to ensure continuing treatment to break the cycle of repeated relapse and readmission in 'revolving-door' patients. How this is phrased varies, but in many jurisdictions it is made explicit in the eligibility criteria for CTOs. For instance, in most US and Australian states and Canadian provinces a documented history of repeated involuntary admissions is required, often stipulating the time recently spent in hospital. Sometimes a diagnosis of psychosis with active positive symptoms is required. This is not, however, the whole picture.

In many cases the real political momentum for introducing CTOs has come from concerns about public safety and the need to strengthen confidence in mental health services. Often this has crystallized out around high-profile homicides carried out by mentally ill individuals. These patients have usually been known to services, most often having been treated for schizophrenia, but at the time of the offence were refusing to continue with medication. Legislation following such tragedies often takes the name of the victim [Kendra's Law in New York (2005), Laura's Law in California (2001), Brian's Law in Ontario, Canada (2000)]. UK legislation (in 2007) did not acquire such a name but was undoubtedly initiated in response to the killing of Jonathan Zito by Christopher Clunis in 1992 (Ritchie 1994). Where legislation is driven by such considerations the public consultation is often long and fraught. The UK legislation was preceded by nearly 20 years of often heated debate, and the legislation in Victoria, Australia (in 1986) by 5 years of consultation. Where the introduction is not fuelled by such concerns about public safety but entirely by those of patient welfare then public debate is often minimal and acceptance readily obtained. Sjöström et al. (2011) have compared the introduction of CTO legislation in Scandinavia with that in the USA and UK and linked concerns with patient welfare and solidarity with an easy acceptance. In New Zealand, where CTO legislation in 1992 simply consolidated routine clinical practice based on the use of long leave, public opinion was highly supportive from the start.

International use of CTO legislation

International experience in the use of CTOs has been thoroughly summarized in a systematic review by Churchill et al. (2007) and in a narrative review by Dawson (2005) with a focus on the legal and constitutional aspects. There are now over 70 jurisdictions that have CTO regimes established, and there is every indication that legislation for them will continue to spread. There is remarkable variation in the rate of use of CTOs (Lawton-Smith 2005). In the US states, despite being so long established, there is no consistency in their use. Australasia has the highest rates, but even within Australia the rates vary by over 100%. Victoria, with a highly developed community service, is the most enthusiastic exponent with a rate of one CTO per thousand population. New South Wales is half that and Western Australia lower still. Even within regions different hospitals have markedly differing rates of use, and within those hospitals clinicians also display inexplicable variations in practice. In the two assertive outreach teams in the Oxford, UK, services, each with around 70 patients, one had no patients on a CTO and the other had over 20.

Patient characteristics

In contrast to the random variation in international utilization of CTOs the characteristics of patients placed on them is reassuringly consistent. Churchill et al.'s (2007) review of 72 CTO publications identified a common theme. Patients were middle aged

(35–40 years old), more often men (60%) and suffered from psychotic illnesses (80% with schizophrenia). They were in the mid phase of their illness with usually about 10 years of service contact and had multiple previous admissions, mostly involuntary. They often had some history of violence, but the current clinical picture was more one of isolation and neglect with minimal insight.

Published studies contain some surprising observations, such as widely varying rates of substance abuse and personality disorder. The latter shows the most extreme variation [24.5% in Western Australia (Xiao et al. 2004) and 0.8% in New Zealand (Dawson and Romans 2001)]. However, it is difficult to be sure how much this demonstrates differences in clinical practice or how much it reflects differences in recording. US publications indicate a very high rate of use with African Americans—between twice and three times the proportions in the local population [New York 42% cf. 15% (New York State Office of Mental Health 2005), North Carolina 66% cf. 22% (Hiday et al. 1999)]. In Australasia, Maori and Aboriginal patients are over-represented by more than 100% (Maori 14% cf. 6%, Aboriginals 7% cf. 3.2%) (Dawson and Romans 2001; Xiao et al. 2004).

Imposition, conditions, and enforcement

CTOs can either be imposed by clinicians and subject to scrutiny and confirmation by tribunals, as in the UK, or they may be imposed by judges or magistrates at the request of clinicians, as in the USA and most other jurisdictions. Generally, clinicians emphasize a longitudinal perspective, basing their judgement on the patient's history, whereas judges and magistrates reportedly focus more on the current condition of the patient. Clinician-imposed CTOs tend to last longer while those imposed by judges are generally shorter (US CTOs are sometimes for less than 3 months). However, this is not always the case—Australian CTOs are imposed by judges but are reputedly very long lived. In New York, where the provisions of Kendra's Law direct extra resources to CTO patients, only 36% of CTOs lasted under 6 months and the average was 16 months (New York State Office of Mental Health 2005). It is important to note that it is very difficult to obtain reliable figures for the duration of CTOs: national figures tend to focus on the number of CTOs instigated each year and the number of CTOs in operation on any given census date.

All CTOs require patients to make themselves available to mental health teams for monitoring, most require them to take stipulated medication, and many require patients to live at a fixed address (although this is controversial). The importance of a more ambitious care plan offering something other than just medication has been stressed by many family members in the spirit of reciprocity. It has been equally resisted on the ethical grounds that the compulsory elements of the care plan should be as few as possible and only those interventions absolutely essential to keep the patient well should be imposed. As the care plan, and consequently any changes to it, has to be ratified by a judge or tribunal in several jurisdictions it is common practice to keep the care plan to the bare essentials so that it is flexible enough to cope with changing circumstances. Most clinicians have abandoned complex conditions (e.g. abstaining from drugs or alcohol, not harassing family members, attending day centres) simply because they have been found to be unenforceable.

No CTO legislation authorizes the use of force to medicate patients in the community. What power they have is exercised through the provision for recall. Patients who fail to cooperate with treatment can be brought back to hospital or some other clinical setting for a period (usually up to 72 hours). During that period they can decide to cooperate and thus be discharged back out on their CTO. If they continue to refuse the clinician has to decide whether to discharge them as voluntary patients or to revoke the CTO and treat them compulsorily as inpatients. It is remarkably difficult to obtain figures on how often this actually happens.

The Queens CTO team in New York, which keeps good records on their 300 CTO patients, average about 250 recalls a year—equivalent to one per patient per year, although they are not equally distributed. Clinicians give very conflicting observations. Some insist that CTOs only really begin to work after a patient has been recalled several times and 'learnt their lesson'. Others consider recall ineffective and a sign that CTOs are not working. Recall of an asymptomatic individual can also be difficult, especially when he or she is competing against very ill patients for a local bed.

In some regimes recall is automatic—for example, after any refusal of a depot injection or a set number of missed appointments—but in most it is a clinical judgement. In the US, police are routinely involved in recalls, sometimes even without a mental health professional being in attendance. In New York the 'clinical assistance team' carries out recalls and comprises four law officers (armed) plus one clinical member. In most settings police assistance can be asked for, although (particularly in Europe) it may not be forthcoming if the patient is not presenting any current risk or obvious disturbance.

Prioritization of CTO patients

Should CTO patients have priority in access to scarce resources such as case managers and accommodation? The UK legislation takes a very firm line that they should not. It was felt that CTOs should not be imposed unless the patient was already in receipt of the best possible care and still demonstrated a need for it. CTOs were not to be a substitute for adequate care but an addition to it. Civil rights groups were concerned any priority would bias clinicians towards imposing CTOs which were not clinically indicated in order to access scarce resources. The impact on access for non-CTO patients also had to be considered. This is not the stand taken in most regimes, however.

In the USA proponents of Laura's Law in California and Kendras' Law in New York have defended them on the grounds that they guarantee effective treatment for a particular group that would otherwise not be provided. In two US randomized controlled trials (RCTs) (Swartz et al. 1999; Steadman et al. 2001) multidisciplinary case management was made available in both arms of the trials, although this was not generally available for such patients. Kendra's Law in New York brought with it an extra $32 million in the first year to provide enhanced outreach specifically targeted to these patients (New York State Office of Mental Health 2005). Within New York City only those patients on CTOs can be sure of persisting comprehensive care. Case workers viewed CTOs as a legal commitment on the service providers as much as on the patient. Even when there is no clear ring-fencing of resources or declared prioritization there is a de facto prioritization in most services.

There is a substantial body of research demonstrating that relapse and readmission in severely ill psychotic patients is reduced by multidisciplinary case management with outreach (Burns et al. 2007). Not surprisingly, both the RCTs that provided this extra care found a significant reduction in readmission rates in the period after randomization compared with that before in both groups. When interpreting the research findings about CTOs it is important to carefully distinguish the possible bias introduced by enhanced care.

Summary

CTOs have become a feature of most developed mental health services in the last 30 years. The political motivation for their introduction has usually been a mixture of reassuring the public about the risk of violence from the mentally ill, a drive to continue to reduce reliance on expensive inpatient care, plus a genuine desire to improve the lot of the 'revolving-door' psychosis patient. Their introduction has often been viewed with suspicion by psychiatrists and mental health professionals but once in place they have rapidly been accepted as a normal part of practice, and often viewed as essential. Other chapters in this book will explore their effectiveness and their acceptability to a wide range of stakeholders.

CTOs generate very strong feelings in all those involved, both for and against. The more extreme prophesies have not come to pass. They have not revolutionized psychiatry and abolished relapse, leaving us with empty beds. Nor have they profoundly damaged our relationships with our current patients or driven away potential patients fearful of a mental health service transformed into an agent of state control. They mark a phase in the development of psychiatry, a practice that is always changing as the society it serves continues to change. CTOs are an innovation that requires a detailed, thorough, and rational examination before final decisions about their place in mental health care can be made.

References

Bachrach LL (1982). Assessment of outcomes in community support systems: results, problems, and limitations. *Schizophrenia Bulletin*, **8**:39–61.

Barton R (1959). *Institutional neurosis*. Bristol: John Wright.

Burns T, Firn M (2002). *Assertive outreach in mental health: a manual for practitioners*. Oxford: Oxford University Press.

Burns T, Catty J, Dash M, et al. (2007). Use of intensive case management to reduce time in hospital in people with severe mental illness: systematic review and meta-regression. *British Medical Journal*, **335**:336.

Burns T, Yeeles K, Molodynski A, et al. (2011). Pressures to adhere to treatment ('leverage') in English mental health care. *British Journal of Psychiatry*, **199**:145–150.

Churchill R, Owen G, Singh S, et al. (2007). *International experiences of using community treatment orders*. London: Institute of Psychiatry.

Dawson J (2005). *Community treatment orders: international comparisons*. Dunedin: Otago University Print. Available at: http://www.otago.ac.nz/law/research/otago036152.pdf

Dawson J, Romans S (2001). Uses of community treatment orders in New Zealand: early findings. *Australian and New Zealand Journal of Psychiatry*, 35:190–195.

Department of Health (1969). *Report of the Committee of Inquiry into allegations of ill-treatment of patients and other irregularities at the Ely Hospital, Cardiff, presented to Parliament by the Secretary of State of the Department of Health and Social Security.* London: Department of Health.

Eastern District of Wisconsin (1972). Lessard v. Schmidt, 349F. Supp. 1078.

Eastman N (1994). Mental health law: civil liberties and the principle of reciprocity. *British Medical Journal*, 308:43–45.

Gibbs A, Dawson J, Ansley C, et al. (2005). How patients in New Zealand view community treatment orders. *Journal of Mental Health*, 14:357–368.

Goffman I (1960). *Asylums: essays on the social situation of mental patients and other inmates.* Harmondsworth: Penguin Books.

Gostin LO (1975). *A human condition: The Mental Health Act from 1959 to 1975; observations, analysis and proposals for reform*, Vol. 1. London: Mind.

Hiday VA, Swartz MS, Swanson JW, et al. (1999). Criminal victimization of persons with severe mental illness. *Psychiatric Services*, 50:62–68.

Katsakou C, Priebe S (2006). Outcomes of involuntary hospital admission—a review. *Acta Psychiatrica Scandinavica*, 114:232–241.

Lawton-Smith S (2005). *A question of numbers. The potential impact of community-based treatment orders in England and Wales.* London: King's Fund.

Leff J, Trieman N, Knapp M, et al. (2000). The TAPS Project: a report on 13 years of research, 1985–1998. *Psychiatric Bulletin*, 24:165–168.

Mangen S (1989). The politics of reform: origins and enactment of the Italian 'experience'. *International Journal of Social Psychiatry*, 35:7–20.

Miller RD (1985). Commitment to outpatient treatment: a national survey. *Psychiatric Services*, 36(3):265–267.

Monahan J, Redlich AD, Swanson J, et al. (2005). Use of leverage to improve adherence to psychiatric treatment in the community. *Psychiatric Services*, 56:37–44.

Mueser KT, Bond GR, Drake RE, et al. (1998). Models of community care for severe mental illness: a review of research on case management. *Schizophrenia Bulletin*, 24:37–74.

New York State Office of Mental Health (2005). *Kendra's Law: final report on the status of assisted outpatient treatment.* New York: Office of Mental Health New York State.

Priebe S, Hoffmann K, Isermann M, et al. (2002). Do long-term hospitalised patients benefit from discharge into the community? *Social Psychiatry and Psychiatric Epidemiology*, 37:387–392.

Ritchie JH (1994). *The report of the enquiry into the care and treatment of Christopher Clunis presented to the Chairman of the North East Thames and South East Thames Regional Health Authorities.* London: HMSO.

Salize HJ, Dressing H (2004). Epidemiology of involuntary placement of mentally ill people across the European Union. *British Journal of Psychiatry*, 184:163–168.

Sjöström S, Zetterberg L, Markström U (2011). Why community compulsion became the solution—reforming mental health law in Sweden. *International Journal of Law and Psychiatry*, 34:419–428.

Steadman HJ, Gounis K, Dennis D, et al. (2001). Assessing the New York City involuntary outpatient commitment pilot program. *Psychiatric Services*, 52:330–336.

Swartz M, Swanson JD, Wagner H, et al. (1999). Can involuntary outpatient commitment reduce hospital recidivism?: findings from a randomized trial with severely mentally ill individuals. *American Journal of Psychiatry*, **156**:1968–1975.

Szasz TS (1972). *The myth of mental illness: foundations of a theory of personal conduct.* London: Paladin.

Szmukler G, Appelbaum PS (2008). Treatment pressures, leverage, coercion, and compulsion in mental health care. *Journal of Mental Health*, **17**:233–244.

Talbott JA (1978). *The death of the asylum: a critical study of state hospital management, services, and care.* New York: Grune and Stratton.

Talbott JA, Clark GH, Jr, Sharfstein SS, et al. (1987). Issues in developing standards governing psychiatric practice in community mental health centers. *Hospital and Community Psychiatry*, **38**:1198–1202.

Wright C, Catty J, Watt H, et al. (2004). A systematic review of home treatment services. Classification and sustainability. *Social Psychiatry and Psychiatric Epidemiology*, **39**:789–796.

Xiao J, Preston NJ, Kisely S (2004). What determines compulsory community treatment? A logistic regression analysis using linked mental health and offender databases. *Australian and New Zealand Journal of Psychiatry*, **38**:613–618.

Zinkler M, Priebe S (2002). Detention of the mentally ill in Europe—a review. *Acta Psychiatrica Scandinavica*, **106**:3–8.

Chapter 3

Community treatment order legislation in the Commonwealth

John Dawson

Introduction

This chapter gives a general account of the legislation that governs the use of community treatment orders (CTOs) in the UK, Canada, Australia, and New Zealand—countries that share the common law tradition due to their having been part of the British Empire.[1] No more than an overview of the legislation can be given, because even within this selected group of countries there are roughly 20 CTO regimes. These regimes defy ready synthesis or comparison. In particular, in countries with a federal legal system, such as Canada and Australia, legislation for CTOs is enacted by parliaments at the provincial or state level of government not at the national level, with the result that different CTO (or outpatient commitment) schemes exist in at least seven provinces of Canada and in all eight states and territories of Australia. In addition, England and Wales, Scotland, and New Zealand, have their own CTO schemes (see Figure 3.1).

In these jurisdictions, legislation governing compulsory outpatient treatment is the major legal product of the deinstitutionalization of psychiatric care. A wave of CTO legislation was passed in Australasia from the late 1980s through to the 1990s, followed by the enactment of similar schemes in Canada and the UK in the early 2000s. It is not possible to compare every aspect of these schemes. This chapter reviews the major themes in the CTO statutes of these jurisdictions, draws attention to certain contrasting approaches, and highlights interesting provisions of certain regimes.[2]

This review indicates that the general structure of the CTO legislation in these Commonwealth jurisdictions is very similar to that of the outpatient commitment regimes established by state statutes in the USA. Roughly 45 states of the USA (see Figure 3.2) authorize outpatient commitment (as it is usually called there), even if

---

[1] The main legislation reviewed is that of Scotland, England and Wales, Saskatchewan, Ontario, Nova Scotia, Newfoundland and Labrador, Victoria, New South Wales, and New Zealand. See also Dawson (2005).

[2] Many notes later in the chapter cite the provisions of CTO statutes, to illustrate the positions discussed. No attempt is made to cite every statute in the Commonwealth that takes the relevant position.

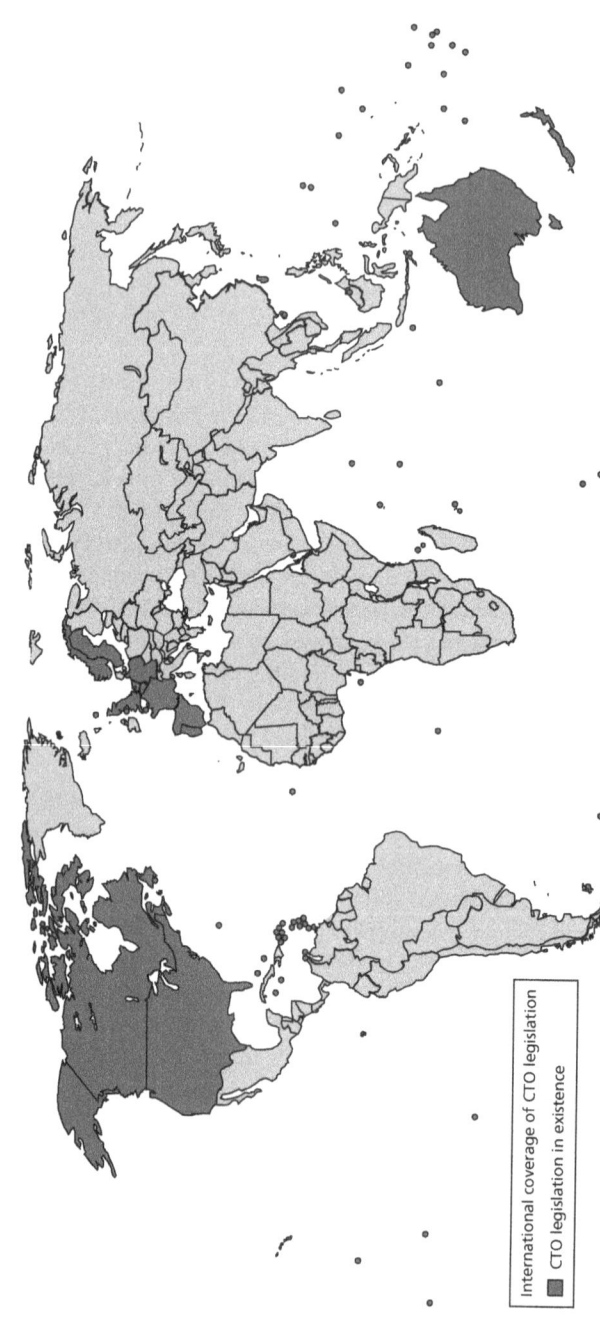

Figure 3.1 International coverage of CTO legislation.

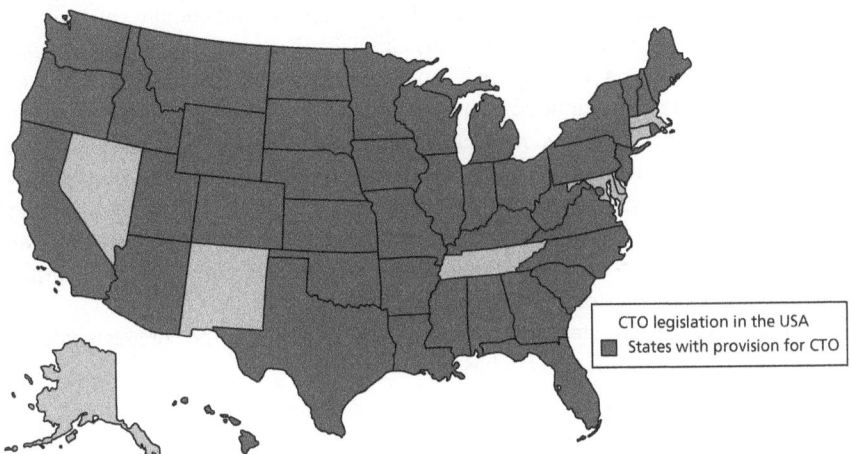

Figure 3.2 CTO coverage in the USA.

many of these statutes seem to be very lightly used. A full review of those state statutes would be a formidable task (Bazelon Center for Mental Health Law 2000), but a brief review of American law, plus study of the well-developed outpatient commitment legislation of New York,[3] Hawaii,[4] and Arizona,[5] suggests that considerable overlap exists between the Commonwealth and the US jurisdictions in the central legal principles followed: that is, in the administrative structure under which compulsory outpatient treatment proceeds, in the criteria and process for such a treatment order, and in the powers conferred.[6]

From a legal point of view, perhaps the most distinctive feature of a CTO scheme is the particular cluster of duties and powers it confers for the purposes of supervising a person's outpatient care. The person under the order (who will be referred to here simply as 'the person') is usually required to accept continuing psychiatric treatment—especially medication—under the terms of a community treatment plan. They are required to maintain contact with members of a community mental health team, either by accepting visits at their residence or attending a clinic or hospital. They may be required to live in a community facility that provides a certain level of care. They

---

[3] New York Mental Hygiene Law, Article 9.60, Assisted outpatient treatment. A constitutional challenge to New York's outpatient commitment regime was turned down in *KL v A-G of New York* (2004) 1 NY 3d 362 (NYCA).

[4] Hawaii Revised Statutes, Division 1, Title 19, Chapter 334, Part VIII, Involuntary outpatient treatment.

[5] Arizona Revised Statutes, Title 36.540, Conditional outpatient treatment.

[6] Perhaps the major difference between the approaches in the statutes of the USA and those of the Commonwealth is the more extensive use of courts (as opposed to tribunals) in the US regimes. In the USA, the initial order for a person's outpatient commitment is usually made by a court, and a court order may be required to recall the person to inpatient care.

may be swiftly returned to hospital should they relapse or not comply with essential elements of the treatment plan. Police assistance with that recall process is authorized, if required. On recall, the person will usually be reassessed, may be treated without consent, and may be readmitted to hospital if they meet the usual criteria for compulsory inpatient care. 'Forced medication' in a community setting is not authorized, however, except perhaps in an emergency. Administration of medication using physical restraint could only proceed lawfully therefore, if at all, in a properly supervised clinic or hospital. It is the threat of swift recall to hospital for non-compliance with community treatment—not forced medication in the community—that is the principal means of enforcing compulsory outpatient care.

This chapter concentrates on legal provisions that establish the core elements of a CTO regime, i.e. on those that establish:

+ the authority to issue a CTO;
+ the criteria and process for making a CTO;
+ the functions of statutory treatment plans;
+ the conditions, or requirements, that may be imposed on a person under a CTO;
+ the powers available to enforce those conditions, especially via recall to hospital;
+ any protections from liability accorded those who treat a person on a CTO;
+ the duration of a CTO.

The broader legal context

This is to take a fairly narrow view of what constitutes 'the law on CTOs'. A broader view could be taken, one that emphasized how CTOs operate within the context of a surrounding body of law, particularly within the framework of a jurisdiction's wider Mental Health Act (MHA) or civil commitment scheme. That wider legislation usually specifies the forms of 'mental disorder' or 'mental illness' that qualify a person for compulsory treatment. It confers authority on certain persons (such as the 'responsible clinician') to intervene or prescribe a course of compulsory care. It establishes the necessary procedures—before a court or tribunal—for review of compulsory status. It may regulate the administration without consent of certain forms of treatment, such as ECT, and require mandatory peer review of the long-term use of medication without consent. In total, these provisions constitute the infrastructure for compulsory treatment and provide many of the foundations for a CTO regime.

In addition, broader principles of the legal system bear on CTOs, including principles designed to promote the protection of human rights against improper exercises of state power (Dawson 2010a). These human rights principles are often relevant to the lawfulness or interpretation of a CTO scheme, including—in relevant jurisdictions—principles drawn from the Canadian Charter of Rights and Freedoms, the European Convention on Human Rights, and the Human Rights Act 1998 (UK). Moreover, the general law of consent to treatment is implicated, particularly law governing treatment without consent and covering situations in which a substitute decision-maker (SDM) may be authorized to approve another person's psychiatric care. The law on powers of entry is relevant when access must be obtained to private premises to make contact with a person on a CTO. The law on privacy and confidentiality applies when information about a person's health is to be shared with a wider circle of carers (including family members) engaged in their community care. Certain principles of criminal law and procedure apply if a criminal court can place a person directly on a CTO. Negligence (or malpractice) law governs the liabilities of clinicians and health services who treat people on CTOs; and so on. All these broader principles could be considered part of the law on CTOs. Nevertheless, specific statutory provisions that bear directly on the use of CTOs are the main focus of this chapter.

Questions of authority

One initial question about a CTO regime concerns its organizational structure. Who carries the authority (and responsibility) for its administration? Upon whom are the essential powers conferred? Two major spheres of authority are usually established. These might be called the sphere of clinicians and the sphere of independent review. In addition, the laws of some jurisdictions, like those of Ontario and Nova Scotia, recognize a third sphere—that of the SDM, whose approval is required to place a person on a CTO. Interaction between people operating within these different spheres of authority is then critical to administration of the scheme.

Certain powers and responsibilities in relation to CTOs are usually exercised by clinical teams, especially community mental health teams. Clinicians propose patients for CTOs. They undertake the necessary consultations, including consulting the person concerned, family members, any SDM appointed to act on the person's behalf, and any community agencies or independent practitioners who provide elements of the treatment plan. Clinicians also exercise the central powers to manage the person's outpatient treatment under the scheme.

The law usually places most of these management functions formally on the shoulders of a responsible clinician (or responsible psychiatrist) who is appointed to manage the person's care, in collaboration with a multidisciplinary team.[7] In addition, certain powers, such as the power to 'take and convey' a person to hospital following recall from a CTO, are often conferred on certain classes of approved health professionals, such as nurses, psychologists, social workers, and ambulance officers, who are specially trained for the task. Moreover, the clinicians are usually under a duty to assess the person's position, on a regular basis, against the ruling criteria for a CTO, and to discharge them from compulsion if those criteria cease to apply. Separate authority to conduct regular, independent review of the need for a CTO is then conferred on a court, tribunal, or board—usually the same body that reviews the need for compulsory inpatient care.

---

[7] In some jurisdictions, certain key functions, such as proposing a person for a CTO, can only be exercised with the formal agreement of another designated health professional. The agreement of an approved mental health professional is required, for instance, in England and Wales, and of a mental health officer in Scotland, the aim being to guarantee multidisciplinary input into decisions.

In some jurisdictions the CTO is formally issued by clinicians (usually one or two psychiatrists) and only then reviewed by a court or tribunal (as in Ontario, and England and Wales). In other jurisdictions, clinicians propose the making of the order, and advocate this before the review body, but the order is issued by a court or tribunal, following a hearing at which the person is entitled to be present, to be legally represented, and to question the need for the order. An intermediate position is for clinicians to issue a temporary order, which may then be confirmed or continued by the review body.[8] The differences between these positions should not be over-stated as in each case the clinicians and the review body must ultimately agree for the order to continue to authorize a person's compulsory care.

In some jurisdictions, a CTO can also be made directly by a criminal court as a form of disposition from the trial process, when that is recommended by clinicians and the usual criteria for a CTO are met. In New Zealand, for example, a criminal court can put a person on a CTO—diverting them directly to compulsory outpatient treatment—following a conviction (as an alternative to a criminal sentence), and following a finding that the person is not guilty by reason of insanity or unfit to stand trial.[9]

CTO legislation then exhibits two main approaches to conferral of community treatment powers. Under one approach, the issue of a CTO confers a pre-established cluster of powers (and associated responsibilities) on community teams: to maintain contact with the person, to provide certain treatment, to return the person to hospital, to enter private property, and so on. Under the other approach, a more individually tailored set of powers is conferred: only those that are necessary to give effect to the particular regime of care listed in the person's treatment plan. That latter approach—conferring only a calibrated set of powers 'proportionate' to the person's needs—may comply more closely with the requirements of human rights law.

Under the latter approach, the key structural device employed is the mandatory outpatient treatment plan. The legislation will specify the minimum requirements of that plan, plus the range of consultations and approvals required in its formulation. The plan must be 'signed off' by particular parties—by the responsible clinician, for instance, and by other community care providers who agree to be involved—as well as being 'signed off', in some cases, by the person concerned (if they retain the capacity to do so) or by a SDM acting on their behalf. In practice, the plan's contents are likely to be stated in rather broad terms, to avoid the need to vary or amend the plan frequently should the person's needs change, but, in this manner, the main 'conditions' or 'requirements' of the plan are specified and agreed. Any means available to enforce that plan that would involve restrictions on the person's usual legal rights would then have to be clearly authorized by law. But once the terms of the plan are finalized and approved the person will be expected to comply with that plan.

---

[8] As under the Mental Health Act 2014 (Victoria) (hereafter 'Victoria').

[9] Criminal Procedure (Mentally Impaired Persons) Act 2003 (NZ), ss 25(1)(a), 26(1), 34(1)(b)(i), 36.

Of course, CTOs are not the only legal device that can be used to enforce outpatient care. Other devices can be used to similar effect. In various jurisdictions extended inpatient 'leave', treatment orders made under adult guardianship (or incapacity) legislation, community forensic orders, or treatment as a condition of parole, probation, or bail are used to require a person to accept outpatient treatment. Some process of enforcement, such as re-hospitalization, re-sentencing, or activation of outstanding criminal charges, might then be used should the person fail to comply.

The criteria for a CTO

In the jurisdictions studied, several distinct sets of legal criteria usually apply to a person's placement on a CTO. Some criteria apply to compulsory psychiatric treatment in general under the MHA, while others apply specifically to compulsory outpatient care. In all jurisdictions, four distinct sets of criteria usually apply. These concern: the presence of 'mental disorder' or 'mental illness'; the 'risks' or 'dangers' that a person's condition must pose; the idea that the CTO must be 'necessary' or 'proportionate'; and the requirement that the outpatient approach to treatment be viable. In addition, some jurisdictions require the consent of the person to their placement on a CTO, or a finding that they lack the capacity to consent to their outpatient care. Some limit the use of CTOs to people about to be discharged from hospital,[10] while others permit those already living in the community to be placed directly on a CTO.

The legislation usually applies the same criteria of 'mental disorder' or 'mental illness', and the same (or similar) standards of risk or danger, to both compulsory inpatient and compulsory outpatient care. However, the relevant standards of risk usually refer not only to direct dangers to the health or safety—of the person or others—but also to a person's 'seriously diminished capacity for self-care',[11] or to 'serious deterioration' in their health, including their mental health.[12]

When applied to CTOs in particular, these standards of risk are usually drafted so as to require a prediction that one of the relevant harms *would* (or would be likely)[13] to befall the person or others if they *were not* placed under compulsory outpatient care. The key technique employed is to express these risk criteria in the conditional tense (or, alternatively, to read the criteria as if they were written in that tense). That is, the law will say (or be read to say) that a person can be placed on a CTO provided the relevant risks 'would be' posed if they were not under compulsory outpatient care.[14]

---

[10] For example, England and Wales, under the Mental Health Act 1983 (UK) (hereafter 'England and Wales'); see Gostin et al. (2010).

[11] For example, under the Mental Health (Compulsory Assessment and Treatment) Act 1992 (NZ), s 2 (hereafter 'New Zealand'); see Dawson and Gledhill (2013).

[12] Mental Health Act (Ontario), RSO 1990, c M.7 (hereafter 'Ontario'), s 15(1.1).

[13] Mental Health Act 2007 (NSW) (hereafter 'NSW'), s 53(3A): 'would be likely to' relapse into an active phase of illness.

[14] Some state statutes in the USA say the person must not be 'dangerous' when under outpatient treatment (see Bazelon Center for Mental Health Law 2000).

Drafting the criteria in that way has the advantage of suggesting that CTOs should only be used as a genuine alternative to compulsory hospital care.

Necessity or proportionality

Several extra legal standards then apply to the use of CTOs specifically. First, the criteria usually say that the CTO must be a necessary or proportionate intervention, in the circumstances. So, continuing treatment, care, or supervision in the community must be 'necessary' to avoid serious harm, or serious deterioration, or adverse consequences of relapse, or the CTO must be likely to prevent the person's condition getting worse or alleviate their symptoms.[15] In addition, the criteria may say that voluntary care must be unsuitable, or ineffective, or has been refused or not reliably followed, or that the person is unlikely, due to illness, to comply.[16] The attitude of the person to their treatment,[17] the history of their illness and its consequences,[18] and any previous refusal of treatment leading to relapse,[19] may be listed as factors to take into account. Some laws say it must be necessary to have certain powers available (that are provided by the CTO). In England and Wales, for instance, it must be 'necessary' to be 'able to exercise the power to recall the patient to hospital'.[20] In addition, the CTO must generally be the least restrictive approach.[21] All these rules give content to the general notion that the CTO must be a 'necessary' or 'proportionate' response.

Some criteria used for these purposes are quite prescriptive, especially in Canada. In effect, they require the person to have recently experienced a 'revolving door' pattern of care. They stipulate that the person must have been previously admitted to hospital—often compulsorily—on a certain number of occasions, or for a certain time, during a prior period of years.[22] In Nova Scotia, for example, the person must have been 'detained in a psychiatric facility' for either 'a total of sixty days or longer' or 'on two or more separate occasions', in the previous 2 years, or have previously been on a CTO.[23]

---

[15] The 'efficacy' of 'any previous order' may have to be considered when renewing a CTO: NSW, s 53.

[16] NSW, s 53(3)(c); Mental Health Care and Treatment Act (Newfoundland and Labrador), SNL 2006, c M-9.1 (hereafter 'Newfoundland and Labrador'), s 40(2)(a)(iii).

[17] Victoria, ss 46(2)(a)(i), 55.

[18] England and Wales, s 17A(6); NSW, s 14(2).

[19] NSW, s 133.

[20] England and Wales, s 17A(5)(d).

[21] NSW, s 53(3)(a).

[22] For example, Nova Scotia, Saskatchewan, Ontario, and Newfoundland and Labrador; see Gray et al. (2008). Some state statutes in the USA have similar requirements (e.g. New York Mental Hygiene Law, Article 9.60(c)).

[23] Involuntary Psychiatric Treatment Act (Nova Scotia) SNS 2005, c 42 (hereafter 'Nova Scotia'), s 47(3)(b).

These strict requirements provide some assurance that CTOs will be used only to prevent readmission to hospital. However, they can be quite inflexible in practice. A prior hospitalization requirement may not be satisfied by the person spending a period in prison while mentally ill, or in a community facility providing a high level of care, or even in a hospital in another province,[24] and the requirement may prohibit use of a CTO following a person's first compulsory admission regardless of their level of insight into their need for care. The concerns behind these prescriptive requirements might be better expressed through the use of the general legal principles already discussed: that is, through a requirement that the voluntary approach to treatment not be viable, that the CTO be necessary to prevent hospitalization, or that compulsory outpatient treatment be the least restrictive option—giving greater flexibility in application.

Viability of community care

Further criteria require that outpatient care be viable. This means, first, that appropriate community services exist and are available to the person, and secondly, that the person could survive safely outside hospital under such care. For example, New Zealand law stipulates that the mental health services must be able to provide 'care and treatment on an outpatient basis that is appropriate to the needs of the patient', and requires that 'the social circumstances of the patient' would be 'adequate for his or her care in the community'.[25] Many statutes require the preparation of a CTO treatment plan, listing the services to be provided and signifying that the relevant service providers agree to provide them (particularly where the providers will be drawn from the charitable or private sectors, or be independent practitioners, not under the direct control of a public health authority). In addition, the law may say that the person must be 'capable of' complying,[26] or 'able to' comply,[27] even—in the case of Newfoundland and Labrador—requiring an 'undertaking by the person' to comply.[28]

Consent or incapacity

Finally, some statutes require that the use of CTOs must conform to certain general legal principles that govern all forms of medical treatment in that jurisdiction, especially legal principles concerning consent to treatment, and substitute decision-making for health care. In some Canadian provinces this means, for instance, that, where a person retains their capacity (or competence) to consent to psychiatric care, a CTO cannot be made without their consent; and, where they lack that capacity, approval must be sought from their SDM. Furthermore, their SDM, when acting on

---

[24] Some Australian statutes provide for interstate transfer of CTO patients, or interstate recognition of CTOs: Victoria, ss 318–325; NSW, ss 181–184.

[25] New Zealand, s 28(4).

[26] Newfoundland and Labrador, s 40(2)(a)(v).

[27] Ontario, s 33.1(4)(c)(iv).

[28] Newfoundland and Labrador, s 41(1)(g); see Ontario, s 33.

their behalf, may be obliged to give effect to any clear views they have expressed previously about their psychiatric care (for a discussion see Dawson 2006, pp. 485–8).

Ontario law illustrates this position. In that province, a separate Health Care Consent Act[29] provides a code of rules governing consent to medical treatment in general, including psychiatric treatment (Hiltz and Szigeti 2005; Gray et al. 2008). Those rules then apply to treatment under the MHA, including use of CTOs. This means—for a CTO to be made—that the consent of the person must be obtained, if they have capacity, or, if they lack capacity, the consent of their SDM.

There is great variation between jurisdictions, however, in the manner in which capacity principles are incorporated into laws governing compulsory psychiatric care (Dawson and Kampf 2006). Generally, within a jurisdiction, the same capacity principles will apply to both compulsory inpatient and compulsory outpatient care—but not always. The law in England and Wales, for example, grants people on CTOs the right to refuse medication (if they retain their capacity) during their treatment as an outpatient, but not during their recall from a CTO to inpatient care. This means different capacity principles apply to inpatient and outpatient care, and it permits a person to be given medication at a hospital or clinic—on recall from a CTO—regardless of their capacity to consent to that treatment.

Generally speaking, in Australasia, no finding of incapacity is required to put a person on a CTO or treat them under the authority of the order. In some other jurisdictions, like Saskatchewan, the opposite position obtains. There a person must lack capacity[30] (or, in Scotland, have 'substantially impaired capacity')[31] to be placed under any form of compulsory psychiatric care, including a CTO. Between those poles, several intermediate positions exist. In some jurisdictions, a finding of incapacity is *not* required to put a person on a CTO if they pose a risk of harm to *others*, but *is* required where they pose a risk to *self*.[32] In others, a finding of incapacity is *not* required to put a person on a CTO, or to exercise some of the powers it confers, but *is* required to administer medication under the order's authority without the person's consent.[33]

To apply the same capacity principles to psychiatric treatment as apply to most other forms of medical care has the advantage of reducing discrimination in the law against people with mental disabilities (Campbell and Heginbotham 1991). It may also prevent people being kept on CTOs for extended periods whose capacity fluctuates in the

---

[29] Health Care Consent Act 1996, RSO 1996, c 2.

[30] Mental Health Services Act (Saskatchewan), SS, c M-13 (hereafter 'Saskatchewan'), s 24.3(1)(a)(v) ('as a result of the mental disorder, the person is unable to fully understand and to make an informed decision regarding his or her need for treatment or care and supervision') (see Gray et al. 2008).

[31] Mental Health (Care and Treatment) (Scotland) Act 2003 (hereafter 'Scotland') (see Franks and Cobb 2005; McManus and Thomson 2005).

[32] Mental Health Act (Alberta), RSA 2000, c M-13 (hereafter 'Alberta'), s 9.1(1)(f)(ii).

[33] See the account of New York law given in the court's decision on the constitutional challenge to that state's outpatient commitment scheme: *In re KL* 806 NE 2d 480 (2004) (NYCA).

course of their condition, if it means they must be released from the CTO as soon as their capacity returns (see Dawson 2006, pp. 485–8).

Powers of enforcement

Two main legal questions arise about the 'enforcement' of CTOs. The first concerns the mandatory 'conditions' or requirements that may be imposed on a person's outpatient treatment under a CTO. What conditions are authorized? The second concerns enforcement. What powers are provided to enforce the conditions set, bearing in mind the principle that any exercise of state power that affects a person's rights must be clearly authorized by law?[34]

The statutes studied illustrate four main approaches to the imposition of mandatory conditions on a CTO:

* directly stipulating in the legislation that certain conditions apply to everyone on a CTO;

* permitting certain mandatory conditions to be imposed, as a matter of discretion, when a CTO is made;

* use of statutory treatment plans that may include some mandatory and some optional elements;

* providing a general statement in the legislation of the purposes for which conditions may be imposed.

Some mixture of these approaches may be also used. Mechanisms for enforcing the CTO are then usually linked—directly or implicitly—to compliance with the conditions imposed.

Using the first approach, New Zealand law specifies that every CTO 'shall require the patient to attend at the patient's place of residence, or at some other place specified in the order, for treatment by employees of the specified service, and to accept that treatment'.[35] It then empowers the responsible clinician to recall a person to hospital from a CTO whenever they 'cannot continue to be treated adequately as an outpatient'.[36] These spare provisions do not say precisely that non-compliance with treatment justifies immediate recall, but they clearly suggest that recall could be used as the mechanism for enforcing the mandatory 'attendance' and 'treatment' conditions automatically imposed on every person under a CTO.

Other statutes describe in general terms the obligations that may be included in a mandatory treatment plan, and then say the person 'shall' meet those obligations. New South Wales law provides that the CTO plan shall provide 'an outline of the proposed treatment, counselling, management, rehabilitation or other services to be provided', and shall state 'in specific terms, the methods by which, the frequency with which, and the place at which the services' will be provided.[37] The person is then required 'to be

---

[34] *Entick v Carrington* (1765) 19 St Tr 1029; 95 ER 807 (KB).

[35] New Zealand, s 29(1).

[36] New Zealand, s 29(3).

[37] NSW, s 54; and see Ontario, s 33.1.

present, at the reasonable times and places specified in the order' to 'receive' the services listed in that plan,[38] and to 'comply' with the CTO.[39] Non-compliance with such requirements would not constitute a contempt of court, or a civil wrong, or a crime, but the law will usually authorize recall to hospital for failure to comply.

The main approach taken in the legislation for England and Wales, in contrast, is not to require the preparation of a statutory treatment plan but to specify the purposes for which conditions may be imposed on a CTO. It is said that conditions may be imposed that are 'necessary or appropriate' to ensure the person receives treatment for mental disorder, to prevent risk of harm to their health or safety, or to protect other people.[40] Within those broad parameters, the conditions might cover supported accommodation, compliance with medication, availability to the treatment team, and avoidance of risk factors or dangerous situations (Dawson 2010b, pp. 531–2).

Nevertheless, the law does not always provide a direct means to enforce every common condition imposed, such as a requirement to 'take medication', 'live where directed', or 'avoid drink and drugs'. No clear power is usually provided, for instance, to administer medication by force in a community setting should the person refuse. No power is conferred on the managers of community care homes to detain a person in that environment who has been directed to live there under the CTO. Nor are the police or other third parties empowered to 'apprehend and return' the person to such a care home should they depart. Nor will a power be provided to physically prevent a person taking drink or drugs when outside hospital.

What the law usually provides is a small cluster of powers for the *indirect* enforcement of such conditions. It provides the power to maintain contact with the person in the community (to monitor their condition) and the power to recall them to hospital if they do not meet the conditions of their treatment or require further inpatient care. Even so, these powers are not unlimited in scope, and may not always be available. They are usually conferred on a limited category of persons, such as the responsible clinician (or community team), not on group home managers, family members, or the world at large. Moreover, their use is usually governed by further legal criteria and a specified process and must be consistent with the purposes of the CTO regime. Something of a gap may open, therefore, between the apparently mandatory conditions of a CTO and the circumstances in which those conditions can be enforced in detail,[41] particularly if recall to hospital is not immediately authorized for failure to comply with every element of the treatment plan.

Under some statutes, non-compliance with mandatory conditions immediately permits use of the recall power, allowing clinicians to direct the person's re-examination,

---

[38] NSW, s 56(1)(b).

[39] NSW, s 57(1).

[40] England and Wales, s 17B(2).

[41] As a result, it may be wise for clinicians to impose only conditions whose breach would readily lead them to recall the person to hospital, as recall will often be the only realistic means of enforcement available (see Smith et al. 2014).

or readmission, whenever they have 'failed to comply'.[42] Difficulties can arise, however, if the law permits recall *only* for non-compliance of that kind with the plan. That approach may prevent the person's readmission, under the authority of the CTO, should their condition deteriorate, requiring hospital care, despite their full compliance with the plan. In that situation, to secure the person's readmission, they may have to be recertified under the front end of the compulsory treatment process, despite already being under a CTO, with no obvious advantage to them or their clinicians.

The alternative approach, therefore, is not to make non-compliance with the treatment plan a necessary condition for exercise of the recall power. Instead, separate legal criteria are established to govern recall that do not require non-compliance. The legislation for England and Wales, for example, says recall can proceed when '(a) the patient requires medical treatment in hospital for his mental condition; and (b) there would be a risk of harm to the health or safety of that patient or to other persons if the patient were not recalled to hospital for that purpose'.[43] In that case, non-compliance with treatment is only one factor to consider when deciding whether those recall standards are met, and a person meeting those standards can be recalled whether or not they have complied with the plan.

Nevertheless, setting separate standards for recall can present its own problems. This is because it requires clinicians to be satisfied that the separate standards for recall are genuinely met. Under the already quoted recall criteria in England and Wales, for example, clinicians have to be satisfied that the person needs hospital treatment and presents certain risks. The question then arises whether failure to comply with a mandatory condition of a CTO—failure to attend a clinic to receive an injection, perhaps—is sufficient to satisfy those recall criteria, if no serious deterioration has yet occurred in the person's condition. If the separate criteria governing recall were not met, no immediate process would be available to enforce the apparently mandatory requirements of the plan.

Setting separate recall standards also has advantages. It usually limits recall to situations in which the person urgently needs treatment in hospital, for current clinical reasons, and may—for that reason—comply more closely with the principles governing detention for mental health purposes, under human rights law.[44]

Specific enforcement powers

To express the force of a CTO more clearly, the legislation then usually adds a list of carefully crafted powers, conferred on certain persons. These powers may then be

---

[42] For example Ontario, s 33.1.

[43] England and Wales, s 17E(1). In addition, in England and Wales, a CTO automatically imposes certain mandatory requirements on the person that are necessary to ensure continuation of the process: notably, to be available for examination by a psychiatrist whenever extension of the order is contemplated or a second opinion on treatment is required. Breach of those conditions automatically authorizes recall: s 17E(2).

[44] *Winterwerp v Netherlands* (1979–1980) 2 EHRR 387; 4 EHRR 288 (ECHR); *Matter of Luttrell* 633 NE 2d 74 (Ill. 1994).

supplemented by additional forms of authority or justification for intervention that are conferred by separate legislation or the common law (Dawson 1999).

Entry for treatment purposes

How, for instance, are community mental health staff to obtain access to a person under a CTO who is living outside hospital, in a private residence perhaps, or a community care home, in order to monitor their condition and continue discussions about their treatment? No doubt entry to the premises could be obtained by consent in most cases. It could be obtained through the consent of the person, or of family members, other occupiers, or staff of the facility in which the person resides. If sufficient consent were not forthcoming, however, some recognized form of authority or justification for entry would be required.

Not all CTO statutes confer a power of entry for treatment purposes, in light of the intrusions on property and privacy involved. Nevertheless, the person is under some pressure to stay in contact with the treatment team, because in the background lies the threat of their recall to hospital if contact cannot be secured. For the purpose of activating that recall process, a clear power to enter—even by force—*is* invariably provided, with police assistance available.

Some statutes expressly confer a power of entry for such treatment and contact purposes. New South Wales law formerly authorized entry to the 'land but not the dwelling' of a person on a CTO, to facilitate contact.[45] New Zealand law goes further, expressly conferring a power of entry on staff of the service responsible, who may 'at all reasonable times, enter the patient's place of residence or other place so specified for the purpose of treating the patient'.[46] No equivalent power seems to be conferred by the statutes in Canada or England and Wales.

There are other means through which community staff could obtain lawful entry, without an occupier's consent. The wider mental health legislation may confer a relevant power. In England and Wales, an approved mental health professional may, for instance, enter any premises and inspect where there is 'reasonable cause to believe' that a 'mentally disordered patient' is 'not under proper care'.[47] That power might be used, on relevant occasions, whether or not the person on the premises was on a CTO. The police, ambulance officers—or indeed any person—may also be authorized to enter in emergencies by other legislation,[48] or by the common law principle of necessity.[49] However, many mental health statutes only authorize entry without consent—under the authority of the CTO—for the purposes of exercising the recall power.

---

[45] Mental Health Act 1990 (NSW), s 146.

[46] New Zealand, s 29(2). The Scottish legislation also requires a person under a Compulsory Treatment Order to 'allow visits' at their residence: Scotland, s 66(1)(g).

[47] See, for example, England and Wales, s 115.

[48] See, for example, Search and Surveillance Act 2012 (NZ), s 14; Police and Criminal Evidence Act 1984 (UK), s 17(1)(e).

[49] *Dehn v Attorney-General* [1988] 2 NZLR 564 (HC).

Directing the person's residence

Residential placement conditions are sometimes added to a CTO. The person might be required to live in a certain kind of residence, or one providing a certain level of support ('24-hour supervision'), or at a specified address. A clinician considering such a condition should ensure that the residence provides an acceptable level of care and that its staff has the necessary skills. Moreover, imposing very stringent conditions, such as an '18-hour curfew', or 'never leaving without supervision from staff', could be viewed as producing de facto detention in a community facility. That might not be authorized by the CTO and could readily be challenged on human rights grounds.[50]

A CTO statute can authorize a residence condition in a number of ways. First, the statute may expressly say this condition can be imposed. Saskatchewan's law says a CTO can stipulate 'that the person is required to stay at a residence specified by the psychiatrist'.[51] In Scotland, a person can be required to 'reside at a specified place'.[52] In Quebec, residence may be controlled through a community care order made by the Superior Court under the incapacity provisions of the Civil Code (Nakhost et al. 2012). In New Zealand, on the other hand, the courts have ruled that the requirement to 'attend' at a certain residence for treatment does not permit a person to be ordered to reside at a specified address.[53]

Secondly, directing a person's residence may fall within the scope of the conditions includable in a CTO plan, or of the 'purposes' for which conditions can be imposed. Thirdly, a residence condition may be approved by the person's SDM, where such approval is required to implement the CTO. In Ontario, for instance, the Health Care Consent Act specifically declares that one form of 'treatment' that a SDM can approve is a 'community treatment plan' under the mental health legislation.[54] Applying that provision, the Consent and Capacity Board of Ontario has ruled that a SDM can consent to the imposition of a residence requirement in the plan when that is consistent with the purposes of the CTO regime.[55]

In practice, the proposed accommodation provider must agree to accept the person in the residence, and the person must at least acquiesce in the living arrangements, because, if the person were to refuse to remain at a residence that was considered essential to their care, their outpatient treatment would no longer be viable and they would cease to qualify for a CTO.

Enforcing a residence requirement can be problematic in practice. No power is usually conferred on staff of a community residence, or on police, neighbours, or the

---

[50] *Guzzardi v Italy* (Application no. 7367/76) (1980) ECHR 5, (1981) 3 EHRR 333; *Pleso v Hungary* (Application no. 41242/08) (2012) ECHR 1767.

[51] Mental Health Services Act, SS, c M-13, s 24(3)(1)(d.1), as amended by Bill 27, An Act to Amend the Mental Health Services Act, 2014.

[52] Scotland, s 66(1)(e).

[53] *Department of Health v D* (1999) 18 FRNZ 233, [1999] NZFLR 514 (FC).

[54] Health Care Consent Act 1996, RSO 1996, c. 2, s 2.

[55] *In the matter of MGB* CanLII (2003) n.14360 (ON, CCB).

public, to enforce it by directly interfering with the physical freedom of the person should they try to leave a specified address. Nor does a CTO confer direct authority to apprehend the person and return them to that address. The principal means of enforcement is therefore recall to hospital, at the discretion of the responsible clinician, for failure to comply with the plan.

Treatment without consent under the CTO

Many complex issues can arise about the lawfulness of treatment provided under the aegis of a CTO without a person's consent—too many issues to be considered fully here. The solutions will often turn on the detailed interpretation of the treatment provisions of the particular regime, and on whether separate rules are provided for outpatient treatment under a CTO. How far does the concept of 'treatment' extend, in this context? How many elements of a person's life can be controlled that directly affect their mental health? Does the CTO authorize the administration of medication—by injection, for example—to which the person acquiesces (or does not object) but does not consent? Is treatment outside hospital ever authorized by 'force' or physical restraint? Can a person be 'taken' to hospital and given treatment authorized by the plan, then released the same day, with no intention of admitting them to inpatient care? On recall, can treatment be immediately provided without consent, or must the person first undergo compulsory reassessment, against the usual standards for inpatient care? Considerable variation exists between jurisdictions in all these arrangements.

Generally, mental health legislation authorizes only treatment 'for mental disorder', but a CTO imposes a duty on a person to accept treatment of that kind, outside hospital, under the treatment plan. The imposition of such a duty may then be considered by the courts to confer a correlative power on staff to administer the treatment without the person's consent, at least where it can be 'administered without the use of more force than would be required if the person had consented'—as the law of New South Wales put it.[56] Furthermore, the law may authorize staff to take 'all reasonable steps to have medication administered',[57] or use 'reasonable force' when exercising their powers.[58]

Nevertheless, except perhaps in an emergency, CTO statutes do not generally authorize the 'forced' administration of medication outside a hospital or clinic through the use of physical restraint. That practice is not authorized, first, because the law on CTOs does not permit 'detention' of a person for the purposes of administering treatment outside hospital, and—as administering medication by physical restraint would usually involve such detention, even if only for a short time—that practice would then be unlawful (unless authorized by some other rule of law).

Secondly, it would not usually be considered a safe or ethical health practice to administer medication via use of physical restraint in a community setting where the person cannot be adequately observed and assessed and where proper clinical

---

[56] NSW, s 57(3). For discussion of this position see Dawson (2010b, pp. 542–3).

[57] NSW, s 57(2).

[58] New Zealand, s 122B; NSW, s 81(2).

assistance is not available. Moreover, manhandling of that kind would clearly have a heavy impact on the person's home and privacy rights. It would go beyond mere administration of treatment, and would not be a 'reasonable' use of force. The proper practice is to return the person to hospital, if necessary, where urgent treatment may usually proceed.

Some CTO statutes authorize the use of force or physical restraint for treatment in an emergency. English law provides that 'force' may be used 'against' a person on a CTO who lacks the capacity to consent when this is 'immediately necessary', required 'to prevent harm to the patient', and 'the force is a proportionate response' to the likelihood and seriousness of that harm.[59] The common law of necessity would probably justify the same approach.

Some statutes also authorize the person to be 'taken' to a hospital or clinic for treatment under the terms of the CTO, even when the formal recall to hospital process has not been activated.[60] Other statutes would insist that the full criteria and process for recall be followed. Most laws authorize immediate treatment on recall, provided this is consistent with the treatment plan and any second opinion required has been obtained.[61] Further statutes—like Ontario's law—require the person to be reassessed initially, by the responsible physician, against the usual standards for compulsory hospital admission, and only when the person meets those standards can treatment proceed without consent.[62]

Recall to hospital

Recall is a further critical and sensitive aspect of the process. Many clinicians might favour a fast-track system, under which a person on a CTO could be smoothly readmitted to hospital without excessive 'paperwork', and they would see having access to such a process as a major reason for putting a person on a CTO. But recall leads to re-detention in hospital, even in secure conditions. It is therefore a particular focus of human rights concern. It should never be 'arbitrary'. It should be governed by clear criteria and a fair process, and should be based on objective medical assessment of the person's need for hospital care. Following recall, the person should have ready access to independent review.

There is a common core to the recall process followed in most jurisdictions, with some variations around that core. Recall is usually authorized either for failure to comply with mandatory elements of the treatment plan,[63] or where the person's outpatient treatment is no longer viable and they require further hospital care. The provisions of some statutes are quite spare, simply authorizing recall on such grounds, at the discretion of the responsible clinician, with no prior process stipulated. In other

---

[59] England and Wales, s 64G.

[60] New Zealand, ss 40, 41.

[61] NSW, s 60(1)(a); England and Wales, Part 4.

[62] Ontario, s 33.3.

[63] In Nova Scotia, 'substantial or deleterious' failure to comply: s 56.

jurisdictions, a series of procedural steps is laid down that must be followed for recall to occur.[64] Clinicians may be required to make reasonable prior efforts to verify that the person could comply (that the necessary services were available, for instance), and to inform the person of their failure to comply. Consultation with the person and other health professionals may be mandatory. Notice to the person of their impending recall is often required. Moreover, in the USA, many state statutes require a court order for recall to occur (Bazelon Center for Mental Health Law 2000).

Once the recall criteria are met and the process has been followed, a cluster of powers is conferred on designated health professionals—assisted by the police or other 'authorized persons'[65]—that permit entry to premises, apprehension or detention of the person, transportation, readmission, and treatment at the hospital. The use of 'reasonable force' is usually authorized, and some statutes spell this out in detail, permitting physical restraint,[66] immediate sedation,[67] search of the person,[68] and seizure of dangerous objects.[69] Some statutes confer an independent power to direct a person's recall—in certain circumstances—on the police, or the courts, as well as on clinicians.[70] Some require a warrant to be obtained from a judicial officer to authorize entry, except in an emergency.

The statute should then carefully specify the consequences of recall for the person's treatment. Immediate treatment at a hospital or clinic is usually authorized under the terms of the treatment plan, and many people would see the threat of such immediate treatment on recall as the key enforcement mechanism for a CTO. The staff must then decide whether to release the person back into the community on the CTO, admit them to hospital, or release them completely from compulsory care. Some statutes make this a two-stage process, initially authorizing a certain period of compulsory reassessment (such as 72 hours[71] or 14 days[72]), and only then requiring staff to take decisions about revocation (or cancellation) of the CTO and the person's return to compulsory inpatient status. Some jurisdictions permit voluntary readmissions during the course of a CTO.

The statute must also carefully specify the consequences of recall for continuation of the CTO. It should indicate precisely when the order is suspended or revoked, for example, as that will often determine the timing of the person's subsequent entitlements, such as their right to a hearing before a court or tribunal or a second opinion on their treatment. There are many pitfalls in this area for the statute to avoid,

---

[64] Ontario, s 33.3; Nova Scotia, s 56; NSW, s 58.

[65] Victoria, ss 3, 353; NSW, s 81(1).

[66] Victoria, s 350; NSW, s 81(2).

[67] Victoria, s 350; NSW, s 81(3).

[68] Victoria, ss 354, 355; NSW, s 81(4).

[69] Victoria, s 356; NSW, s 81(5).

[70] Alberta, ss 10, 12.

[71] England and Wales, s 17F.

[72] New Zealand, s 29(3)(a).

such as imposing a complex process for reissue of a CTO after a brief period of recall. One legislative approach is to use an overarching Compulsory Treatment Order that authorizes both compulsory inpatient and outpatient care. That headline order can continue in force, conferring regular review entitlements on the person, whether their care proceeds inside or outside hospital.

Liability of staff

There is some potential for health professionals who manage people on CTOs to be exposed to civil liability in novel circumstances. In particular, it might be alleged that they have failed properly to exercise their powers of supervision or control over a person under the scheme, or provide them with adequate outpatient care, and 'but for' that failure some harm to the person or a third party would not have occurred. Such allegations are especially likely, of course, when serious violence has occurred (see Dawson 2006, pp. 491–2).

Aspects of the drafting of CTO legislation could enhance such liability concerns—if, for example, the legislation were to say that the services listed in the treatment plan 'must' be provided, or if clinicians 'signing off' the plan seemed to agree to guarantee a certain level of care, which was later not forthcoming. Negligence (or malpractice) actions might be more likely to succeed, in other words, if aspects of the legislation reinforce the clinicians' duty of care.

However, there is no evidence so far that the courts in the Commonwealth are more likely to impose liability on clinicians for such reasons. Nor does it appear that successful actions have been brought for negligence in the conduct of a CTO regime. It has been held, in England, for example, that the requirement of the MHA that local authorities provide after-care for discharged patients does not give rise to an action for damages if that duty is not fulfilled,[73] and the High Court of Australia recently held—in a case concerning discharge of a compulsory patient into the care of a friend, with tragic consequences—that hospital clinicians owed no duty of care under the law of negligence that would conflict with their obligation to take the least restrictive approach to a patient's care.[74]

Some mental health statutes directly address the liability concerns. Typically, they confer a limited protection from liability on staff who exercise statutory powers in 'good faith',[75] without affecting their liability for negligent clinical care. The Ontario legislation specifically addresses one aspect of liability in the use of CTOs. It recognizes that many independent agencies may agree to provide services under a CTO plan, none of whom should be expected to assume responsibility for the others' default. It therefore confers protection from liability on any party to the plan who 'believes, on

---

[73] *Clunis v Campden and Islington Health Authority* [1998] QB 978 (CA).

[74] *Hunter and New England Local Health District v McKenna* [2014] HCA 44; and see *Hunter Area Health Authority v Presland* [2005] NSWCA 33.

[75] NZ, s 122; NSW, s 191(1).

reasonable grounds and in good faith' that the [other] parties who 'are responsible for providing' services 'are doing so in accordance with the plan'.[76]

Duration, review, discharge

The maximum duration of a CTO before renewal is required is usually 3, 6, or 12 months. Six months is perhaps the most common, though a 'sliding scale' is often used, with orders lasting 6 months initially, then going to 12 months on the first or second renewal.

The person is generally entitled to independent review of the order by a court or tribunal at least once during its term, particularly at (or within a month or two of) the time when the order is made, and then when it is renewed, though these reviews may also occur on a sliding scale, being more frequent early in the order's life and less frequent later. A mix of automatic reviews, and reviews on application by the person or other interested parties, is frequently employed. The same (or similar) procedures are usually followed as for inpatient reviews. The review body has (and must have) the power to discharge the person from the CTO.[77]

Too frequent reviews may over-burden the system and become superficial, or be conducted 'on the papers', or on the phone. If the number of reviews is too high, it may be difficult to recruit sufficient professional members of the tribunal (especially psychiatrists) to conduct the process, with the result that single-member tribunals may be adopted (usually involving a lawyer, to manage the procedure). That may produce an inferior form of review.

There are many other routes to discharge from a CTO. Most commonly, discharge would occur on expiry of the CTO without its renewal, or on the person's release by their responsible clinician—who has a continuing power (and duty) to discharge them when they no longer meet the criteria. Some statutes confer an additional power of discharge on hospital managers or senior mental health administrators.[78] The superior courts usually retain a power of discharge.[79] In England and Wales, in certain situations, the person's nearest relative has the power.[80] The CTO is usually cancelled by imposition of a more restrictive form of legal control, such as a sentence of imprisonment or an order for forensic care, though shorter periods of imprisonment—on remand, prior to trial, for instance—may only suspend the order.

Conclusion

This review of CTO legislation shows, above all, that a certain legal framework is required for a well-developed CTO regime. A particular legal agenda must be addressed

---

[76] Ontario, s 33.6.

[77] A regular 'legislated review' (or evaluation) of the CTO regime itself is required by some statutes: Ontario, s 33.9; Nova Scotia, s 59; Newfoundland and Labrador, s 6.

[78] England and Wales, s 72.

[79] New Zealand, s 84.

[80] England and Wales, ss 23(2)(c), 25.

to produce a well-crafted scheme. This produces common features to the CTO regimes in different jurisdictions. It is therefore no surprise that there is considerable overlap between the legal principles exhibited by the Commonwealth schemes studied here and those found in state statutes in the USA. A clear administrative structure must be established that allocates responsibilities—for issuing and reviewing a CTO, supervising compulsory outpatient treatment, and deciding on recall to hospital care. The criteria and process must be set under which these decisions are made. There must be a mechanism for settling the mandatory conditions for a person's outpatient care. The powers of enforcement must be fashioned with special care, due to the implications for the person's rights. The duration of the order must be established, avenues must be set for discharge, and the consequences must be indicated for the person's compulsory status of their recall to hospital care.

When rights to liberty, to privacy, and to refuse treatment are so obviously implicated, all these issues must be carefully addressed. This produces a common core to the statutory scheme. Within this general structure there is room for considerable variation in detail, and notable variations are found between the laws of the different Commonwealth jurisdictions in the strictness of the criteria for placing a person on a CTO, whether consent or incapacity is required to put a person on a CTO, the role played by mandatory treatment plans, the range of conditions that can be imposed on a person's community tenure, and the powers available to enforce the order, especially the details of the recall power.

More recent statutes tend to be more detailed, especially in their treatment of the conditions that can be imposed on outpatient care and the powers of enforcement available. This is the flip side of heightened human rights concern—a trend towards more elaborate codes of rules that specify more clearly and precisely the circumstances in which limits may be placed on the rights of a person under compulsory outpatient care.

References

Bazelon Center for Mental Health Law (2000). *Involuntary outpatient commitment: summary of state statutes.* Washington, DC: Bazelon Center for Mental Health Law. Available at: http://www.bazelon.org/LinkClick.aspx?fileticket=CBmFgyA4i-w%3D&tabid=324

Campbell T, Heginbotham C (1991). *Mental illness: prejudice, discrimination, and the law.* Aldershot: Dartmouth Publishing.

Dawson J (1999). The law of emergency psychiatric detention. *New Zealand Law Review* 1999:275–303.

Dawson J (2005). *Community treatment orders: international comparisons.* Dunedin: Otago University Print. Available at: http://www.otago.ac.nz/law/research/otago036152.pdf

Dawson J (2006). Fault-lines in community treatment order legislation. *International Journal of Law and Psychiatry*, 29:482–494.

Dawson J (2010a). Compulsory outpatient treatment and the calculus of human rights. In: *Rethinking rights-based mental health laws* (ed. B McSherry, P Weller), pp. 327–354. Oxford: Hart Publishing.

Dawson J (2010b). Community treatment orders. In: *Principles of mental health law and policy* (ed. L Gostin, P Bartlett, P Fennell, et al.), pp. 513–554. Oxford: Oxford University Press.

Dawson J, Gledhill K (eds) (2013). *New Zealand's Mental Health Act in practice.* Wellington: Victoria University Press.

Dawson J, Kampf A (2006). Incapacity principles in mental health laws in Europe. *Psychology, Public Policy and Law,* **12**:310–331.

Franks R, Cobb D (2005). *Mental Health (Care and Treatment) (Scotland) Act 2003.* Edinburgh: W Green.

Gostin L, Bartlett P, Fennell P, et al. (eds) (2010). *Principles of mental health law and policy.* Oxford: Oxford University Press.

Gray J, Shone M, Liddle P (2008). *Canadian mental health law and policy,* 2nd edn. Markham, ON: LexisNexis Canada.

Hiltz D, Szigeti A (2005). *A guide to consent and capacity law in Ontario.* Markham, ON: LexisNexis Butterworths.

McManus J, Thomson L (2005). *Mental health and Scots law in practice.* Edinburgh: W Green.

Nakhost A, Perry J, Frank D (2012). Assessing outcome of compulsory treatment orders on management of psychiatric patients at 2 McGill University-associated hospitals. *Canadian Journal of Psychiatry,* **57**:359–365.

Smith M, Branton T, Cardno A (2014). Is the bark worse than the bite? Additional conditions used within community treatment orders. *Psychiatric Bulletin,* **38**:9–12.

Part 2

The evidence

Chapter 4

Descriptive and epidemiological studies

Stéphane Morandi

Introduction

The deinstitutionalization that would be the hallmark of psychiatry in industrialized countries during the second half of the twentieth century began in the USA in the 1960s. This movement made it possible for numerous individuals suffering from mental illness to leave hospital and reintegrate into their communities (Zusman et al. 1988). Emphasis was placed on greater respect for individual freedoms, a reduction of coercion in psychiatric care, and less recourse to involuntary hospitalization. This 'rhetorical quest for community' described by Cohen (1985), which juxtaposed 'the bad exclusionary institution' and 'the good, open, benevolent and accepting community', was quickly confronted with reality and unexpected challenges (McDonnell and Bartholomew 1997). Outpatient treatment and support in the community did not systematically respond to the needs of patients leaving their institutions (Lamb and Bachrach 2001). The frequent rehospitalization of individuals who were seriously ill and did not have access to suitable outpatient care became known as the 'revolving door'.

Community treatment orders (CTOs) were developed in several jurisdictions and first commonly used in the USA in the 1960s and 1970s. They were quickly adopted by other countries, especially in the English-speaking world (Hiday 2003). By authorizing outpatient care within the structure of a CTO, the aim was to offer a less restrictive alternative to involuntary hospitalization. It was hoped that CTOs would make it possible to keep people in care outside of hospital, to avoid any decline in their state of health and social situation, and crucially to limit recourse to institutional placements (least restrictive CTOs). Several countries further adapted their legislation to authorize the use of CTOs on a preventative basis (preventative CTOs).

The nature of the evidence considered in this chapter

There have been a number of studies and reports regarding CTO regimes following the introduction of different frameworks. This chapter will focus on descriptive and non-experimental studies that have observed and described the effects of the introduction of such regimes. Experimental studies comparing a population placed under a CTO with a control group are dealt with in Chapter 5.

Thirty-nine articles or reports are included in this review. Fifteen were conducted in the USA, 11 in Australasia, 5 in Canada, and 3 in Israel. Although CTOs exist in many other countries, there is little literature regarding their use. In Europe, CTOs exist in Italy, Norway, Sweden, the UK, Luxembourg, Belgium, France, Spain, and Switzerland. Only three descriptive studies (two in Spain and one, as-yet unpublished, in France) and three reports related to CTOs (from the UK) could be identified. We consider the evidence relating to CTOs under three broad headings: their practical application and processes of use, the characteristics of those they are used for, and their outcomes.

CTOs in practice

Rates of use of CTOs

The introduction of CTOs raised concerns that the number of individuals placed under compulsion would progressively increase. The available evidence from descriptive studies does not confirm an increase in the use of CTOs over time. However, some national reports regarding the use of community compulsion suggest that there are increases.

In 1983, a revision to the law on commitments authorized recourse to a CTO in the state of Arizona, USA. Van Putten et al. (1988) examined the impact of this new legal statute on the total number of commitments in the state. Data were collected during the 6 months before and 12 months after the introduction of CTOs. The total number of involuntary treatments (CTOs and involuntary admissions) dropped from 133 to 104 in the first 6 months following the introduction of new statutes, but then rose in the second 6 months to 147. The authors explained the decrease in the number of commitments observed during the first 6 months by caution on the part of professionals in using the new legislation, possible modification of care practices, and a seasonal fluctuation in the number of constraint measures. The increase over the following 6 months was explained by the fact that initial enthusiasm to limit the number of hospitalizations was possibly too strong during the first 6-month period. The use of CTOs was proportionately greater in the first 6 months than in the second (60% versus 44%, respectively, of total commitments).

Miller and Fiddleman (1984) observed whether the introduction of new conditions regarding community compulsion had any effect on the practice of existing (less restrictive) CTO laws. The main changes were the introduction of automatic readmission of patients who did not comply with their CTO and the requirement that both hospital and ambulatory care staff concurred with the proposed CTO. Their study was conducted in 1979 in North Carolina. It was carried out on 67 patients and considered the 6 months following the revision of the law. The proportion of CTOs dropped from 4.7% to 3.1% of the total number of commitments following the introduction of the new conditions. While none of the 67 patients had been hospitalized before the revision of the law, 32% of the sample were hospitalized in the following 6 months.

Miller (1992) studied the impact of the addition of 'criteria based need for treatment' to the commitment code in seven US states (South and North Carolina, Alaska, Hawaii,

Kansas, Texas, and Colorado) between 1975 and 1990 on the total number of hospitalizations. This new legal disposition authorized recourse to CTOs as a preventative measure and, more unusually, as an alternative to hospitalization. An increase in the number of hospitalizations was expected. For each state, observations were conducted during the 2 years before and after the introduction of the new law. Despite predictions, there was no dramatic increase in the number of hospitalizations and no overall trend could be defined. The number of hospitalizations increased in Hawaii and South Carolina following the legislative changes, while they decreased in North Carolina, Colorado, and Alaska. The number of hospitalizations remained stable in Texas and Kansas.

The hypothesis of 'net widening' was explored by Geller et al. (2006). According to this concept, compulsion becomes progressively more used when it is available despite the criteria remaining constant. In order to confirm this hypothesis, the authors documented the number of CTOs ordered in the state of Massachusetts between 1991 and 2002. In this state, guardianship law stated that an individual might be placed under a CTO simply by the court determining that he or she was not competent to make treatment decisions. Geller reported an increase in the use of CTOs during the first 4 years, with a subsequent decrease. During the period studied, CTOs represented 3% of all measures of constraint in psychiatry. As this rate remained very low and fluctuated only slightly, the authors concluded that the concept of 'net widening' should not be an argument for limiting the use of CTOs. Others have investigated why CTOs were little used in certain areas.

Torrey and Kaplan (1995) conducted a survey to determine the extent of CTO use in the USA. They called upon people who were 'knowledgeable about CTO use' (attorneys in the state office of mental health and officials at the state alliance for the mentally ill) in the 35 states (and the District of Columbia) that had relevant legislation. In 12 states and the District of Columbia CTO use was rated 'very common' or 'common'. It was 'occasional', 'rare', or 'very rare' in 23 states. The reasons cited for not using CTOs included concerns about civil liberties, liability for crimes committed by patients, the financial burden on community services, professionals' lack of information and interest in CTOs, failure of some states to set enforceable consequences for non-compliance, a lack of hospital beds to accommodate non-compliant patients, and the fact that criteria were too restrictive.

Sixty-nine psychiatrists in Saskatchewan, Canada, were surveyed in 2000 to determine their pattern of CTO use (O'Reilly et al. 2000); 72% ($n = 50$) responded. Just over half of them had not used CTOs since their introduction 3 years previously. Reasons cited included: no suitable patients (53%), insufficient information (19%), insufficient powers (19%), and, for one (4%), that the powers provided by CTOs were excessive and unnecessary.

Community compulsion was enabled in Florida in January 2005. Only 71 orders were issued during the following 3 years. During that period, 41,997 individuals had two or more emergency examinations under Florida's civil commitment law and were thus eligible for a CTO. Petrila and Christy (2008) explained this low rate (0.17%) as due to problems of implementation, lack of resources, and lack of enforcement.

Several national reports regarding CTO use paint a different picture though. A 2005 report attempted to estimate the number of individuals who would be placed under a CTO in England and Wales when powers were introduced (Lawton-Smith 2005). The report concluded that, regardless of jurisdiction, the number of people placed on a CTO almost universally increased year on year. Internationally, several reports confirm this increase in prevalence over time. In New Zealand, community compulsion was introduced in 1992 (Dawson 2005). The number of CTOs documented in the country was 1207 in 1998 (Lawton-Smith 2005), 1943 in 2004, and 2493 in 2012. CTOs were introduced in England and Wales in 2008 (Department of Health 2008). Over the course of the year 2009–10, there were 4107 CTOs documented (Prior and Behan 2013). For 2012–13, the number of CTOs initiated increased to 4647. In Ontario, Canada, legislation has enabled the establishment of CTOs since 2000 and their prevalence has consistently increased (RA Malatest and Associates 2012) from less than 5 per 100,000 inhabitants in 2003 to 36 per 100,000 in 2010–11. In countries where the legislation is applicable in a fairly similar manner across an entire territory, the rate of recourse to CTOs can vary considerably between regions. Light et al. (2012) documented usage rates in different Australian states. Rates varied from 30 per 100,000 inhabitants in Tasmania to 99 per 100,000 in Victoria. The authors attributed these differences to the attitude of clinicians (powers provided by a CTO, perceived liability for patient's conduct in the community, perceived impact of coercion on therapeutic relationships, risk management, proportionality of coercion), subtle legal variations, resource variation, and differing statutory bodies.

Implementing CTOs

This subsection describes aspects related to the implementation of CTOs: justification for and aims of a CTO, conditions stipulated, duration, and appeal processes and rates.

Justifications, aims, and content

Information about justifications for CTOs, their aims, and content is scarce in descriptive studies. Only four publications in our review detail the reasons why the order was used (O'Keefe et al. 1997; Bar El et al. 1998; Rohland 1998; Canete-Nicolas et al. 2012). The main justifications were potential danger to self or others and non-compliance with medication. The aims of CTOs were specified in only one paper (Ozgul and Brunero 1997) and their content described in two studies (McDonnell and Bartholomew 1997; Ozgul and Brunero 1997). The results of these studies are summarized in Table 4.1.

Duration of compulsion and its cessation

Most reports found that CTOs were usually renewed at the end of the initial period. McDonnell and Bartholomew (1997) reported that 80% of initial CTOs were for between 10 and 12 months, the maximum allowed by Victorian legislation. Nearly a third of the people in the sample were on orders that had been extended for a period beyond the initial 12 months. The total number of CTOs and renewals for the 35 patients included in the Sydney study was 141 for a 3-year period (Ozgul and Brunero 1997). Twenty-six patients were on their fourth order and 90% of CTOs were renewed. The New York State Office of Mental Health Audit (2005) reported on the implementation of CTOs in New York State during the 5 years following the introduction of Kendra's Law in 1999. Thirty-six per cent of the sample spent between

Table 4.1 Justifications, aims, and content

Study	Location	Period of observation	Sample size	Justifications for CTO	Aims of CTO	Content of CTO
USA						
O'Keefe et al. (1997)	New Hampshire	Not specified	26 CTOs	54% indirect self-harm 12% direct self-harm 35% harm to others		
Rohland (1998)	Iowa	1991–6	274 CTOs	81.1% danger to self 17.9% danger to others 26.6% medication non-compliance 51.5% severely mentally impaired		
Australasia						
McDonnell and Bartholomew (1997)	Victoria	Not specified	130 CTOs			98% compulsory medication (for over half this was the sole form of treatment) 44% counselling or psychotherapy

(continued)

Table 4.1 (Continued)

Study	Location	Period of observation	Sample size	Justifications for CTO	Aims of CTO	Content of CTO
Australasia						
Ozgul and Brunero (1997)	Sidney	1993–6	141 CTOs (46 individuals)		100% medication compliance	100% compulsory medication
					99% regular appointment with case manager or doctor	99% appointments with care provider
					53% reduced relapse and hospital admission	46% support, education, and counselling
					43% support and education	30% involvement in rehabilitation activities
					These objectives were generally identified as having been achieved	4% education regarding substance use
Israel						
Bar El et al. (1998)	Jerusalem	1991–2	65 CTOs (50 individuals)	61% non-compliance with treatment		
				15% danger to self		
				23% danger to others		
				23% danger to others but not immediate		
Spain						
Canete-Nicolas et al. (2012)	Valencia	2003–12	140 CTOs	63% frequent relapses due to stopping medication		
				24% poor compliance		
				13% aggressive behaviours		

0 and 6 months under a CTO, the maximum duration of the initial order. The CTO order was renewed in 64% of cases. Nineteen per cent of people spent between 6 and 12 months, 21% between 12 and 18 months, 17% between 18 and 30 months, and 7% over 30 months under community compulsion. The average time under a CTO was 16 months. To assess the outcome of CTOs in Quebec, Nakhost et al. (2012) included all patients who had their primary CTO from July 1998 until August 2007. The mean duration of the CTO was 24.3 months and there was a progressive increase in the average length of compulsion from 12 to 36 months.

Although being placed under a CTO is a source of dissatisfaction for many, only a minority engage in legal opposition to their implementation. O'Brien and Farell (2005) examined this in a sample of psychiatric patients discharged from the Royal Ottawa Hospital in Ontario and placed on a CTO between 2001 and 2003 ($n = 25$). No patients chose to contest the CTO. Data for all patients who received a CTO over a 2-year period (May 1995 to June 1997) in north Jerusalem were reviewed ($n = 26$) (Greenberg et al. 2005). Only one person appealed. In the larger Victorian sample, rates of appeals were also low at 19% (McDonnell and Bartholomew 1997).

Patient profile

The socio-demographic characteristics of patients included in each study are depicted in Table 4.2 and their clinical profile is reported in Table 4.3.

These different studies were conducted on four continents in countries with considerable variations in legislation. Despite this there is remarkable homogeneity of those who are subject to orders. The typical portrait of an individual placed under a CTO is a single man in his forties who suffers from schizophrenia, has experienced repeated hospitalizations in a psychiatric setting, and presents behavioural challenges in the form of substance abuse or aggressive behaviour. While it is clear that this is a generalization and many different types of people are subject to orders, the proportion of people 'matching this description' is high and fairly constant.

Dawson and Roman (2001) in one jurisdiction in New Zealand included all 259 patients treated under a CTO between 1992 and 1998 ($n = 259$). They divided the sample into three categories: 47 'short-term' patients who had been under a CTO for less than a year, 117 'long-term' patients who were readmitted during the year, and 53 'long-term stable' patients whose CTO ran for more than a year without readmission. Comparisons showed significantly more patients with alcohol problems, schizophrenia, and aggression in the long-term groups.

In Victoria, Australia, Brophy et al. (2006) examined the clinical, social, and demographic characteristics of 164 people on CTOs in 1989. They divided people into 'clusters'. In the first 'connected' cluster ($n = 27$) there was a high rate of female patients with better social functioning. Criteria for a CTO emphasized the risk of deterioration, caregiver burden, and the impact of relapse on dependent children. The second 'young males' cluster ($n = 33$) included young patients with a diagnosis of paranoid schizophrenia. They were typically of low socio-economic status and appeared disconnected from the community. A CTO was generally used with these patients due to poor compliance, potential for relapse, lack of social support, additional diagnosis of drug and

Table 4.2 Socio-demographic characteristics of patients placed on CTOs and included in descriptive studies

Study	Mean age (years)	Male	Ethnicity	Marital status	Years of education	Employment	Living conditions
USA							
Fernandez and Nygard (1990)	36.8	59%	51.3% White 47.4% Black	53.2% single 17.5% married 28% separated, divorced or widowed			
Munetz et al. (1996)	41.4 (SD 14.3)	55%	100% White	90% unmarried	11.8 (SD 1.9)		
O'Keefe et al. (1997)	43 (SD 11)	54%		38% never married 22% married 38% separated, divorced, or widowed			
Rohland (1998)	37.3 (range 13–76)	53.7%	59.2% Black 40.7% White	48.5% single 23.9% married	45.8% between 0 and 11 years 36.3% had been in high school		
Rohland et al. (2000)	36.9 (range 18–76)	62%	87.7% White	61.7% never married 13.6% married		13.6% employed	87.7% own home

	Age		Ethnicity	Marital status	Housing
New York State Office of Mental Health (2005)	37.5	66%	34% White 42% Black 21% Hispanic 2% Asian 1% other	75% single or never married 8% married or cohabiting 17% divorced	
Australasia					
Power (1992)	40 (SD 14.9; range 11–99)	58%	66% Australian born	54% single 11% married 30% divorced or separated	90% private housing 6% supported housing 4% homeless
McDonnell and Bartholomew (1997)	>40	55.8%			70.8% private housing 48.5% living with family or friends 41.5% living alone
Ozgul and Brunero (1997)	36 (SD 13.74)	67%	67% Australian born	31% single	
Dawson and Roman (2001)	40 (SD 13.45)	60.2%	77.2% European 14.3% Maori (Maori were 4.8% of Otago population) 1.9% Pacific Islanders 0.8% Asian		

(continued)

Table 4.2 (Continued)

Study	Mean age (years)	Male	Ethnicity	Marital status	Years of education	Employment	Living conditions
Australasia							
Brophy et al. (2006)	40.5 (SD 11.6)	69.5%	68.9% Australian born	59.1% single 12.6% married 28.3% separated, divorced, or widowed		11.6% employed, student, or on home duties	79.8% were living alone or with family
Ingram et al. (2009)	39.4 (range 16–66)	70.2%		64.9% never married			
Canada							
O'Brien and Farell (2005)	45 (range 20–70)	60%		72% never married 12% living with a partner		4% received no monetary support	
Frank et al. (2005)	48.4 (SD 16.4)	52%	100% White				
Nakhost and Perry (2012)	46.3% (SD 15.5)	51.3%	52.7% White 16.6% Black 19.4% Asian or Arab	86.1% single, separated, or divorced 12.5% married 1.4% widowed 1.4% unknown		1.4% employed	44.4% living alone 43.1% living with relatives 4.2% living in group home or supervised apartment 4.2% homeless 4.2% other facilities

Israel

Study	Age	%	Religion	Marital status	Employment	Living situation
Bar El et al (1998)	37.5 (SD 10.9) (range 18–68)	68%	98% Jewish 2% Muslim	69% single 18% married 12% divorced 1% unknown		
Durst et al. (1999)	40.5 (SD 11.9)	71.8%		59.7% single 22% married 18.2% separated, divorced, or widowed		
Greenberg et al. (2005)	40 (range 19–76)	50%				34.6% living alone 65.4% living with relatives

Spain

Study	Age	%	Religion	Marital status	Employment	Living situation
Vallespir et al. (2008)	39.5 (SD 15.5)	70.2%			60.8% inactive 7.8% protected job 3.9% incapacitated 2% retired	58.7% living with relatives 20% living alone 6.7% living in a couple 6.7% living in an institution
Canete-Nicolas et al. (2012) (Valencia)	40	66%				

(continued)

Table 4.3 Clinical characteristics of patients placed on a CTO and included in descriptive studies

Study	Diagnosis	Other clinical features	Risk	Hospitalizations prior to CTO	Forensic history
USA					
Fernandez and Nygard (1990)	48.1% schizophrenia 11.1% bipolar disorder	10.6% alcohol or substance abuse as principal diagnosis			
Munetz et al. (1996)	75% schizophrenia	60% histories of drug or alcohol abuse		Mean 12.9 (SD 12.8)	40% arrested or incarcerated
O'Keefe et al. (1997)	58% schizophrenia 31% bipolar disorder				
Rohland (1998)	23.6% schizophrenia 11.2% other psychotic disorders 19.5% bipolar disorder				
Rohland et al. (2000)	45.7% schizophrenia 33.3% bipolar disorder	50.6% substance abuse			
New York State Office of Mental Health (2005)	71% schizophrenia or other psychotic disorder	52% concurrent diagnosis of drug or alcohol abuse		Mean 3.08 (range 0–13) during the 3 years prior to CTO 97% at least one hospitalization during the 3 years prior to CTO	

Australasia

Study	Diagnosis		
Power (1992)	78% schizophrenia	24% concurrent diagnosis, principally drug or alcohol abuse	18% at risk to themselves 89% at risk to the others	Mean 6.95 (range 1–41) 51% at least one admission during the year prior to CTO
McDonnell and Bartholomew (1997)	73% schizophrenia			
Ozgul and Brunero (1997)	89% schizophrenia			Mean 1.51 (SD 0.75) during the year prior to CTO
Dawson and Roman (2001)	54.8% schizophrenia 25.9% affective psychosis 5.4% schizoaffective psychosis			16.6% forensic history
Ingram et al. (2009)	100% schizophrenia (other diagnosis excluded)	30.1% concurrent diagnosis of substance misuse 17% concurrent diagnosis of alcohol misuse Mean length of illness 13 years (range 1–39)		Mean 4.82

Canada

Study	Diagnosis		
O'Brien and Farell (2005)	64% schizophrenia	44% concurrent diagnosis of substance dependence		
Frank et al. (2005)	55% schizophrenia 21% bipolar disorder			
Nakhost and Perry (2012)	85.5% diagnosis of schizophrenia or schizoaffective disorder			

(continued)

Table 4.3 (Continued)

Study	Diagnosis	Other clinical features	Risk	Hospitalizations prior to CTO	Forensic history
Israel					
Bar El et al. (1998)	85% schizophrenia	60% aggressive behaviours 60% active psychotic symptoms		61% more than five 17% between two and four 9% one 11% none	66% police history
Durst et al. (1999)	68.1% schizophrenia 15% schizoaffective disorder	88% aggressive behaviours 63.9% delusions		66% more than five 42% between two and four 24% one 5.7% none	62.4% police history
Greenberg et al. (2005)	76.9% schizophrenia			92.3% at least one 57.7% had never received an ambulatory treatment prior to CTO	
Spain					
Vallespir et al. (2008)	57% schizophrenia 16.5% delusional disorder 8.9% bipolar disorder	31% concurrent diagnosis of multiple drug abuse			53.4% violent behaviours against others reported
Canete-Nicolas et al. (2012) (Valencia)	68.6% schizophrenia	A third of people with schizophrenia also had a concurrent diagnosis of substance abuse disorder			

alcohol abuse, and/or caregiver burden. The 'chaotic' cluster ($n = 68$) included people with difficulties in relationships and living situation, a history of violence, multiple diagnoses, drug abuse, and a long duration of illness with numerous hospitalizations. This population had complex needs and represented high levels of risk. The authors concluded that people in each cluster had specific needs for assistance and required planning for more targeted treatment.

In an Australian review, Power (1999) proposed that the best clinical outcomes of CTOs were for patients over 28 years old, in the mid-phase of their overall illness, who had worse compliance with community treatment prior to their CTO.

Durst et al. (1999) examined the profile of all patients placed on a CTO in the southern districts of Jerusalem between 1991 and 1995. Two hundred and eight patients were included (a total of 326 CTOs). During the same period, 5264 involuntary admissions were issued. The population was divided into three outcome groups: 'success' was defined as continuous treatment for the entire CTO period or as voluntary hospitalization; 'failure' was defined as a need for compulsory admission; 'partial success' was defined as the inability to conform to the CTO terms but without compulsory hospitalization. One hundred and forty-one patients had a 'success' outcome, 106 a 'failure', and 72 a 'partial success'. A single previous hospitalization was associated with a more successful outcome than either no previous admissions or more than one previous admission. Beyond 2 years, the effectiveness of the CTO decreased. Successful outcomes were significantly associated with less aggressive behaviour and fewer delusions.

Outcomes

The 20 studies discussed in this section compared data from each patient population during a period before and after the introduction of a CTO. They are described briefly in Table 4.4. The results of each study are summarized in Table 4.5.

The overwhelming majority of studies focused on the impact of compulsion on the rate and duration of hospitalization. Treatment compliance, contact with outpatient care services, and violence were also considered, but less uniformly. Clinical changes and functioning were reported on less often, presumably reflecting the resource implications of this form of research.

Length of hospital stay and hospitalizations

All 13 studies which focused on the impact of CTOs on hospitalization rate noted a decrease in the number of hospitalizations after patients were placed under a CTO.

Of the 13 studies examining the number of days spent in hospital, 11 reported a significant decrease in time spent in hospital following the introduction of a CTO. Two found a non-significant reduction.

In North Carolina in the late 1970s, Hiday and Goodman (1982) followed all 408 CTO patients for the maximum time of an initial commitment, 3 months. Involuntary rehospitalization within 90 days decreased. In Washington DC, state hospitals experimented with CTOs beginning in 1971. Twelve years later, Zanni and Deveau (1986) investigated the effect of CTOs on hospitalization rate 1 year before and after commitment for 42 patients whose status changed from voluntary to requiring a CTO.

Table 4.4 Naturalistic follow-up studies of patients placed on CTO

Study	Location	Period of observation	Sample size	Data collection
USA				
Hidey and Goodman (1982)	North Carolina	1978–9	250 patients on CTO during the first year 158 patients on CTO during second year	3 months (maximum time of the initial CTO) after introduction of the CTO
Zanni and Deveau (1983)	Washington, DC	1983	42 patients placed on CTO	1 year before and after introduction of the CTO
Miller and Fiddleman (1984)	North Carolina	1979	67 patients placed on CTO	6 months before and after revision of a new statute law on CTO
Van Putten et al. (1988)	Arizona	1983–4	All the 384 psychiatric patients hospitalized in Tucson	6 months before, 6 months after, and between 6 and 12 months after introduction of CTO
Fernandez and Nygard (1990)	North Carolina	1985–8	4179 patients	1000 days before and after introduction of CTO
Munetz et al. (1996)	Ohio	1992–3	20 patients discharged on a CTO from state psychiatric unit for at least 12 months on the measure	1 year before an after assignment to a CTO
O'Keefe et al. (1997)	New Hampshire	Not specified	26 patients discharged on a CTO from state hospital	1 year before and 2 years after introduction of the CTO
Rohland et al. (2000)	Iowa	1991–6	81 patients placed on a CTO and with psychotic illness from outpatient clinic	1 year before and after introduction of the CTO

Study	Location	Years	Sample	Comparison
New York State Office of Mental Health (2005)	New York State	1999–2004	4041 referrals resulting in CTOs	Time spent on CTO
Geller et al. (2006)	Massachusetts	1991–2	21 patients (104 CTOs) placed on a CTO	1 year before and 2 years after introduction of the CTO
Esposito et al. (2008)	Florida	2005	21 patients placed on CTO (pilot program)	Time spent on a CTO and the equivalent time before CTO
Australasia				
Power (1992)	South Melbourne, Victoria	1987–91	125 patients placed on CTO 31 patients were followed up after discharge from the CTO during the same period spent on CTO	Time spent on a CTO and the equivalent time before CTO
Ozgul and Brunero (1997)	Sydney, New South Wales	1993–6	46 patients (141 CTOs) randomly selected among 74 severely ill people placed on CTO	1 year before and after introduction of the CTO
Muirhead and Harvey (2000)	Melbourne, Victoria	1996–8	58 patients with schizophrenia and placed on a CTO	1 year before and after introduction of CTO
Ingram et al. (2009)	Melbourne, Victoria	1996–9	94 patients with schizophrenia and placed on a CTO for at least 10 months	1 year before and after introduction of CTO

(continued)

Table 4.4 (Continued)

Study	Location	Period of observation	Sample size	Data collection
Canada				
O'Brien and Farell (2005)	Ottawa, Ontario	2001–3	25 patients discharged from Royal Ottawa Hospital and placed on a CTO	1 year before and after introduction of CTO
Frank et al. (2005)	Montreal, Quebec	1998–2000	42 patients discharged from hospital and placed on a CTO	5 years before the pre-index admission (two hospitalizations prior to CTO) and at least to the first rehospitalization post CTO
Nakhost et al. (2012)	Montreal, Quebec	1998–2007	72 patients with complete data, discharged from 2 hospitals and placed on CTO	5 years before the pre index admission (two hospitalizations prior to CTO) and at least to the first rehospitalisation post CTO
Israel				
Durst et al. (1999)	Jerusalem and southern districts of Jerusalem	1991–2	208 patients (326 CTOs) placed on a CTO	6 months after introduction of the CTO
Greenberg et al. (2005)	North Jerusalem	1995–7	26 patients placed on a CTO	Observation times before, during, and after introduction of CTO not specified
Spain				
Canete-Nicolas et al. (2012)	Valencia	2003–12	140 patients placed on a CTO	Not specified

Table 4.5 Outcomes of naturalistic follow-up studies of patients placed on CTO

Study	Hospitalizations	Length of stay	Contacts with ambulatory care	Compliance	Violent behaviours	Clinical status	Emergency visits	Substance abuses	Employment	Housing conditions	Forensic problems
USA											
Hidey and Goodman (1982)	↓										
Zanni and Deveau (1983)	↓	n.s.									
Miller and Fiddleman (1984)	↑										
Van Putten et al. (1988)	↓	↓		↑[2]							
Fernandez and Nygard (1990)	↓	↓									
Munetz et al. (1996)	↓	↓	↑				↓				
O'Keefe et al. (1997)		↓[1]		↑	↓			↓	↑[1]	+[1]	
Rohland et al. (2000)	↓	↓	↑				↓				

(continued)

Table 4.5 (Continued)

Study	Hospitalizations	Length of stay	Contacts with ambulatory care	Compliance	Violent behaviours	Clinical status	Emergency visits	Substance abuses	Employment	Housing conditions	Forensic problems
USA											
New York State Office of Mental Health (2005)	→		↑	↑	→					+	→
Geller et al. (2006)	→	→									
Esposito et al. (2008)		→									→
Australasia											
Power (1992)	→	→		↑[3]	→	+					
Ozgul and Brunero (1997)	→	n.s.									
Muirhead and Harvey (2000)	→	→			→						
Ingram et al. (2009)					→					+	
Canada											
O'Brien and Farell (2005)	→	→	↑							+	

Study		
Frank et al. (2005)	→	
Nakhost et al. (2012)	→	
Israel		
Durst et al. (1999)		↑[2]
Greenberg et al. (2005)	→	↑
Spain		
Canete-Nicolas et al. (2012)		

n.s., not significant.

[1] Significant improvement during the first but not during the second year of observation.

[2] Increased voluntary use of mental health services after CTO had ended.

[3] Medication compliance decreased significantly after patients had been discharged from CTO.

↑, Increased; ↓, Decreased; +, Improved; −, worsened.

The authors found a non-statistically significant reduction in the length of inpatient stays. The reduction in number of hospitalizations was significant. All 384 psychiatric patients hospitalized and made subject to outpatient commitment in Tucson, Arizona, between February 1983 and August 1984 were followed up to ascertain hospital use (Van Putten et al. 1988). Before being placed on a CTO, patients were held for longer in hospital (a median of 21 days during the preceding 6 months, 11 days during the first 6 months after that and 8 days during the next 6 months). Fernandez and Nygard (1990) determined the impact of the revised preventative CTO laws of North Carolina on the 'revolving-door syndrome'. Data were collected for all 4179 patients placed on a CTO between 1985 and 1988. A reduction of 82% in the number of hospital admissions and of 33.3% in the length of hospital stay was reported.

Patterns of service use were observed by Munetz et al. (1996) in the year prior to and following assignment to a CTO in Ohio in the early 1990s. Individuals had to be subject to a CTO for at least 12 months. Significant reductions in the number of hospital admissions and length of stay were reported. Long-term effects of CTOs on service use were also observed by Rohland et al. (2000). Eighty-one patients with psychotic illnesses from an Iowa outpatient clinic were selected between 1991 and 1996. Outcome was measured for the 12 months before and 12 months after the individual was placed on a CTO. Significant decreases were found in admissions. A subgroup analysis of 25 patients with a CTO duration of more than 5 years showed similar patterns. A 77% reduction in psychiatric hospitalizations was also reported by the New York State Office of Mental Health (2005) audit. In central Massachusetts, Geller et al. (1997) reported the effects of CTOs on admission rates for the first 20 patients placed on orders in 1991. The 2 years following the introduction of the measure were divided into periods of 6 months and compared with the 6 months prior to CTOs. Mean numbers of hospital days and admissions decreased during the observation time.

In Australia, Power (1992) followed all patients living in south Melbourne who were placed on a CTO between 1987 and 1991 (n = 125). When periods before and after the CTO were compared, significant reductions were found in the number of admissions and days spent in hospital. Ozgul and Brunero (1997) investigated the outcomes of CTOs and reported a drop in admissions. The effectiveness of CTOs for patients with schizophrenia was examined by Muirhead and Harvey (2000) in Melbourne between 1996 and 1998. The study included 58 patients (74 were excluded because their medical records were not available or because they had a diagnosis other than schizophrenia, so results must be interpreted with great caution). Measurements were made during the 12 months before and after the CTO started. The authors observed significant decreases in the number of admissions and in the length of stay in days. The same pattern of changes was seen with those on oral and depot medication.

A Canadian study by O'Brien and Farell (2005) compared the year before and after CTO involvement and reported a significant reduction in the average number of admissions and a significant decrease in the number of days in hospital. Frank et al. (2005) examined the effect of CTOs on time spent out of hospital during a 5-year period before and at least 21 months after initiation of a CTO in Montreal, Quebec, for all consecutive patients placed on a CTO between July 1998 and June 2000. That study included 42 patients with a total number of 238 admissions. After some fairly complex subdivisions of patients they concluded that CTOs were associated with significantly increased periods free of hospitalization. After dividing patients per hospitalizations as in Frank et al.'s study, Nakhost and Perry (2012) found that CTOs were associated with a significant reduction in the number of admissions and an increase in the median time to readmission.

All patients who received a CTO over a 2-year period (May 1995 to June 1997) in north Jerusalem (*n* = 26) were reviewed and followed up from 3 to 5 years (Greenberg et al. 2005). Fifteen per cent were rehospitalized during the 6-months of their CTO. Fifty-eight per cent of the patients were readmitted during the time period after their CTO. Comparing the follow-up period with the same duration before the order, the number of psychiatric hospitalizations and the number of days in hospital were significantly reduced.

Contacts with outpatient care and compliance

All of the studies that reported on treatment compliance noted an increase in the number of contacts with outpatient care services and/or better compliance with medical treatment during the time the patient was under a CTO compared with the preceding period. A significant increase in outpatient contacts was observed after patients were placed under a CTO in two studies (Munetz et al. 1996, Rohland et al. 2000). O'Keefe et al. (1997) observed a significant improvement in compliance with medication in both the first and second year after patients were placed on a CTO. The New York State Office of Mental Health (2005) audit described increased participation in case management and other services during the first 6 months after introduction of CTOs. O'Brien et al. (2005) reported the same.

The positive effect of CTOs on compliance does not, however, seem to be systematically maintained once the order is completed. Van Putten et al. (1988) reported an increase in voluntary use of mental health services by patients whose CTO had ended. In Durst et al.'s (1991) study, 21% of the patients continued treatment on a voluntary basis after the CTO had ended. Greenberg et al. (2005) observed that of the 18 patients in regular treatment or hospitalized during the CTO (70% of the total sample), 95% continued to attend after the CTO expired. Power (1992) also reported a significant increase in compliance with outpatient attendance to appointments and outpatient medication during the CTO, but once completed, compliance with outpatient medication decreased significantly.

Clinical, social, and forensic outcome

Surprisingly, only a single descriptive study looked at the clinical condition of patients following the introduction of a CTO (Power 1992). This study reported an overall improvement in symptoms of 70%, though it is unclear how this was measured.

As concerns wider outcomes, accommodation was the main focus. Four studies reported a greater stability of residence (O'Keefe et al. 1997), more appropriate housing, especially supported housing (O'Brien et al. 2005), and a significant reduction in homelessness (New York State Office of Mental Health 2005; Ingram et al. 2009).

Five studies reported a significant decrease in violent behaviour in patients once they had been placed under a CTO (Power 1992; O'Keefe et al. 1997; Muirhead and Harvey 2000; New York State Office of Mental Health 2005; Ingram et al. 2009). Only one study noted a reduction in substance misuse (O'Keefe et al. 1997). The New York State Office of Mental Health (2005) audit reported that beyond the first 6 months on a CTO incarcerations were reduced by 87% and arrests by 83%. Esposito et al. (2008) also reported a significant decrease in the number of days spent in jail when periods before and after a CTO were compared.

Discussion and conclusion

This chapter has looked at the different descriptive studies reporting on the implementation of CTOs internationally. Although the legal framework and services varied by time and geography, there were important similarities in terms of the patterns of use, target population, and outcomes of these orders. Many of these studies were set up following the introduction of legal regimes allowing compulsion in community settings.

Studies examining the prevalence of CTOs did not confirm initial fears of widespread use. However, as we have discussed, international comparisons have suggested increases and 'net widening' over time. Most studies considered were local, time-limited, and had small sample sizes, undoubtedly reflecting the difficulties of this kind of research. As a result they may not be representative. The main stated goal of CTOs was to improve a patient's compliance with treatment (especially medication) and to reduce relapse and hospitalization. Though the goals of CTOs were often mentioned, only two studies described the methods used to arrive at them. Medication was a central theme, and practically 100% of patients were obliged to take some. This was often the sole obligation. This may justify the fears of certain professionals, family groups, and patients who see CTOs as leading to an over-reliance on drug treatment. Ozgul and Brunero (1997), however, noted that a patient's dose of antipsychotic medication decreased when the patient was placed under a CTO and that the dose significantly decreased as the number of CTOs for that individual increased.

The majority of CTOs last the full first period and are renewed. These observations and the progressive increase in the average duration of CTOs over time strongly support the 'lobster pot' hypothesis that makes it difficult for a patient to break free of legal constraint. This hypothesis suggests that the criteria for initiating a CTO may be less stringent than the requirements to be taken off one, leading to people being 'stuck' like a lobster in a pot. If a patient is doing well then the care team are reluctant to change and if they are doing badly it can be seen as justification for ongoing compulsion. This may be further compounded by the fact that appeals are rarely undertaken and are often unsuccessful when they are.

The profile of people placed under a CTO has remained remarkably similar over time and across regions. Certain authors have described specific subtypes of individuals placed under a CTO as shown by illness and socio-demographic characteristics. Some have suggested that such differences may predict outcome, but there are no hard data to back up such claims.

The works reviewed in this chapter attempted to study the impact of CTOs on individuals before and after the introduction of a CTO. They conclude fairly unanimously that CTOs reduce the number of psychiatric hospitalizations and length of hospital stay, increase compliance with care plans, reduce aggressive behaviours, and improve clinical, social, and forensic outcomes.

However, these findings need to be viewed with extreme caution given the nature of the majority of the studies and their inherent methodological flaws. While they provide a richness of detail and understanding, they must be looked at together with Chapter 5 that details more robust forms of evidence. The majority of the studies in this chapter were carried out retrospectively, a well-known flaw in services research when it comes to interpreting results. Limited outcomes were considered, with few studies concentrating on important clinical and social outcomes. Most studies used hospitalization data, but the meaning of readmission can be contested. In some it is a 'negative' event signifying failure of treatment, while in others it is a 'positive' aspect of treatment signifying improved engagement (O'Brien et al. 2009). Issues such as the coerciveness of legislation, perceived leverage, or stigma were not considered.

Every single one of these studies was conducted without a control group. This methodology makes it impossible to define whether a favourable result is the consequence of the CTO itself or if other factors were involved. For example, upon the introduction of Kendra's Law in the state of New York, significant sums of money were invested to develop outpatient care services (New York State Office of Mental Health 2005). Without a control group, it was not possible to establish whether the improvements observed in persons placed under a CTO were because of the order or because of the increased amount of care they received. This was particularly relevant, as being subject to compulsion was one of the important criteria for receiving enhanced care. The phenomenon of regression to the mean must also be taken into consideration. According to this, any event with a fluctuating course that is observed at a critical moment will tend to stabilize over time. In this context, a person placed under CTO is generally at a very difficult phase of their illness and life. It is reasonable to suppose that this state will not continue indefinitely and will end up improving. Without a control group, it is impossible to determine whether the favourable evolution that appeared upon the introduction of the CTO is the consequence of this measure or whether it reflects the natural course of the psychological disorder.

The different studies presented in this chapter may not be held as valid arguments to justify the use of CTOs because of their methodological weaknesses. They do, however, represent a first research step related to engaging with this relatively new form of legal intervention and provide significant richness of detail. More methodologically robust studies looking to evaluate the effectiveness of CTOs while controlling for environment or comparing CTO groups with control groups have been conducted.

Acknowledgement

I would like to thank Benedetta Silva who helped me with the literature review and Michelle Bailat-Jones for her advice regarding translation.

References

Bar El YC, Durst R, Rabinowitz J, et al. (1998). Implementation of order of compulsory ambulatory treatment in Jerusalem. *International Journal of Law and Psychiatry*, 21:65–71.

Brophy LM, Reece JE, McDermott F (2006). A cluster analysis of people on community treatment orders in Victoria, Australia. *International Journal of Law and Psychiatry*, 29:469–481.

Canete-Nicolas C, Hernandez-Viadel M, Bellido-Rodriguez C, et al. (2012). Involuntary outpatient treatment (iot) for severe mental patients: current situation in Spain. *Actas Espanolas de Psiquiatria*, 40:27–33.

Cohen S (1985). *Visions of social control: crime, punishment and classification*. Cambridge: Polity Press.

Dawson J (2005). *Community treatment orders: international comparisons*. Dunedin: Otago University Print. Available at: http://www.otago.ac.nz/law/research/otago036152.pdf

Dawson J, Romas S (2001). Uses of community pretreatment orders in New Zealand: early findings. *Australian and New Zealand Journal of Psychiatry*, 35:190–195.

Department of Health (2008). *Mental Health Act 2007: patients on aftercare under supervision (ACUS): transitional arrangements*. London: Department of Health.

Durst R, Teitelbaum A, Bar-El Y, et al. (1999). Evaluation of compulsory ambulatory treatment in Israel. *Psychiatric Services*, 50:698–700.

Esposito R, Westhead V, Berko J (2008). Florida's outpatient commitment law: effective but underused. *Psychiatric Services*, 59:328.

Fernandez GA, Nygard S (1990). Impact of involuntary outpatient commitment on the revolving-door syndrome in North Carolina. *Hospital and Community Psychiatry*, 41:1001–1004.

Frank D, Perry JC, Kean D, et al. (2005). Effects of compulsory treatment orders on time to hospital readmission. *Psychiatric Services*, 56:867–869.

Geller JL, McDermeit M, Grudzinskas AJ, Jr, et al. (1997). A competency-based approach to court-ordered outpatient treatment. *New Directions for Mental Health Services*, Fall(75):81–95.

Geller JL, Fisher WH, Grudzinskas AJ, Jr, et al. (2006). Involuntary outpatient treatment as 'desintitutionalized coercion': the net-widening concerns. *International Journal of Law and Psychiatry*, 29:551–562.

Greenberg D, Mazar J, Brom D, et al. (2005). Involuntary outpatient commitment: a naturalistic study of its use and a consumer survey at one community mental health center in Israel. *Medicine and Law*, 24:95–110.

Hiday VA (2003). Outpatient commitment—the state of empirical research on its outcomes. *Psychology, Public Policy, and Law*, 9:8–32.

Hiday VA, Goodman RR (1982). The least restrictive alternative to involuntary hospitalization, outpatient commitment—its use and effectiveness. *Journal of Psychiatry and Law*, 10:81–96.

Ingram G, Muirhead D, Harvey C (2009). Effectiveness of community treatment orders for treatment of schizophrenia with oral or depot antipsychotic medication: changes in problem behaviours and social functioning. *Australian and New Zealand Journal of Psychiatry*, 43:1077–1083.

Lamb HR, Bachrach LL (2001). Some perspectives on deinstitutionalization. *Psychiatric Services*, 52:1039–1045.

Lawton-Smith S (2005). *A question of numbers: the potential impact of community-based treatment orders in England and Wales*. London: King's Fund.

Light EM, Kerridge IH, Ryan CJ, et al. (2012). Out of sight, out of mind: making involuntary community treatment visible in the mental health system. *Medical Journal of Australia*, 196:591–593.

McDonnell E, Bartholomew T (1997). Community treatment orders in Victoria: emergent issues and anomalies. *Psychiatry, Psychology and Law*, 4:25–36.

Miller RD (1992). Need-for-treatment criteria for involuntary civil commitment—impact in practice. *American Journal of Psychiatry*, 149:1380–1384.

Miller RD, Fiddleman PB (1984). Outpatient commitment—treatment in the least restrictive environment. *Hospital and Community Psychiatry*, 35:147–151.

Muirhead D, Harvey C (2000). *Involuntary treatment of schizophrenia in the community: clinical effectiveness of community treatment orders with oral or depot medication in Victoria*. Melbourne: Royal Australian and New Zealand College of Psychiatrists.

Munetz MR, Grande T, Kleist J, et al. (1996). The effectiveness of outpatient civil commitment. *Psychiatric Services*, 47:1251–1253.

Nakhost A, Perry JC, Frank D (2012). Assessing the outcome of compulsory treatment orders on management of psychiatric patients at 2 McGill University-associated hospitals. *Canadian Journal of Psychiatry–Revue Canadienne de Psychiatrie*, 57:359–365.

New York State Office of Mental Health (2005). *Kendra's Law. Final report on the status of assisted outpatient treatment*. New York: New York State Office of Mental Health.

O'Brien AMA, Farrell SJ (2005). Community treatment orders: profile of a Canadian experience. *Canadian Journal of Psychiatry–Revue Canadienne de Psychiatrie*, 50:27–30.

O'Brien AJ, McKenna BG, Kydd RR (2009). Compulsory community mental health treatment: literature review. *International Journal of Nursing Studies*, 46:1245–1255.

O'Keefe C, Potenza DP, Mueser KT (1997). Treatment outcomes for severely mentally ill patients on conditional discharge to community-based treatment. *Journal of Nervous and Mental Disease*, 185:409–411.

O'Reilly RL, Keegan DL, Elias JW (2000). A survey of the use of community treatment orders by psychiatrists in Saskatchewan. *Canadian Journal of Psychiatry–Revue Canadienne de Psychiatrie*, 45:79–81.

Ozgul S, Brunero S (1997). A pilot study of the utilisation and outcome of community orders: client, carer, case manager and mental health review tribunal perspective. *Australian Health Review*, 20:70–83.

Petrila J, Christy A (2008). Florida's outpatient commitment law: effective but underused—reply. *Psychiatric Services*, 59:328–329.

Power P (1992). A controlled study of the clinical effectiveness of community treatment orders in Australia: a 'mirror-image' analysis. Unpublished.

Power P (1999). Community treatment orders: the Australian experience. *Journal of Forensic Psychiatry*, 10:9–15.

Prior D, Behan D (2013). *Monitoring the Mental Health Act in 2011/12*. Newcastle upon Tyne: Care Quality Commission.

RA Malatest and Associates (2012). *The legislated review of community treatment orders (final report)*. Toronto, ON: Ministry of Health and Long-Term Care. Available at: http://www.health.gov.on.ca/en/common/ministry/publications/reports/mental_health/cto_review_report.pdf

Rohland BM (1998). *The role of outpatient commitment in the management of persons with schizophrenia*. Iowa City, IA: Iowa Consortium for Mental Health, Services, Training, and Research.

Rohland BM, Rohrer JE, Richards CC (2000). The long-term effect of outpatient commitment on service use. *Administration and Policy in Mental Health*, **27**:383–394.

Torrey EF, Kaplan RJ (1995). A national survey of the use of outpatient commitment. *Psychiatric Services*, **46**:778–784.

Van Putten RA, Santiago JM, Berren MR (1988). Involuntary outpatient commitment in Arizona—a retrospective study. *Hospital and Community Psychiatry*, **39**: 953–958.

Zanni G, Deveau L (1986). Inpatient stays before and after outpatient commitment. *Hospital and Community Psychiatry*, **37**:941–942.

Zusman J, Friedman RM, Levin BL (1988). Moving treatment into the community: Implications for psychiatry. *Psychiatric Quarterly*, **59**:140–149.

Chapter 5

Assessing the effectiveness of compulsory community treatment

Steve Kisely

Introduction

This chapter initially considers methodological issues that arise in the assessment of the effectiveness of compulsory community treatment (CCT). It then reviews the evidence from uncontrolled, controlled, and randomized studies for various types of CCT. Finally the implications of the findings are discussed.

CCT is highly controversial among mental health policy-makers, clinicians, and patient advocate groups. In theory, CCT, when properly regulated, can ensure the safety of patients in the community, prevent recurrent admissions by decreasing the likelihood of decompensating, and ensure continuity of care. However, critics argue that, under CCT, compulsion is used where intensive case management or assertive community treatment would be effective, and they are concerned that any potential therapeutic benefits of court-ordered treatment are negated by their coerciveness and associated stigma, and damage to therapeutic relationships (Pinfold and Bindman 2001). By contrast, proponents of CCT contend that it is a means to avoid or minimize hospital admission, arrest, or imprisonment, allowing individuals to remain in their communities during treatment (Pinfold and Bindman 2001).

What types of compulsory community treatment are there?

Any consideration of the effectiveness of CCT has to take into account the wide range of measures covered by the term. These include mandatory outpatient treatment, involuntary outpatient commitment (OPC), community treatment orders (CTOs), extended leave, extended release, or supervised discharge. It does not cover individuals who have committed an offence and are required to follow a treatment plan as a condition of probation, or have been found not to be criminally responsible for a crime. These patients are covered by criminal as opposed to civil law and are looked after by the prison health service, forensic psychiatry services, or the probation service. There are three main types of CCT: extended leave, CTOs, and court-ordered OPC.

Extended leave

Extended leave provisions or supervised discharges apply at the time of discharge from compulsory inpatient treatment. They are used in New Hampshire (Torrey and Kaplan 1995) and some Canadian provinces (Gray and O'Reilly 2001, 2005) and give mental health professionals the right to return a patient to hospital against their wishes if the patient does not comply with treatment.

Community treatment orders

CTOs are used in countries such as Canada (Gray and O'Reilly 2005), Australia (Vaughan et al. 2000), New Zealand (Romans et al. 2004), and the UK (Lawton-Smith 2005). They give mental health professionals the right to place an individual on an order whether they are in hospital or not. This is in contrast to provisions for extended leave or supervised discharge, which only apply to patients who are being discharged from inpatient care (Gray and O'Reilly 2001, 2005). CTOs are designed to divert people from possibly having to be admitted as inpatients. In addition, unlike leave, the individual may not have to meet the same criteria for treatment as an inpatient (Gray and O'Reilly 2001).

Court-ordered outpatient committal

Involuntary or mandatory outpatient treatment is the preferred term in the USA and covers court-ordered OPC (Gray and O'Reilly 2001). In this case, a judge, not a health-care professional, decides on the appropriateness of the order. These orders require patients to attend outpatient appointments at specified times and places.

Methodological issues

There are five methodological issues that must be considered when assessing the effectiveness of CCT (Kisely and Campbell 2007); these are considered in the following subsections.

What is the purpose of compulsory community treatment?

The purpose of a CTO is important when deciding how effectiveness should be gauged. For instance, contact with mental health services is usually increased in individuals who are on CTOs, but while this is necessary for individuals to receive treatment it can be argued that contact is a process variable and not the ultimate desired outcome.

By contrast, if the primary purpose is to provide a less restrictive alternative to hospitalization, consideration should be given to the degree of coercion experienced by individuals placed on CTOs. Again the meaning of success is unclear. Does a least restrictive alternative mean that the person spends fewer days as an involuntary patient in hospital, or should the total time as an involuntary patient, whether in hospital or in the community, be considered?

If the purpose of a CTO is to reduce violence, direct measurement of violent behaviour, such as conviction for violent offences, is needed.

Finally, a wider range of additional outcomes may be needed to measure whether CTOs can promote stability and recovery. These outcomes may include mortality, physical health, severity of psychiatric symptoms, self-harm, arrest and incarceration rates, freedom from victimization, ability to work, quality of life, and stability and independence of type of residence.

How do we measure success?

A question related to the lack of clarity about purpose is uncertainty about how to measure success following the use of CCT. Does CCT reduce admission rates, allowing individuals to remain in their communities during treatment, or are rates increased as a result of earlier identification of relapse? For example, 'recall' or 'breach' admissions, where a patient is brought briefly to the hospital for assessment or medication, under the powers conferred by a CTO may be considered part of the CTO process, while admissions resulting in revocation of a CTO may be considered as an outcome (Kisely and Campbell 2007; Rugkåsa and Burns 2014). Without such distinctions, a patient's readmission could be variously interpreted as the CTO working (i.e. early detection of non-adherence) or failing (i.e. relapse) (Rugkåsa and Burns 2014). Would length of stay be a more appropriate measure, on the basis that increased admission would still be the least restrictive alternative if individuals spent less time in hospital? Is diversion from the criminal justice system in the form of reduced arrests or imprisonment another possible outcome?

Are we assessing the same intervention?

As indicated previously, the range of different interventions makes it even harder to interpret the literature. The situation is complicated by the fact that in some jurisdictions different forms of community treatment such as extended release and involuntary outpatient treatment exist in parallel.

Are we assessing the same patients?

There are also variations in the type of patients being placed on CCT. Canadian jurisdictions such as Ontario require patients, or their substitute decision-makers, to consent to CCT (Gray and O'Reilly 2001). These requirements are not generally found elsewhere. Some jurisdictions allow the use of CTOs in early episode presentations while others require prior evidence of treatment recidivism. These are therefore very different patient groups.

Efficacy or effectiveness?

Another issue is the trade-off between efficacy and effectiveness. Efficacy means the evaluation of an intervention under ideal conditions, such as in rigorously conducted randomized controlled clinical trials. Effectiveness means an evaluation of an intervention as it happens in routine practice. This might include less restrictive inclusion criteria for subjects.

Uncontrolled and controlled before and after studies

Many early studies evaluated effectiveness and often used patients as their own controls in a 'mirror image' design of outcomes before and after the initiation of a CTO. These uncontrolled before and after (UBA) studies generally reported significant decreases in hospital use in terms of the number of hospital readmissions, accumulated days in hospital, or offending (Hough and O'Brien 2005; Muirhead et al. 2006; Christy et al. 2009; Nakhost et al. 2012). However, the weakness of these designs is that it is difficult to determine the reason for any change in outcome. Apart from the potential effect of the intervention of interest, other possible explanations include the effect of other interventions, life events or changes in social circumstances, as well as regression to the mean. The latter refers to the statistical tendency of data to gravitate towards the centre of a distribution, provided they start on either end of the distribution and are free to fluctuate. Children of very tall parents, for example, tend to be taller than the average child—but shorter than the average of the parents' heights (Last 1988). All these factors often overestimate the effect of the intervention of interest.

Subsequent controlled before and after (CBA) studies have given more equivocal results (Table 5.1). CBA studies avoid problems caused by temporal changes and regression to the mean. However, a major criticism of these studies is that while it is possible to obtain appropriate controls matched for age, gender, and diagnosis, it is not possible to match or adjust for other important factors, such as the degree of insight or overt treatment refusal. Most of these studies have also not adjusted for historical non-adherence to treatment. Case-matched studies are also vulnerable to the possibility that individuals on a CTO may have received enhanced services not provided to the controls.

CBA studies have used three main datasets: population-based linked epidemiological data from Victoria and Western Australia derived from the psychiatric case register from each jurisdiction, as well as longer-term outcome data from the New York State Office of Mental Health (Table 5.1).

Victoria

In Victoria, conditional discharge was associated with an overall mean increase of 15 bed-days, despite a reduction in the days per admission or care episode (Segal and Burgess 2006a). The interpretation of this is unclear, but it could represent an increase in 'revolving-door' care whereby individuals have more admissions and spend longer in hospital. These results were consistent with a second study using the same Victorian database where the risk of readmission increased following initial placement on a CTO (Burgess et al. 2006). However, in certain circumstances CTOs were associated with reductions in bed-days. These were in patients experiencing their first episode (Segal and Burgess 2006b) and for CTOs lasting longer than 6 months (Segal and Burgess 2006c). A further study from Victoria found that patients on conditional release from hospital had lower mortality rates than expected, taking into account community care use, age, gender, inpatient experience, and diagnosis (Segal and Burgess 2006d).

Table 5.1 Results from controlled before and after outcome studies

Outcome	Studies reporting a reduction	Studies reporting an increase	Studies reporting no difference
Readmission	Bursten (1986), Tennessee, n = 156 Swartz et al. (2010), NY, n = 5601 Segal et al. (2006b), Victoria, n = 24,973[1] Segal et al. (2006c), Victoria, n = 1182[2] Hunt et al. (2007), Toronto, n = 316[2]	Burgess et al. (2006), Victoria, n = 12,842[7] Segal et al. (2006a), Victoria, n = 24,973 Kisely et al. (2004), n = 754[3] Kisely et al. (2005), WA versus Canada, n = 539 Zanni and Stavis (2007), District of Columbia, n = 193	Bursten (1986), Tennessee, n = 75 Hiday and Scheid-Cook, n = 1226 (1987, 1989, 1991)[4] Geller et al. (1998), Massachusetts, n = 72[5] Preston et al. (2002), n = 456 Vaughan et al. (2000), NSW, n = 246
Duration of readmissions	Vaughan et al. (2000) (initial readmission only) Segal and Burgess (2006b), Victoria, n = 24,973[1] Kisely et al. (2013a), WA, n = 5916 Hunt et al. (2007), Toronto, n = 316 Segal et al. (2009), WA, n = 246[6]	Segal and Burgess (2006a), Victoria, n = 24,973[7] Zanni and Stavis (2007), District of Columbia, n = 193	Bursten (1986), Tennessee, n = 156 Hiday and Scheid-Cook, n = 1226 (1987, 1989, 1991)[4] Geller et al. (1998), Massachusetts, n = 72[5] Preston et al. (2002), WA, n = 456 Segal andn Burgess (2006c), Victoria, n = 1182 Kisely et al. (2005), WA versus Canada, n = 539[8]

(continued)

Table 5.1 (Continued)

Outcome	Studies reporting a reduction	Studies reporting an increase	Studies reporting no difference
Community service use	Hunt et al. (2007), Toronto, $n = 316$	Bursten (1986), Tennessee, $n = 156$ Hiday and Scheid-Cook, $n = 1226$ (1987, 1989, 1991)[4] Geller et al (1998), $n = 72$ Preston et al. (2002), WA, $n = 456$ Kisely et al. (2013a), WA, $n = 5916$ Kisely et al. (2005), WA versus Canada, $n = 539$	Segal and Burgess (2006a), Victoria, $n = 24,973$ Segal and Burgess (2006b), Victoria, $n = 1182$

Adapted from *Social Psychiatry and Psychiatric Epidemiology*, 49(12), Rugkåsa J, Dawson J, Burns T, CTOs: what is the state of the evidence?, pp. 1861–1871, Copyright (2014), with permission from Springer.

Victoria, based on a large register in Victoria, Australia, containing information on 128,427 cases including 16,216 CTOs (1990–2000); NY, based on a large register of Medicare claims in the state of New York, USA, containing information on large numbers of cases including 8752 CTOs (1999–2006); WA, Western Australia, based on a large register in Western Australia including up to 2958 CTOs (1998–2010).

[1] Significant reductions for patients placed on a CTO within 30 days of first contact with services.

[2] Significant only if duration of CTO > 6 months.

[3] Adjusted for forensic history: 265 CTO cases, 265 matched controls, 224 consecutive controls.

[4] Many of the analyses used subsets of this sample.

[5] No significant differences were found between the CTO and demographically and clinically matched control groups on admission at 6 months or 2-year follow-up. However, CTO cases had a greater average decrease in admissions.

[6] Significant only for CTOs from hospitals. For community-initiated CTOs duration increased.

[7] Increase in total inpatient days, reduced average duration of inpatient episodes and inpatient days per 100 days in care.

[8] No decrease in duration overall. Decrease in admissions lasting > 100 days.

Western Australia

Data from Western Australia gave similarly equivocal results. An initial study in the first year of operation of CTOs reported no difference in bed-days or admissions compared with controls matched for age, sex, discharge date, and diagnosis (Preston et al. 2002). However, this approach was criticized for not taking into account an important reason for CTOs—to shorten future lengths of stay compared with pre-order levels. Using this outcome instead, a secondary analysis limited to those cased discharged from hospital found that CTO cases had 19 fewer days in hospital from before the order compared with controls, a statistically significant result ($n = 574$) (Segal et al. 2009). A subsequent study, covering 10 years of experience in using CTOs, reported smaller but significant reductions ($n = 5918$) (Kisely et al. 2013a).

However, when it was possible to adjust for forensic history by linking health and criminal justice data, the CTO group had increased readmission rates compared with both controls matched on either discharge date from inpatient care or on sociodemographic characteristics, diagnosis, past psychiatric history, and treatment setting (Kisely et al. 2004).

No matter how careful and comprehensive the matching process of possible confounders is, there is always the suspicion that selection of controls from the same jurisdiction as the CTO cases may be subject to confounding from other known or unknown variables. A further study therefore compared Western Australia with another jurisdiction that did not have CCT. As there was no Australian jurisdiction that did not have CTOs, it was necessary to use an international comparison, Nova Scotia, Canada (Kisely et al. 2005). Although in different countries, Western Australia and Nova Scotia had mental health services that were free at the point of delivery and with similar characteristics in terms of staffing and the balance of inpatient and outpatient care. Importantly, neither had jurisdiction-wide assertive community treatment that could act as a confounding variable. Moreover, at the time of the study, Nova Scotia had never had any form of CCT, including extended leave from hospital. This was unlike most other provinces and territories in Canada. Both jurisdictions also had linked administrative databases that covered the use of mental health services across the whole state or province, including inpatient, outpatient, and community contacts (Kisely et al. 2005). This made it possible to match all patients who had been subject to CCT in Western Australia with controls from Nova Scotia. To ensure comparability of the two samples the sample was restricted to those patients placed on a CTO on discharge from hospital. One hundred and ninety-six patients placed on CTOs on discharge from hospital in Western Australia were matched with the same number of patients from Nova Scotia, controlling for the same demographic and clinical characteristics as the study restricted to Western Australia, by matching or multivariate analyses. The findings were equivocal. On one hand, CTOs did not prolong survival in the community for patients in Western Australia compared with controls in Nova Scotia. On the other hand, the same CTO cases were less likely to have long hospital stays (100 days or longer) in the year after the index date than the Nova Scotian controls. The major weakness of the design was that the use of an international comparison group rather than one from the same country may have introduced additional confounders for which the authors were unable to control (Kisely et al. 2005).

In terms of other outcomes, CTOs had no effect on psychiatric symptomatology as measured by the Health of the Nation Outcome Scales (HoNOS) compared with matched controls at 6- and 12-month follow-up (Kisely et al. 2014). Again, this used a subset of the original dataset from the time that routine use of the HoNOS was introduced in 2005 (n = 1433). As in Victoria, CTOs were associated with reductions in preventable deaths from physical disorders such as cancer or cardiovascular disease at 1-, 2-, and 3-year follow-up compared with controls (Kisely et al. 2013b). One explanation was that increased contact with mental health clinicians might have allowed the identification and management of co-morbid physical illness. This was consistent with a finding from the same study that the effect on mortality was attenuated after adjusting for outpatient contacts following CTO placement.

New York

Several authors have used linked administrative data from the New York State Office of Mental Health and Medicaid to examine whether patients on OPC experienced reduced rates of hospitalization, shorter hospital stays, and improvements in other outcomes. Controls were not matched but were patients receiving assertive community treatment (ACT).

One study investigated the effect of adding CCT to ACT in comparison with a group on ACT alone. Addition of a CTO to ACT significantly reduced the likelihood of readmission compared with patients on ACT alone, as well as significantly increasing community contacts, especially if the order extended beyond 6 months (Swartz et al. 2010). A further study found that patients on OPC were significantly more likely to be in possession of guideline-recommended medication than those on ACT or neither of these interventions (Busch et al. 2010).

In terms of forensic outcomes, two studies compared the arrest records of New York outpatients, of whom some had been on OPC and some on entirely voluntary treatment (Gilbert et al. 2010; Link et al. 2011). Both reported that the controls had nearly double the odds of arrest compared with the OPC group in the period during and shortly after commitment (Gilbert et al. 2010; Link et al. 2011).

Other databases and/or jurisdictions

Most studies have come from the USA (Table 5.1). An early study from Tennessee compared two CTO groups with two of matched controls (Bursten 1986). In one comparison (n = 156) patients on CTOs showed a significant reduction in hospital admissions compared with controls (20%), while in the other (n = 75) there was virtually no difference (3% reduction). The reason for this disparity is unclear, but given the degree of difference it is unlikely to have been due to an underpowered second comparison.

Studies from Massachusetts and North Carolina found no significant differences between patients on OPC and controls in terms of admissions or bed-days (Hiday and Scheid-Cook 1987, 1989, 1991; Geller et al. 1998). By contrast, a before and after study from the District of Columbia indicated that CTO cases had a reduced number of admissions per year compared with controls. These patients also had fewer seclusion episodes and hours, and fewer restraint episodes and hours than the controls (Zanni and Stavis 2007). In all cases, outpatient and community contacts were increased compared with controls.

There was also one further Australian study from New South Wales (Table 5.1). It found that CTO cases were more likely to be admitted on an involuntary basis, although there were no significant differences between CTO and non-CTO groups in the length of an initial readmission (Vaughan et al. 2000). However, the authors were unable to match on key variables and so these findings have to be treated with caution.

Elsewhere, a Toronto-based study ($n = 316$) reported better outcomes for CTO patients where equal access was provided to case management, particularly when CTOs were extended beyond 6 months (Table 5.1) (Hunt et al. 2007).

Conclusions from the results of uncontrolled and controlled before and after studies

Initial uncontrolled studies suggested that CCT led to increased follow-up with clinical services, a reduction of inpatient admissions, and reduced length of stay in hospital. In general, controlled studies have also reported increased follow-up with mental health services, but in relation to other health service outcome results are more equivocal and dependent on the method used. However, when it was possible to adjust for forensic history by linking health and criminal justice data or to make comparisons with a jurisdiction without any such legislation, CTO patients experienced significantly greater readmission rates (Kisely et al. 2004).

CTOs may reduce health service outcomes in certain subgroups—these include early episode cases and people on orders for more than 180 days (Segal and Burgess 2006c; Hunt et al. 2007; Swartz et al. 2010). The implication of the latter finding is unclear. It could be due to long-term benefits (Swartz et al. 1999), or that those on the order long term were maintained on it because things were going well clinically and the CTO was presumed to be responsible (Szmukler and Hotopf 2001).

In terms of other outcomes, CBA evidence shows promise in areas such as arrests or maintenance on treatment, but as will become apparent these findings have not been confirmed in randomized controlled trials (RCTs). Two recent studies using different databases have also reported reduced mortality on CTOs (Segal and Burgess 2006d; Kisely et al. 2013b), possibly by improving physical care through increased contact with community psychiatric services. It is worth noting that some important outcomes, such as mortality, cannot easily be assessed by a RCT.

Randomized controlled trials

RCTs are the most rigorous study design but are rare due to the inherent ethical, legal, and political conflicts involved. In consequence, there have only been three RCTs. Two were conducted in the late 1990s in the USA (New York and North Carolina) (Swartz et al. 1999; Steadman et al. 2001) and one more recently in the UK (Burns et al. 2013). None of these RCTs demonstrated a significant reduction in the primary outcome of readmission to hospital, or bed-days, in the 12 months following CTO placement. Where reported, there was also no randomized evidence for differences in any psychosocial outcomes, compliance with medication, or contacts with the criminal justice system.

Studies from the USA

As we have noted, there were no significant differences in admissions, bed-days, psychosocial functioning, medication compliance, or forensic outcomes between CTO cases and randomized controls in either the New York or North Carolina studies (Swartz et al. 1999; Swanson et al. 2000; Steadman et al. 2001; Compton et al. 2003). However, patients on CTOs did have increased outpatient contacts (Wagner et al. 2003) and felt less victimized (Hiday et al. 1999), although this was at the price of feeling more coerced (Swartz et al. 2002).

The RCT from North Carolina also undertook a post-hoc analysis of individuals who were maintained on CTOs for 6 months or more (Swartz et al. 1999). This study reported decreased hospitalization, decreased violence, and a number of other positive outcomes in comparison with the controls on voluntary treatment (Swartz et al. 1999). The relevance of these results has been questioned, as the analysis potentially introduced a selection bias that randomization is designed to avoid—individuals may have been maintained on a CTO because they were showing improvement.

The two trials from the USA have been the subject of much debate. Both explicitly excluded patients with a history of violence. Although understandable from an ethical and legal standpoint, this limits their generalizability, as recent dangerousness, particularly violence against others, is often the reason for compulsory treatment in hospital or the community. Selection bias was further compounded by high dropout rates. Of the 577 patients identified as eligible for participation in the New York and North Carolina studies, only 331 (57%) were followed up 1 year later. This included a non-randomized arm of the North Carolina study judged too violent to be in the RCT (Swartz et al. 1999). While the North Carolina study had a higher completion rate among randomized patients at the final follow-up than the New York study (82% versus 45%), data were not available for all patients for all of the outcomes (Swartz et al. 1999; Steadman et al. 2001). For example, only 70% of participants could be included in the analysis of victimization due to attrition or missing data. The rate of attrition was also higher among those in the non-randomized violent subgroup. Of the 67 participants for whom baseline measures were available, only 46 (69%) remained in the study at the 12-month end-point. The 1-year follow-up was therefore of a highly selected, and potentially unrepresentative, population that was not dangerous and sufficiently compliant to participate in baseline and follow-up assessments. In the case of the New York study (Steadman et al. 2001) there was also the suggestion that members of the control group and their case managers thought that they were actually on OPC (Rugkåsa and Burns 2014).

In addition, the two trials were of OPC. This is a court-ordered compulsory treatment plan and the findings may not be applicable to other jurisdictions where CCT is initiated by clinicians.

The Oxford study

The most recent RCT was conducted in England, and is known as the Oxford Community Treatment Order Evaluation Trial (OCTET) (Burns et al. 2013). OCTET was a study of clinician-initiated treatment rather than the court-ordered treatment studied in the RCTs in the USA, and is thus more relevant to jurisdictions such as Scotland, Canada, Australia, and New Zealand.

OCTET randomized 336 patients discharged from hospital to an experimental group (CTO) or a control group (extended leave under Section 17 of the Mental Health Act) and compared their outcomes at 12 months (Burns et al. 2013). 'Leave of absence' under Section 17 of the Act allows patients to leave hospital for some hours or days, or even exceptionally weeks, while still being subject to recall. Unlike the two US studies, there were no exclusions for dangerousness. Attrition was low (0% in the case of the primary outcome), and where it did occur the two groups were comparable.

As in the two studies from the USA, there were no differences in the number of patients readmitted or in lengths of stay between the CTO patients and controls. Neither were there differences in terms of psychiatric morbidity or social functioning as measured by standardized instruments.

Given the study's recency the exact place of OCTET has yet to be determined, but commentators have focused on two issues: potential bias and the nature of the control condition.

As regards the first issue, treating physicians were able to make clinical decisions irrespective of initial randomization. This was necessary for the trial to be lawful but resulted in over a quarter of the individuals initially randomized to conditional leave eventually being placed on a CTO during the study period. In addition, 35 patients (22%) randomized to CTOs did not actually receive the intervention. Sensitivity analyses to remove these protocol violations did not alter the findings, although it is possible that this may have reduced the power of the study. However, the similarity between the two groups in terms of subsequent outcomes suggests that increasing the numbers would have been unlikely to change the non-significant nature of the results. A further source of potential bias arose from the pragmatic nature of the trial and the fact that randomization involved allocation to two different types of legal status. This meant it was both impossible and unlawful to mask research assistants, treating clinicians, or patients. A final consideration is generalizability. Around 20% of the sample were ineligible or refused to take part. These subjects may have been the most unwell or insightless, and therefore the ones most likely to benefit from CTOs.

The second main issue is whether OCTET was a comparison of CCT with voluntary care or two types of compulsory treatment, as in theory Section 17 allows patients to leave hospital for weeks. In practice, protracted use of Section 17 is discouraged by the courts, and clinicians are now required to consider using a CTO when extending leave beyond a week (Rugkåsa and Burns 2014). This is reflected in the findings from OCTET, where clinicians discharged patients on Section 17 to voluntary status after a median of only 8 days. However, although the length of *initial* compulsory outpatient treatment differed significantly between the two groups (medians of 183 days versus 8 days), Section 17 patients averaged 3 months on some form of compulsory treatment over the course of the study. Alternatively, it could be argued that Section 17 patients were on voluntary treatment for the bulk of the time (medians of 8 versus 257 days, respectively, for initial randomized legal compulsion and 103 versus 262 over the course of the study) (Burns et al. 2013). There is also debate about whether total time on compulsory treatment was a process or outcome measure. These topics will doubtless be the subject of ongoing debate, as will the exact interpretation of the findings. It might be that patients on CCT do not achieve better results than controls who received voluntary treatment for the bulk of the time. An alternative view is that short periods of conditional leave may be sufficient for some patients.

Conclusions from the RCT results

This is a difficult area to research using a RCT and so all three studies contained a number of potential biases. One issue in all three RCTS was selection bias and consequent generalizability. Depending on the study, patients with a history of dangerousness were excluded and around 20% of eligible patients lacked the capacity to consent to the study, or refused to take part. This limits their applicability, as recent dangerousness, particularly violence against others, is often the reason for compulsory treatment in hospital or the community (Swartz et al. 2002). Only two of the three studies describe the process of randomization in detail (Steadman et al. 2001; Burns et al. 2013). There is also a risk of bias when outcome data are not assessed blind to group status and the results of people who were not randomized or post-hoc analyses are included in papers. All three studies used included intention-to-treat analyses for all (Swartz et al. 1999; Burns et al. 2013) for at least some of the outcomes of interest (Steadman et al. 2001).

In the case of the North Carolina study (Swartz et al. 1999), it was sometimes difficult to separate the results of the randomized trial from those of the follow-up of an additional non-randomized group of patients with a recent history of violence who were also placed on OPC. In the case of the New York study, there was a relatively small number of participants and the suggestion that members of the control group and their case managers thought that they were actually on OPC (Steadman et al. 2001). These factors would minimize any effect of the intervention (Kisely et al. 2011). There were also fewer data on psychosocial outcomes as measured by standardized instruments.

Reviews and meta-analyses

Although RCTs remain the most robust study design for the evaluation of any intervention, logistical and ethical considerations have hampered their utility in this area. This has been compounded by the small numbers in some studies and consequent lack of power. In this situation, meta-analysis, in which results of small studies are combined in a single analysis, can help address the issue of insufficient power.

Cochrane and Cochrane-like systematic reviews and meta-analyses

A Cochrane review of 416 patients from the two US RCTs found no advantage to CTOs for readmission, health service use, psychiatric morbidity, social functioning, or satisfaction with services (Kisely et al. 2011). In terms of numbers needed to treat (NNT), the authors calculated that it would take 85 OPC orders to prevent one readmission, 27 to prevent one episode of homelessness, and 238 to prevent one arrest. There was some evidence that CTOs reduced the risk of victimization.

As already noted, the generalizability of the US findings may have been limited by the exclusion of violent patients and the court-initiated nature of the intervention (CTOs) (Kisely and Campbell 2007). Accordingly, a subsequent review included non-randomized studies that measured relevant outcomes and were of sufficient quality to be pooled with the RCT data (Kisely et al. 2007). The review was conducted in accordance with guidelines of the Cochrane Effective Practice and Organisational Care (EPOC) group. Eligible methodologies included CBA studies and interrupted time series (ITS). For inclusion in the review, CBA studies had to have contemporaneous data collection and use appropriate control groups. CBA studies also had to contain data on the comparability of intervention and control groups and similar baseline measurements in both groups, protection against contamination, follow-up rates, and reliability of outcome assessment. ITS studies had to include an intervention delivered at a defined point in time and report three or more data points before and after the intervention.

Eight papers covering five studies (the two US RCTs included in the Cochrane review and additional three CBAs) met the inclusion criteria (total $n = 1108$) (Kisely et al. 2007). These included patients with a history of violence and on clinician-initiated CTOs. Statistical significance was not reached for any outcome, including admission rates, duration of admissions, total days in hospital, and treatment/contact adherence (Kisely et al. 2007). No ITS analyses were identified.

Like the Cochrane review, this paper was still limited by the small number of studies that could be included (two RCTs and three CBA studies). As before, the two RCTs were of court-ordered OPC in the USA, which may not be generalizable to other jurisdictions where CCT is initiated by clinicians and excludes patients with a history of violent outcomes (Swartz et al. 1999; Steadman et al. 2001). Of the three CBA papers, two were epidemiological studies from Western Australia that compared patients on CTOs with controls from within the same jurisdiction and internationally ($n = 652$) (Preston et al. 2002; Kisely et al. 2005). However, the two studies were restricted to patients placed on CTOs in the first year of the legislation and may not have reflected subsequent practice as clinicians gained experience in the use of the Act.

The most recent update of the original Cochrane review included the OCTET paper as a separate comparison from the two US papers because of the continuing debate about the status of the control condition. However, it was possible to do a sensitivity analysis of the effect of including the OCTET study in the meta-analysis of the two other papers. This yielded 749 subjects (Kisely and Hall 2014). Compared with controls, CTOs did not reduce admissions to hospital in the subsequent 12 months, neither were there significant differences in psychiatric symptoms or global assessment of functioning in the two papers where these were reported (Steadman et al. 2001; Burns et al. 2013).

Other reviews

The findings of this review are consistent with several other independent narrative reviews of CCT, which all found little evidence that CCT had an effect on outcomes such as hospital admissions, length of stay, or compliance with medication (Ridgely et al. 2001; Churchill et al. 2007). These include a systematic review of 72 papers published up until 2006, which was recently updated by a further review of 18 outcome papers from 2006 to 2013, including the OCTET study (Maughan et al. 2014).

An almost universal plea has been the greater standardization of outcome measures so that more studies could be incorporated and more patients pooled in meta-analyses including greater adherence to CONSORT standards of reporting (Maughan et al. 2014).

Limitations of the research to date

There are of course many difficulties in assessing the effectiveness of CCT. These include variations in the type of intervention being studied and uncertainty as to how to measure success.

In addition, study outcomes have largely been limited to health service use, such as admissions or lengths of stay, rather than on outcomes that might be more relevant to patients and their families, for example symptomatology, social functioning, and satisfaction.

Further limitations have already been discussed in my description of each of the individual papers. In the case of the epidemiological studies, irrespective of how they controlled for confounders, the selection of controls from the same jurisdiction as the CTO patients may be subject to confounding from unmeasured variables such as social disability or characteristics of the treating team (Preston et al. 2002; Kisely et al. 2004). This might explain why some patients, and not others, were placed on CCT. Comparing jurisdictions with and without CCT partially addresses this concern but raises the issue of comparability of the two health systems, especially internationally (Kisely et al. 2005).

Systematic reviews and meta-analyses of the literature were only able to include a limited number of studies with either appropriately matched or randomized controls. RCTs are the most rigorous design but are difficult to undertake in this area because of the associated ethical and legal issues. Two RCTs were of court-ordered OPC in the USA, which may not be generalizable to other jurisdictions where CCT is initiated by clinicians. The third RCT of CTOs in England is more applicable to other jurisdictions but the voluntary or compulsory status of the control group remains a subject for discussion. In addition, studies either excluded patients with a history of dangerousness (Swartz et al. 1999; Steadman et al. 2001) or had a refusal rate of 25% (Burns et al. 2013). These refusers might have been the ones who might have benefited most from a CTO.

Finally, a focus on CCT as a crime prevention measure has the unfortunate effect of emphasizing the dangerousness of people with psychiatric illness and so increasing the stigma experienced by people with severe mental illness. This is despite of the lack of evidence that, in the absence of co-occurring issues of substance misuse, people with mental health problems are necessarily a risky group (Steadman et al. 1998; Davis 2002; Davidson and Campbell 2007).

Implications for practice

Proponents of CCT argue that it is less coercive than the alternatives of compulsory admission to hospital or arrest (Pinfold and Bindman 2001). However, research findings suggest that CCT remains an unproven way of reducing either. Even where changes in outcome have been shown, such as decreased criminal victimization (Hiday et al. 2002), it is not known whether these are due to the legislative framework or greater intensity of contact (McIvor 1998, 2001). Despite the lack of evidence of effectiveness, governments in other jurisdictions are actively considering further legislation in this area. Apart from the effect on individual liberties, such initiatives give the impression that legislators are addressing the needs of patients and carers while in fact they are doing very little at all. CTOs may potentially divert mental health services away from evidence-based interventions for recognized psychiatric disorders towards programmes of social control for people whom society does not wish to deal with. This type of legislation may also detract from the introduction of interventions that are of benefit to individuals with a severe mental disorder such as ACT (Marshall and Lockwood 2000), but which are more expensive than legislative solutions to the problem.

In terms of protecting the public, limited findings of an effect from the non-randomized literature (Hough and O'Brien 2005; Gilbert et al. 2010; Link et al. 2011) have not been confirmed in RCTs where CTOs did not have an influence on arrests or imprisonment (Swartz et al. 1999; Steadman et al. 2001). These RCT findings are consistent with data from England and Wales on other forensic outcomes (Kisely 2009). For instance, CCT appears to have little effect on homicides either, even though the enabling legislation is often named after a high-profile victim who was murdered by someone who happened to have a psychiatric illness: New York has Kendra's Law, California Laura's Law, and Ontario Brian's Law (Kisely and Campbell 2006). Only 10% of people who committed homicide in Britain between 1999 and 2003 were in contact with mental health services in the year before the offence ($n = 249$) (Jethwa and Galappathie 2008; Lawton-Smith et al. 2008). Furthermore, of these 249 cases, 220 were judged to be at low risk of immediate violence (Jethwa and Galappathie 2008; Lawton-Smith et al. 2008). In addition, there is no evidence of any reduction in the rates of homicide by people with a mental illness in countries such as Canada, Australia, or New Zealand where CCT has been available (Lawton-Smith et al. 2008).

Implications for future research

Despite the widespread use of CCT there are relatively few studies with appropriately matched or randomized controls. Another interesting finding was the absence of any work from outside the English-speaking world, even though literature searches for the systematic reviews and meta-analyses were not restricted to publications in English. It is unclear whether this is due to publication bias or because such legislation is either absent or accepted without controversy. Given the difficulties of conducting RCTs in this area, it is unlikely that many other studies will be attempted. Further evaluation will depend on quasi-experimental designs, with the analyses of routine databases as one way of minimizing bias (Bindman 2002). ITS analyses would be particularly appropriate given the difficulties of finding suitable controls.

Further research may also determine if CCT can reduce health service use in the longer term, or whether there are particular people with specific problems that are best managed with CTOs.

Finally, there should be more research into the effect on outcomes that are more relevant to patients and their families, including symptomatology, social functioning, and satisfaction, rather than reliance on measures of health service use alone. In this regard, qualitative techniques may give additional insights into the effect of CCT on patients, carers, and health-care professionals (O'Reilly 2001).

Conclusions

In conclusion, CCT illustrates how health policy remains determined by social or political factors as much as by evidence (Black 2001). Decisions therefore emerge out of a dialogue between government, the professions, lobbyists, the media, and the criminal justice system, rather than evidence. If a more rational approach were ever contemplated, researchers, funding bodies, and policy-makers should at the very least collaborate in evaluating the effects of the proposed legislation. Such studies should ideally include a range of patient, family, and health service outcomes using mixed methods, rather than focus on admission rates and lengths of stay.

In the meantime, it may be more appropriate to openly acknowledge the limits of our knowledge, rather than rely on the illusion that evidence exists. As it also seems unlikely that these difficult issues will be resolved using a rationalist–objectivist model, all that can be hoped for is more honesty about how, when, and if we use research evidence.

References

Bindman J (2002). Involuntary outpatient treatment in England and Wales. *Current Opinion in Psychiatry*, **15**:595–598.

Black N (2001). Evidence based policy: proceed with care. *British Medical Journal*, **323**:275–279.

Burgess P, Bindman J, Leese M, et al. (2006). Do community treatment orders for mental illness reduce readmission to hospital? An epidemiological study. *Social Psychiatry and Psychiatric Epidemiology*, **41**:574–579.

Burns T, Rugkåsa J, Molodynski A, et al. (2013). Community treatment orders for patients with psychosis (OCTET): a randomised controlled trial. *The Lancet*, **381**:1627–1633.

Bursten B (1986). Posthospital mandatory outpatient treatment. *American Journal of Psychiatry*, **143**:1255–1258.

Busch A, Wilder C, Van Dorn R, et al. (2010). Changes in guideline-recommended medication possession after implementing Kendra's Law in New York. *Psychiatric Services*, **61**:1000–1005.

Christy A, Petrila J, McCranie M, et al. (2009). Involuntary outpatient commitment in Florida: case information and provider experience and opinions. *International Journal of Forensic Mental Health*, **8**:122–130.

Churchill R, Owen G, Singh S, et al. (2007). *International experiences of using community treatment orders*. London: Institute of Psychiatry, Kings College London.

Compton SN, Swanson JW, Wagner HR, et al. (2003). Involuntary outpatient commitment and homelessness in persons with severe mental illness. *Mental Health Services Research*, **5**:27–38.

Davidson G, Campbell J (2007). An examination of the use of coercion by assertive outreach and community mental health teams in Northern Ireland. *British Journal of Social Work*, **37**:537–555.

Davis S (2002). Brief report: autonomy versus coercion: reconciling competing perspectives in community mental health. *Community Mental Health Journal*, **38**:239–250.

Geller J, Grudzinskas AJJ, McDermeit M, et al. (1998). The efficacy of involuntary outpatient treatment in Massachusetts. *Administration Policy and Mental Health*, **25**:271–285.

Gilbert AR, Moser LL, Van Dorn RA, et al. (2010). Reductions in arrest under assisted outpatient treatment in New York. *Psychiatric Services*, **61**:996–999.

Gray JE, O'Reilly RL (2001). Clinically significant differences among Canadian mental health acts. *Canadian Journal of Psychiatry–Revue Canadienne de Psychiatrie*, **46**:315–321.

Gray JE, O'Reilly RL (2005). Canadian compulsory community treatment laws: recent reforms. *International Journal of Law and Psychiatry*, **28**:13–22.

Hiday VA, Scheid-Cook TL (1987). The North Carolina experience with outpatient commitment: a critical appraisal. *International Journal of Law and Psychiatry*, **10**:215–232.

Hiday VA, Scheid-Cook TL (1989). A follow-up of chronic patients committed to outpatient treatment. *Hospital and Community Psychiatry*, **40**:53.

Hiday VA, Scheid-Cook TL (1991). Outpatient commitment for'revolving door' patients: compliance and treatment. *Journal of Nervous and Mental Disease*, **179**:83–88.

Hiday V, Swartz M, Swanson J, et al. (1999). Criminal victimisation of persons with severe mental illness. *Psychiatric Services*, **50**:62–68.

Hiday VA, Swartz MS, Swanson JW, et al. (2002). Impact of outpatient commitment on victimization of people with severe mental illness. *American Journal of Psychiatry*, **159**:1403–1411.

Hough WG, O'Brien KP (2005). The effect of community treatment orders on offending rates. *Psychiatry, Psychology and Law*, **12**:411–423.

Hunt AM, da Silva A, Lurie S, et al. (2007). Community treatment orders in Toronto: the emerging data. *Canadian Journal of Psychiatry–Revue Canadienne de Psychiatrie*, **52**:647–656.

Jethwa K, Galappathie N (2008). Community treatment orders. *British Medical Journal*, **337**:a613.

Kisely S (2009). Compulsory community treatment: does it work? *Irish Psychiatrist*, **10**:26–28.

Kisely S, Hall K (2014). An updated meta-analysis of randomized controlled evidence for the effectiveness of community treatment orders. *Canadian Journal of Psychiatry-Revue Canadienne de Psychiatrie*, **59**:561–564.

Kisely S, Campbell LA (2006). Community treatment orders for psychiatric patients: the emperor with no clothes. *Canadian Journal of Psychiatry–Revue Canadienne de Psychiatrie*, **51**:683–685 [discussion 691].

Kisely S, Campbell LA (2007). Methodological issues in assessing the evidence for compulsory community treatment. *Current Psychiatry Reviews*, **3**:51–56.

Kisely SR, Xiao J, Preston NJ (2004). Impact of compulsory community treatment on admission rates: survival analysis using linked mental health and offender databases. *British Journal of Psychiatry*, **184**:432–438.

Kisely S, Smith M, Preston NJ, et al. (2005). A comparison of health service use in two jurisdictions with and without compulsory community treatment. *Psychological Medicine*, **35**:1357–1367.

Kisely S, Campbell LA, Scott A, et al. (2007). Randomized and non-randomized evidence for the effect of compulsory community and involuntary out-patient treatment on health service use: systematic review and meta-analysis. *Psychological Medicine*, **37**:3–14.

Kisely S, Campbell LA, Preston N (2011). Compulsory community and involuntary outpatient treatment for people with severe mental disorders. *Cochrane Database of Systematic Reviews*, **16**(2):CD004408.

Kisely S, Preston N, Xiao J, et al. (2013a). An eleven-year evaluation of the effect of community treatment orders on changes in mental health service use. *Journal of Psychiatric Research*, **47**:650–656.

Kisely S, Preston N, Xiao J, et al. (2013b). Reducing all-cause mortality among patients with psychiatric disorders: a population-based study. *Canadian Medical Association Journal*, **185**:E50–E56.

Kisely S, Xiao J, Crowe E, et al. (2014). The effect of community treatment orders on outcome as assessed by the Health of the Nation Outcome Scales. *Psychiatry Research*, **215**:574–578.

Lawton-Smith S (2005). *A question of numbers. The potential impact of community-based treatment orders in England and Wales.* London: King's Fund.

Lawton-Smith S, Dawson J, Burns T (2008). Community treatment orders are not a good thing. *British Journal of Psychiatry*, **193**:96–100.

Last JM (ed.) (1988). *A dictionary of epidemiology*, 2nd edn. New York: Oxford University Press.

Link BG, Epperson MW, Perron BE, et al. (2011). Arrest outcomes associated with outpatient commitment in New York State. *Psychiatric Services*, **62**:504–508.

McIvor R (1998). The community treatment order: clinical and ethical issues. *Australian and New Zealand Journal of Psychiatry*, **32**:223–228.

McIvor R (2001). Care and compulsion in community psychiatric treatment work. *Psychiatric Bulletin*, **25**:369–370.

Marshall M, Lockwood A (2000). Assertive community treatment for people with severe mental disorders. *Cochrane Database of Systematic Reviews*, (2):CD001089.

Maughan D, Molodynski A, Rugkåsa J, et al. (2014). A systematic review of the effect of community treatment orders on service use. *Social Psychiatry and Psychiatric Epidemiology*, **49**:651–663.

Muirhead D, Harvey C, Ingram G (2006). Effectiveness of community treatment orders for treatment of schizophrenia with oral or depot antipsychotic medication: clinical outcomes. *Australian and New Zealand Journal of Psychiatry*, **40**:596–605.

Nakhost A, Perry JC, Frank D (2012). Assessing the outcome of compulsory treatment orders on management of psychiatric patients at 2 McGill University-associated hospitals. *Canadian Journal of Psychiatry–Revue Canadienne de Psychiatrie*, **57**:359–365.

O'Reilly RL (2001). Does involuntary out-patient treatment work? *Psychiatric Bulletin*, **25**:371–374.

Pinfold V, Bindman J (2001). Is compulsory community treatment ever justified? *Psychiatric Bulletin*, **25**:268–270.

Preston N, Kisely S, Xiao J (2002). Assessing the outcome of compulsory psychiatric treatment in the community: epidemiological study in Western Australia. *British Medical Journal*, **324**:1244–1249.

Ridgely S, Borum R, Pertila J (2001). *The effectiveness of involuntary outpatient treatment. Empirical evidence and the experience of eight states.* California: RAND.

Romans S, Dawson J, Mullen R, et al. (2004). How mental health clinicians view community treatment orders: a national New Zealand survey. *Australian and New Zealand Journal of Psychiatry*, **38**:836–841.

Rugkåsa JDJ, Burns T (2014). CTOs: what is the state of the evidence? *Social Psychiatry and Psychiatric Epidemiology*, **49**:1861–1871.

Segal SP, Burgess PM (2006a). Conditional release: a less restrictive alternative to hospitalization? *Psychiatric Services*, **57**:1600–1606.

Segal SP, Burgess PM (2006b). Factors in the selection of patients for conditional release from their first psychiatric hospitalization. *Psychiatric Services*, **57**:1614–1622.

Segal SP, Burgess PM (2006c). The utility of extended outpatient civil commitment. *International Journal of Law and Psychiatry*, **29**:525–534.

Segal SP, Burgess PM (2006d). Effect of conditional release from hospitalization on mortality risk. *Psychiatric Services*, **57**:1607–1613.

Segal SP, Preston N, Kisely S, et al. (2009). Conditional release in Western Australia: effect on hospital length of stay. *Psychiatric Services*, **60**:94–99.

Sensky T, Hughes T, Hirsch S (1991). Compulsory psychiatric treatment in the community. A controlled study of compulsory community treatment with extended leave under the Mental Health Act: special characteristics of patients treated and impact of treatment. *British Journal of Psychiatry*, **158**:792–799.

Steadman HJ, Mulvey EP, Monahan J, et al. (1998). Violence by people discharged from acute psychiatric inpatient facilities and by others in the same neighborhoods. *Archives of General Psychiatry*, **55**:393–401.

Steadman HJ, Gounis K, Dennis D, et al. (2001). Assessing the New York City involuntary outpatient commitment pilot program. *Psychiatric Services*, **52**:330–336.

Swanson JW, Swartz MS, Borum R, et al. (2000). Involuntary out-patient commitment and reduction of violent behaviour in persons with severe mental illness. *British Journal of Psychiatry*, **176**:324–331.

Swartz MS, Swanson JW, Wagner HR, et al. (1999). Can involuntary outpatient commitment reduce hospital recidivism?: findings from a randomized trial with severely mentally ill individuals. *American Journal of Psychiatry*, **156**:1968–1975.

Swartz MS, Wagner HR, Swanson JW, et al. (2002). The perceived coerciveness of involuntary outpatient commitment: findings from an experimental study. *Journal of the American Academy of Psychiatry and the Law*, **30**:207–217.

Swartz MS, Wilder CM, Swanson JW, et al. (2010). Assessing outcomes for consumers in New York's assisted outpatient treatment program. *Psychiatric Services*, **61**:976–981.

Szmukler G, Hotopf M (2001). Effectiveness of involuntary outpatient commitment. *American Journal of Psychiatry*, **158**:653a–654a.

Torrey EF, Kaplan RJ (1995). A national survey of the use of outpatient commitment. *Psychiatric Services*, **46**:778–784.

Vaughan K, McConaghy N, Wolf C, et al. (2000). Community treatment orders: relationship to clinical care, medication compliance, behavioural disturbance and readmission. *Australian and New Zealand Journal of Psychiatry*, **34**:801–808.

Wagner HR, Swartz MS, Swanson JW, et al. (2003). Does involuntary outpatient commitment lead to more intensive treatment? *Psychology, Public Policy and Law*, **9**:145–158.

Zanni GR, Stavis PF (2007). The effectiveness and ethical justification of psychiatric outpatient commitment. *American Journal of Bioethics*, **7**:31–41.

Chapter 6

Informal coercion: current evidence

Ksenija Yeeles

Introduction

The literature on coercion has focused mainly on the compulsory treatment of psychiatric patients in hospital. Coercion was thus often equated with involuntary status. However, in practice, the distinction between coerced and voluntary status is more complex. Many voluntary patients feel coerced into treatment and many are uncertain of their legal status (Lidz et al. 1995; Hoge et al. 1997; Katsakou et al. 2011). Coercive pressures, often called 'informal coercion', such as the threat of involuntary admission are widely used with voluntary patients and some involuntary patients report feeling less coerced than voluntary patients (Rogers 1993; Hoge et al. 1997). Focusing on involuntary treatment and regarding 'coercion' and 'involuntary treatment' as identical prevents researchers from recognizing other coercive strategies.

Legal compulsion remains the clearest expression of coercion in most health-care systems. Recently increasing numbers of patients have been subject to legal compulsion in the community but the vast majority are still treated voluntarily. It has been argued that purely voluntary or involuntary psychiatric treatments are very rare and there is usually some form of pressure (Susser and Roche 1996). Psychiatric patients are routinely subject to various pressures from their clinicians, family members, friends, housing officers, the welfare and criminal justice systems, and other agencies. Such pressures are assumed to improve patients' adherence to treatment and clinical outcomes, and consequently prevent hospital admissions. These non-legislative forms of coercion are hard to identify or measure. They are not systematically recorded in medical records, and they are not regulated by policies or legislation.

As explained in Chapter 1, community mental health services have developed different approaches to the traditional treatment of patients in hospitals and will often provide services in patients' homes and neighbourhoods. They often collaborate widely with patients' family, friends, carers, and employers, and liaise with welfare, housing, and criminal justice agencies. Current approaches build upon assertive outreach and a close and enduring personal relationship (Godin 2000). Clinicians use various pressures in such relationships aimed at improving patients' adherence to treatment (Lützén 1998; Godin 2000). However, such pressures may pose risks to a patient's trust, and clinicians need a clearer understanding to choose strategies to ensure both the patient's collaboration and a trusting relationship (Lützén 1998).

There is a limited but growing body of evidence on such non-legislative pressures in community treatment. This chapter will review this evidence and identify common themes. The literature on clinicians' experiences of using such pressures is reviewed in Chapter 8. While the ethical issues and justification for treatment pressures are dealt with in Chapter 14, this chapter will present some guidance for practitioners. This chapter is based on a scoping review of publications on informal coercion published between January 1980 and June 2014. The literature search was performed electronically by searching the Ovid MEDLINE, Embase, CINAHL, PsycINFO, and Web of Science Core Collection databases supplemented by a manual search of the reference lists in key papers. All the studies identified were conducted in the USA or Europe and there were no studies from other countries. I will outline the key concepts applied in the literature, present data regarding the prevalence and outcome of reported informal coercion, and finally identify challenges to future research and clinical practice.

What is informal coercion?

Monitoring and encouraging patients to take medication has become a central task in community psychiatry. Both public pressure and professional responsibilities may push clinicians to use unnecessarily coercive strategies to avoid failures in care that might put the patient or public at risk (Watts and Priebe 2002). The shift from a paternalistic to a more collaborative interaction aims to reduce patients' experiences of coercion. To avoid legal compulsion, clinicians have adopted other 'tools' to improve adherence, often using informal coercion. Better understanding of patients' perceptions of coercion can enable clinicians both to minimize the negative consequences of coercion and to improve their practice. This is especially important as the evidence reviewed elsewhere in this book suggests that compulsion in the community has limited effects upon outcome (see Chapters 4 and 5).

The terminology used in the literature is complex and at times confusing with varying terms and concepts used for compulsion, coercion, and treatment pressures. I will use *legal compulsion* for formal or statutory coercion which is regulated by mental health legislation. This includes community compulsion, variously referred to as community treatment order (CTO), outpatient commitment and assisted outpatient treatment. This chapter concentrates, however, on *informal coercion*. This is a broad term covering various *non-statutory treatment pressures* used on a day-to-day basis by clinicians, carers, family members, and the welfare and criminal justice systems to improve patients' stability and treatment adherence. The narrower term *leverage* will be used for a form of treatment pressure which employs a specific explicit treatment *lever* in a declared effort to increase adherence. *Perceived coercion* is the patient's subjective perception of the coerciveness of their treatment.

Informal coercion, like legal compulsion, is primarily employed to encourage patients to do something that they may not want to do. Patients are encouraged or pressured to change their behaviour. While there are various definitions of coercion and informal coercion in the literature (Curtis and Diamond 1997; Lidz et al. 1998; Lützén 1998; Lakeman 2000; Mason 2000; O'Brien and Golding 2003; Szmukler and Appelbaum 2008; Canvin et al 2013) there is no simple, widely accepted concept of coercion. Most conceptualizations include a spectrum of treatment pressures applied either in an open or an indirect manner to influence a patient's behaviour. The most broadly accepted framework of coercion is the Szmukler and Appelbaum (2008) hierarchy of treatment pressures. It comprises five levels: persuasion, interpersonal leverage, inducement, threats, and compulsion (see Chapter 14). While there is wide agreement about the coerciveness at the most coercive end of the continuum of treatment pressures (e.g. physical force, restraint, legal compulsion), there is inconsistency about less coercive measures. Persuasion is non-coercive according to some authors (Mason 2000; Beauchamp and Childress 2001; Szmukler and Appelbaum 2008) but potentially coercive according to others (O'Brien and Golding 2003). Housing leverage can be construed as a relatively non-coercive treatment pressure, yet it can have a major effect on patients (Allen 2003). This remaining lack of clarity on the less manifestly coercive forms of pressure requires more research to inform the current debate.

What is leverage?

The term *leverage*, as applied to research on informal coercion, originated in North America. People with severe mental illnesses often depend on welfare support and are frequently involved with the criminal justice system. Leverage refers to the explicit use of pressure by making needed provisions such as housing and financial support, or the reduction of criminal charges, directly contingent upon adherence to prescribed treatment. Canvin et al. (2013, p. 102) proposed three conditions for leveraged pressures: '(i) consequences contingent upon a specified response (conditionality), (ii) a lever' (e.g. access to services, access to social welfare benefits, depot injection, hospital admission, discharge from services, avoidance of imprisonment or criminal charges), and '(iii) direct communication by someone perceived to have the power to bring about the specified consequences'. Leverage is thus different from both legal compulsion and persuasion (Monahan et al. 2005; Szmukler and Appelbaum 2008). It may compromise the patient's autonomy and the therapeutic relationship (Monahan et al. 2001; Angell et al. 2007) yet not always be perceived as coercive (Susser and Roche 1996). The most researched and described forms of leverage include access to welfare benefits (e.g. access to housing and financial support), the avoidance or reduction of criminal sanctions, access to or custody of children, and the avoidance of involuntary admission via community compulsion. These may be explicitly made conditional on adherence to treatment (Elbogen et al. 2005; Monahan et al. 2005; Robbins et al. 2006; Busch and Redlich 2007; Jaeger and Rossler 2010; Burns et al. 2011).

Some landlords believe that housing leverage will make patients better tenants (because they are adherent). For clinicians and family its purpose is to keep patients stable and in treatment (Allen 2003). Many residential housing programmes in the USA include housing leverage in the contract/lease (Robbins et al. 2009; Wong et al. 2010) although it is not clear whether this is entirely legal (Monahan et al. 2001). Housing leverage is often used at hospital discharge (Diamond 1995; Allen 2003) when moving into specific residential accommodation or into accommodation with restrictive regimes (Monahan et al. 2001; Allen 2003).

Many patients with severe mental illness have few basic financial skills and little experience. Little is known about financial incapacity and there is no structured or evidence-based guidance for its assessment (Marson et al. 2006). However, many patients are assigned someone to support them to manage their finances. This arrangement can be formal (a financial guardian or representative payee, often a clinician) or informal (carer, family member). Representative payee programmes in the USA pay a person's rent and utility bills using their disability benefits. A representative payee may make access to the remaining funds dependent upon adherence. Informal financial management is mostly voluntary but financial leverage is not unusual. The legality of withholding or delaying access to money from patients is not entirely clear in the USA (Monahan et al. 2005) and little is known about the use of informal financial leverage.

Criminal justice leverage has long been used when people with substance abuse and/ or psychosis appear before the criminal justice system in many countries. Practices vary, but patients are often offered the choice of entering treatment instead of criminal sanctions such as imprisonment or conviction. Adherence to mental health treatment is a frequent condition of probation, parole, or for charges to be dropped (Monahan et al. 2005). The USA relies more on designated mental health courts (Monahan et al. 2001, 2005; Griffin et al. 2002; Lamberti 2007) whereas in Europe the practice relies on court diversion schemes. In such schemes patients are screened by mental health staff and many do not progress to a hearing but are diverted to treatment. Drug treatment orders exist in most European countries and operate like the sentences handed down by mental health courts in the USA.

In some US states patients legally eligible for involuntary hospital admission may be directed to have compulsory treatment in hospital or in the community (Monahan et al. 2001, 2005). Avoidance of hospital treatment (leverage) via community compulsion is conditional upon adherence to treatment.

Patients with severe mental illnesses may be reluctant to disclose that they have children or to seek treatment for fear of losing custody (Nicholson et al. 1998). Access to their own children may be made a condition of adherence. Whilst they are a potential powerful motivator, such requirements can be very stigmatizing (Nicholson et al. 2002; Nicholson 2005).

What is perceived coercion?

Patients' subjective perception of coercion does not always match their legal status in the hospital setting (Lidz et al. 1995; Hoge et al. 1997). These findings have encouraged researchers to investigate patients' subjective perceptions of coercion. In a complex clinical setting it is not always obvious when coercion is applied or how it is perceived by patients. Although compulsion is likely to be perceived as coercive, it is also important to consider the 'coercion context' (see Chapter 8) that may render non-compulsory interventions coercive (Sjöström 2006). Patients' views of important subjective issues are particularly revealing when they feel coerced in situations where objective coercion is not applied and there are no legal mechanisms for appeal (Szmukler and Appelbaum 2008).

The research base: current evidence

A significant increase in coercion research stemmed from the establishment of the MacArthur Research Networks on Mandated Community Treatment and on Mental Health and the Law in the USA in the late 1980s. Growing interest in formal and informal coercion among researchers outside the USA has resulted in well-established and productive research groups in Australia, Canada, New Zealand, the Netherlands, Scandinavia, and the UK. In this section I summarize published evidence of what is known about the prevalence and outcomes of informal coercion with attention to issues of perceived fairness and effectiveness, the use of financial incentives, and the place of qualitative studies.

Prevalence of informal coercion

Leverage is probably the most researched form of treatment pressure yet there are only three published studies on its frequency (Monahan et al. 2005; Jaeger and Rossler 2010; Burns et al. 2011). The first, and the largest, study was of lifetime leverage (money, housing, criminal justice, and avoidance of hospitalization) in US public mental health services conducted by the MacArthur group (Monahan et al. 2005). This was a cross-sectional study with 1011 community psychiatric patients recruited from five sites in different states. Between 44% and 59% of patients reported lifetime experience of leverage, with an average of 51%. Housing leverage was the most prevalent at 23–40% ($n = 312$) followed by criminal justice leverage at 15–30% ($n = 230$), financial leverage at 7–19% ($n = 121$), and avoidance of hospitalization at 12–20% ($n = 150$) (Monahan et al. 2005). Variation in the prevalence of different leverages between sites was significant and probably reflected the different programmes and services available. These findings suggest that leverage may be more common than legal compulsion (Monahan et al. 2005).

The ULTIMA ('Use of Leverage To Improve Mental health treatment Adherence') study (Burns et al. 2011) replicated the MacArthur study in England and included 417 patients from four discrete clinical groups [psychosis patients from assertive outreach teams (AOT), psychosis patients from standard community mental health teams (CMHT), non-psychosis patients from CMHTs, and substance abuse patients receiving methadone or subutex treatment]. The prevalence of lifetime leverage was significantly lower at 35% ($n = 145$) than in the USA but the pattern was similar (Figure 6.1). Housing leverage was the most common at 24% ($n = 98$), followed by criminal justice leverage at 15% ($n = 62$). Childcare and financial leverage had very low rates in the ULTIMA sample at 8% ($n = 34$) and 2% ($n = 10$), respectively. When childcare leverage rate was removed (it was not recorded in the MacArthur study), the difference between two studies was even larger at 31% in England and 51% in the USA (Burns et al. 2011). The ULTIMA clinical groups varied markedly, with the substance abuse sample having the highest rates 64/101(63%). This exceeded the highest rates among amongst the US sites. Psychosis patients recruited from AOTs had a similar rate to psychosis patients from CMHT, 33% and 30% respectively. The lowest rates were in the non-psychosis CMHT sample 17/113 (15%). The substance abuse sample had the highest rate for each form of leverage. Multiple forms of leverage were reported by 51

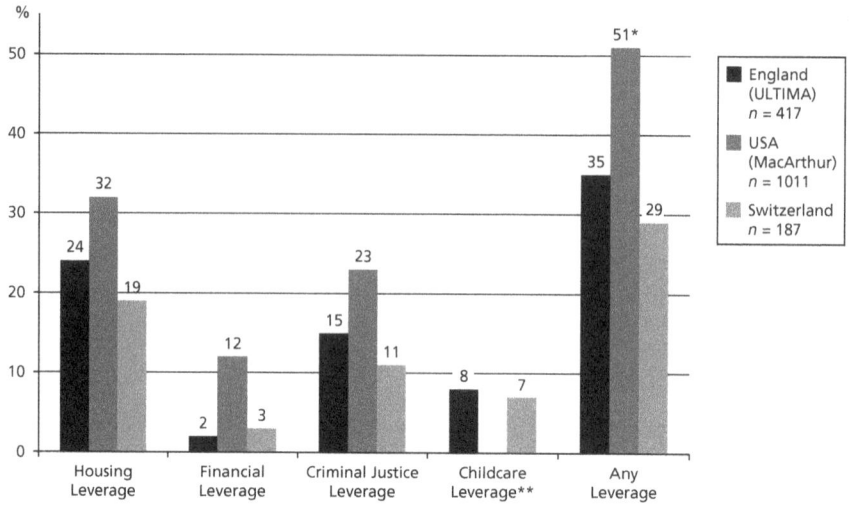

*Includes CTO as leverage to avoid hospital admission.
**Child leverage rates were not reported in the MacArthur study.

Figure 6.1 Leverage rates in England, the USA, and Switzerland.

patients (12%) in the ULTIMA sample; more than half of these were from the substance abuse group (Burns et al. 2011).

A Swiss study recruited 187 patients from both community 69 (37%) and inpatient 118 (63%) settings (Jaeger and Rossler 2010). Of these 187 people, 38% were involuntary. The inclusion criteria and data collected were very similar to the MacArthur (Monahan et al. 2005) and ULTIMA (Burns et al. 2011) studies using the same questionnaire. The Swiss patients reported the lowest prevalence for lifetime leverage at 29%. The pattern of prevalence of different forms of leverage was similar to that in the MacArthur and ULTIMA studies, as shown in Figure 6.1. The most prevalent was housing leverage at 19% (*n* = 36) followed by criminal justice leverage at 11%, childcare leverage at 7%, and financial leverage at 3% (Jaeger and Rossler 2010).

The lower prevalence of lifetime leverage in European studies may reflect differences in clinician attitudes, in social welfare and legal systems, or a combination of the two. Housing and disability benefits are entitlements in Europe, whereas in the USA they may be contingent upon treatment adherence in specific programmes. Similarly individuals with severe mental illness in the UK are often redirected to the mental health system before they enter courts and therefore the leverage is neither noted nor recorded (Griffin et al. 2002). Variation across the different US states (Bonnie and Monahan 2005; Monahan et al. 2005) may also reflect different legal practices and treatments.

Recent or current (last 6 months) experience of housing leverage was assessed in the MacArthur study and 162 (12–18%) patients reported it for leverage related to treatment adherence while 298 (26–35%) reported leverage related to substance abstinence (Robbins et al. 2006). In the study of 27 supported housing programme teams in the

USA Wong et al. (2010) found that in 16 (59%) teams tenants could be excluded for non-adherence to medication, relapse, or alcohol and drug use. It was regular practice in 17 (63%) teams to test tenants for drug and alcohol use. Again it is not clear whether this is consistent with legislation on tenants' rights.

Financial leverage is probably the most researched form of leverage, and most of the literature emanates from the USA. Much of this literature is described in Chapter 11. Elbogen et al. (2003a) reported the first figures on prevalence of financial leverage in 258 patients with psychosis from a trial (Swartz et al. 1999a) of CTOs. Fewer patients (37%) reported having someone who had ever managed their finance than in the MacArthur study (51%; Monahan et al. 2005) and the ULTIMA (40%; Burns et al. 2011), and 24% had their disability benefits paid to a representative payee. Almost 30% (76 patients) reported experience of financial leverage, much higher than in any other studies (Monahan et al. 2005; Jaeger and Rossler 2010; Burns et al. 2011). This may reflect the characteristics of a sample selected for compulsory treatment.

Surprisingly few patients in the two European studies reported financial leverage, with 2% in England (ULTIMA) and 3% in Switzerland compared with 12% in the USA (MacArthur). The leverage rates among those who ever had someone to manage their money were also much higher in the US sample at 121/519 (32%) than in the English one 10/165 (6%) (Monahan et al. 2005; Burns et al. 2011).

Reported rates of recent financial leverage (last 6 months) vary. Appelbaum and Redlich (2006a) found that 7–19% of 321 patients with a current representative payee in the MacArthur study and 14–27% of 390 with someone to manage their money reported recent financial leverage. The highest financial leverage rates were amongst those with clinicians as money managers (Appelbaum and Redlich 2006a; Angell et al. 2007).

Lifetime childcare leverage was only directly investigated by the English and Swiss studies (Jaeger and Rossler 2010; Burns et al. 2011). Using data from the MacArthur study Bush and Redlich (2007) reported that 36 (19%) of 187 patients with underage children felt that their custody or contact with children had been leveraged in the last 6 months.

Redlich and Monahan (2006) reported rates of recent (last 6 months) 'general pressures' in the MacArthur study ($n = 1011$) and compared them with specific pressures. 'General pressures' were related to 'feeling' that someone would take or admit the patient to hospital, stop them seeing or having custody of children, inform the authorities about non-adherence, and deny access to money. This is different from leverage where the contingency has to be explicit. The prevalence of recent general pressures was similar (41–55%) to that of lifetime leverage experience (44–59%) (Monahan et al. 2005) but higher than recent leverage rates (22%) (Redlich and Monahan 2006). The most prevalent 'general pressures' were related to hospitalization (27–43%) and housing (15–21%). Much less frequent were those related to childcare (3–7%) and employment (2–10%). Multiple general pressures were common, with 20% of patients reporting six or more (Redlich and Monahan 2006).

Predictors of informal coercion

Reported associations between lifetime leverage rates and patient characteristics are inconsistent. The MacArthur study reported that lifetime experience of any leverage was significantly more likely in younger patients (< 44 years), those with lower functioning, longer illness, a history of multiple hospitalizations, and a high frequency of contacts with community services. Multiple hospitalizations and lower functioning were significant predictors of all forms of leverage (Monahan et al. 2005). The ULTIMA study failed to find the same set of predictors and only multiple hospitalizations was a significant predictor in both studies. It is unclear whether this was due to a greater sample size and variation in clinical characteristics in the MacArthur study. ULTIMA patients with a substance abuse diagnosis and lower insight were more likely to report lifetime leverage. Those with a substance abuse diagnosis who had a history of imprisonment and those who were living in independent accommodation were more likely to report multiple forms of leverage. In the ULTIMA mental illness group (when substance abuse patients were excluded) lifetime experience of leverage was associated with greater severity of illness (Burns et al. 2011).

Several studies have found that specific forms of pressure were more frequent in patients with adherence problems, poor functioning, or severe symptoms (Neale and Rosenheck 2000; Elbogen et al. 2003b; Monahan et al. 2005; Angell 2006). Using data from 120 patients in the MacArthur study Appelbaum and Redlich (2006b) found no strong association between decisional capacity and reported leverage. This contradicts clinicians' common justification that relies on impairment in decision-making capacity. This was, however, a small sample with a retrospective study design that measured capacity and leverage rates at the same time.

'General pressures' were found to have similar predictors as lifetime leverage in the MacArthur study (Monahan et al. 2005; Redlich and Monahan 2006). Patients who were younger than 44 years, had severe mental illness, more severe symptoms, poor functioning, and co-morbid and historical substance abuse were more likely to report 'general pressures'.

A group of papers have investigated predictors of specific forms of leverage. More than a third of quantitative empirical papers (Appelbaum and Redlich 2006a,b; Redlich and Monahan 2006; Redlich et al. 2006; Robbins et al. 2006; Swanson et al. 2006; Angell et al. 2007) use data from the MacArthur study and several (Elbogen et al. 2003a,b; Swartz et al. 2003a, 2004) take data from other studies (Swartz et al. 1999a, 2003b) conducted by the same group. The associations between patient characteristics and lifetime housing leverage were inconsistent in US studies, with only male gender being regularly identified. Other predictors were diagnosis of psychosis, more severe symptoms, lower functioning, history of multiple hospital admissions, increased number of contacts with services, longer time in treatment (Monahan et al. 2005), experience of living in special housing or group homes, and having social support for treatment (Robbins et al. 2006). Patients who lived in their own homes or in 'housing-first' accommodation were less likely to report housing leverage than those in supported or subsided housing (Robbins et al. 2006, 2009).

Having a representative payee or financial guardian does not necessarily mean experiencing financial leverage. Multiple hospitalizations and substance abuse were common predictors of financial leverage in the MacArthur study (Monahan et al. 2005; Appelbaum and Redlich 2006a). Other significantly associated characteristics were male gender, diagnosis of psychosis, lower functioning, and lower levels of insight

(Monahan et al. 2005). In patients with financial management those with a parent or a partner/spouse managing their finance were more likely to report financial leverage (Appelbaum and Redlich 2006a). Generally poor functioning characterized by drug abuse, lower insight, and multiple hospitalizations predicted financial leverage.

Elbogen et al. (2003a) found that African-American patients, those whose finances were being managed, and those who experienced other forms of leverage were more likely to report financial leverage or 'money warnings'. It appears that patients are more likely to be exposed to financial leverage within a coercive context of other leverages.

Criminal justice leverage was consistently associated with younger age (Draine and Solomon 2001; Monahan et al. 2005; Redlich et al. 2006). Two analyses of MacArthur study data found it was associated with male gender, a history of multiple hospitalizations, and over 20 years of treatment (Monahan et al. 2005; Redlich et al. 2006). More criminal justice leverage was also reported by patients with substance abuse problems (Monahan et al. 2005). In a study of 250 psychiatric patients on probation or parole in the USA fewer threats were reported by those with more severe thought disorder and by those in an acute episode (Draine and Solomon 2001). Analysis of the MacArthur study data by Swanson et al. (2006) found that a combination of violence and non-adherence is likely to impact on the prevalence of reported criminal justice leverage. A history of serious violence was a significant predictor of criminal justice leverage, and any assaultive behaviour was a predictor of both criminal justice and social welfare leverage. Voluntary adherence may moderate the relationship between violence and the use of leverage (Swanson et al. 2006).

Avoidance of hospitalization leverage by the use of community compulsion was more likely to be reported by patients with poor functioning and a history of hospitalization in the MacArthur study (Monahan et al. 2005) and the expanded data analysis by Swartz et al. (2006). The latter also found that various factors were positively associated with the reported avoidance of hospitalization leverage via community compulsion: living in staffed residential accommodation, recent contact with services, dissatisfaction with social support, substance abuse, recent violent behaviour, and recent contact with police (Swartz et al. 2006).

Overall therefore there is little evidence from empirical studies regarding predictors of informal coercion. From what does exist it appears that more disabled patients with a history of multiple hospitalizations, intensive contact with services, substance abuse, and poor functioning are more likely to report various forms of leverage.

Outcomes of informal coercion

Perceived coercion

Subjective reports of coercion are accepted as a main indicator of treatment coerciveness for patients (Lidz et al. 1995; Szmukler and Appelbaum 2008; Newton-Howes and Stanley 2012). Patients' perceived coercion can be considered a 'side effect' of coercive psychiatric interventions (Newton-Howes and Stanley 2012) yet little is known about whether informal coercion reduces or increases patients' experience of coercion. Identifying the least coercive forms of informal coercion and factors associated with patients' perception of coercion may enable clinicians to use the most effective

interventions with the least impact on patients' perception of their influence and control in treatment decisions. Perceived coercion in community treatment is also examined in Chapter 9. Here I present what is known about the perceived coerciveness of
informal coercion.

The development of an instrument to measure perceived coercion (Gardner et al.
1993) enabled researchers to investigate patients' perception of the coerciveness
of both legal compulsion and informal coercion. Gardner et al. (1993) developed
two scales to measure perceived coercion: The MacArthur Admission Experience
Interview (AEI) and the MacArthur Admission Survey (AES). The AES or MacArthur
Perceived Coercion Scale is a structured scale of five questions regarding influence,
control, choice, freedom, and whose idea it was to come to hospital. Two additional
subscales ('negative pressures' and 'procedural justice') were later included in the AES
and were adapted (Lidz et al. 1995; Hiday et al. 1997) and validated for use in a community setting (Gardner et al. 1993; Hiday et al. 1997; Swartz et al. 1999b).

Patients recruited in a trial of community compulsion in the USA (Swartz et al. 1999a)
were more likely to report high levels of perceived coercion when other forms of leverage were used along with 'money warnings' (financial leverage) (Elbogen et al. 2003a).
Patients from the same study who were either under community compulsion or had
a representative payee did not differ in perceived coercion from patients with neither
community compulsion nor a representative payee (Elbogen et al. 2003b). Patients with
both community compulsion and a representative payee were, however, more likely to
report perceived coercion than those with neither of these two control mechanisms.
Similarly, patients with a representative payee and those with both community compulsion and a representative payee were more likely to report higher perceived coercion
than those with no reported financial leverage (Elbogen et al. 2003b). A relationship
between multiple leverages and perceived coercion was also found in the MacArthur
study by Appelbaum and Redlich (2006a). Patients felt more coerced but they also felt
that financial leverage was effective. It seems that the experience of multiple rather than
single forms of financial leverage is associated with perceived coercion.

Housing leverage was strongly associated with perceived coercion, and patients in
the MacArthur study who reported housing leverage were more likely to report other
forms of leverage (Robbins et al. 2006). In another analysis of this data set, patients
who reported multiple forms of leverage were more likely to report barriers to help-
seeking due to a fear of coercive or involuntary treatment (Van Dorn et al. 2006).
Barriers to help-seeking can potentially impact on patients' willingness to comply with
treatment and may lead to disengagement due to fear of coercive treatment experienced in the past (Swartz et al. 2003a; Van Dorn et al. 2006). In the Swiss study on
informal coercion by Jaeger and Rossler (2010), patients who reported any lifetime
leverage were more likely to report higher perceived coercion and lower perceived
fairness of treatment. Perceived coercion was associated with most forms of leverage, coerced voluntarism, a history of involuntary hospitalization, and a diagnosis of
schizophrenia (Jaeger and Rossler 2010). The experience of different forms of leverage
appears to be an important predictor of perceived coercion.

A good therapeutic relationship is generally accepted as crucial for successful psychiatric treatment and adherence (Johansson and Eklund 2003). Procedural justice as

measured in the MacArthur Perceived Coercion scale (Gardner et al. 1993) assesses patient experience of having a 'voice' in treatment decisions. Procedural justice reduces perceived coercion at hospital admission (Lidz et al. 1995; Monahan et al 2001). Community patients in a US study (Swartz et al. 2003b) who perceived financial leverage as coercive were more likely to report poor relationships with the family members or clinicians who applied that leverage (Elbogen et al. 2005). In the MacArthur study perceived coercion and reported barriers to help-seeking led to reduced perceived effectiveness and fairness of the leverages used (Van Dorn et al. 2006). Patients treated with respect and fairness recognize the positive side of pressures and sometimes express gratitude (Lidz et al. 1995; Van Dorn et al. 2005). It seems that transparent communication about the purposes of leverage (Lidz et al. 1998) and fair treatment (Lidz et al. 1995) can reduce the perception of coercion and enhance the recognition of the value of leverage, as reported in the Swiss study on informal coercion (Jaeger and Rossler 2010). Support, respect, and consideration of patients' views by those who apply financial leverage may reduce its negative effects. Current evidence overall suggests that the experience of multiple pressures increases perceived coercion but procedural justice and good therapeutic relationships may reduce it.

Other outcomes of informal coercion

Little is known about the effectiveness of informal coercion on treatment adherence. Two analyses of the data set from the MacArthur study, one looking at any leverage (McNiel et al. 2013) and one at criminal justice leverage (Redlich et al. 2006), failed to find any association with adherence to medication and appointments.

Associations between leverage and satisfaction with services have been investigated in several studies. Patients who reported housing leverage in the MacArthur study did not differ in satisfaction from patients who did not (Robbins et al. 2006). Housing programmes with leverage included in the tenancy did not differ in satisfaction from 'leverage free' (housing-first) housing programmes in the USA (Robbins et al. 2009). Any leverage (McNiel et al. 2013) and criminal justice leverage (Redlich et al. 2006) were not associated with satisfaction with services assessed in the MacArthur study. However, satisfaction was lower in those who reported lifetime multiple leverages alongside community compulsion (Swartz et al. 2006). Leverage in independent housing programmes in the USA reduced patients' stability, making them more likely to leave (Wong et al. 2010). A weak effect was found for informal coercion as a barrier to help-seeking in the US study on patients with schizophrenia. Patients with a history of involuntary hospitalization and recent warnings about poor adherence were more likely to report barriers to treatment (Swartz et al. 2003a).

Financial leverage acted as a mediator for increased conflict in the therapeutic relationship in the analysis of a subsample from the MacArthur study (Angell et al. 2007). Having clinicians in control of patient finances is not disruptive for the therapeutic relationship in itself, but may become so if a patient feels pressured to adhere to treatment by it (Angell et al. 2007).

Currently there is no evidence that the use of any leverage is associated with adherence or satisfaction with treatment, and only weak evidence for other outcomes. Most studies had methodological problems and their cross-sectional designs precluded the establishment of causality.

Perceptions of fairness and effectiveness of treatment pressures

A person's perception of coercion appears to be affected by their beliefs about the fairness of their treatment (Monahan et al. 1995), although there are only a handful of studies that have explicitly investigated this perception of fairness. Two validated scales have been developed—an index of fairness and an index of effectiveness. The perception of fairness and effectiveness of treatment are strongly correlated ($r = 0.50$–0.53) (Swartz et al. 2004; Van Dorn et al. 2006; Jaeger and Rossler 2010). Patients who perceive pressures as effective will probably also see them as fair (Swartz et al. 2004). As perception of the fairness of treatment can minimize perceived coercion, prioritizing pressures perceived as effective by patients may reduce perceived coercion.

Elbogen et al. (2005) found that 68 out of 104 (65%) patients with schizophrenia in the USA perceived financial leverage as an unhelpful tool in keeping them well. In contrast, the majority of patients from the same study and patients with a broader range of diagnoses in the MacArthur study perceived pressures as fair (55–69%) and effective (48–62%) (Swartz et al. 2004; Van Dorn et al. 2005). Greater insight was associated with perceived fairness in the Swiss (Jaeger and Rossler 2010) and two US studies (Swartz et al. 2004; Van Dorn et al. 2005). Lower perceived coercion and more previous hospitalizations were significant predictors of fairness in Van Dorn et al.'s (2005) analysis of the MacArthur study data set. These predictors were not tested in the other studies. Better insight was also found to be a predictor of perceived effectiveness in two US studies (Swartz et al. 2004; Van Dorn et al. 2005), but there was no consistency in other identified associations (Swartz et al. 2004; Elbogen et al. 2005; Van Dorn et al. 2005).

Fairness and effectiveness were not related to lifetime treatment pressures including avoidance of hospitalization via community compulsion in the Swiss and one US study on schizophrenia patients (Swartz et al. 2004; Jaeger and Rossler 2010). This is at variance with previous findings that a history of involuntary treatment makes patients less positive about their care (Kaltiala-Heino 1996). Single rather than multiple forms of leverage and adherence reminders predicted perceived effectiveness of pressured treatment in Van Dorn et al.'s (2005) analysis of MacArthur study dataset. The relationship between experienced informal coercion and perception of fairness and effectiveness may be moderated by other factors.

Better insight and low levels of perceived coercion seem to be important for the positive evaluation of the effectiveness and fairness of treatment pressures including legal compulsion. Patients who believe that they are ill and need treatment, and who feel free in making treatment decisions, are likely to see treatment pressures as beneficial. Although insight may not affect perceived coercion, increasing it may lead to an improved acceptance of pressure(s).

The relationship between formal and informal coercion

With the introduction of community compulsion and the widespread use of informal coercion in the community (Monahan et al. 2005; Jaeger and Rossler 2010; Burns et al., 2011) differences between hospital and community treatments may be diminishing (Godin 2000). For instance, if a severely ill patient in the UK rejects their appointment an assertive outreach worker may continue to visit. Avoidance of treatment, as in hospital, may be almost impossible (Watts and Priebe 2002). Little is known about the relationship between legal compulsion and informal coercion in community mental health care. There is no evidence as to whether legal compulsion increases or decreases the use of informal coercion; either is possible. Clinicians may use more informal coercion with patients under legal compulsion because of a paternalistic mind-set. Conversely legal compulsion may suffice to keep the patient adherent and other forms of pressure may not be needed, with informal coercion being less used. In their 12-month follow-up study Elbogen et al. (2003b) found that having a representative payee while receiving treatment under community compulsion both increased adherence and the chance of an individual reporting financial leverage and perceived coercion. In the trial of effectiveness of community compulsion in England (Rugkåsa et al., 2015) patients who were randomized to treatment under community compulsion did not differ in reported recent leverage from patients in the control arm after 12 months' follow-up. Although the community compulsion group spent longer under compulsion, both groups were subject to involuntary hospitalization during follow-up (Burns et al. 2013). The long-term consequences of combined community compulsion and use of leverage are unknown.

Financial incentives to improve adherence to treatment

There has been a growing interest among clinicians and academics in the use of financial incentives in mental health treatment in the last decade (Claassen 2007; Claassen et al. 2007; Szmukler 2009; Burton et al. 2010; Priebe et al. 2010, 2013; Staring 2010; Highton-Williamson et al. 2015). There is some evidence that such interventions improve adherence to antipsychotic medication in community care in the UK (Priebe et al. 2013). The idea of 'paying' psychiatric patients for taking medication generally provokes strong responses among clinicians in the UK (Claassen et al. 2007; Priebe et al. 2010) and debates regarding its ethics among academics (Burns 2007; Claassen 2007; Szmukler and Appelbaum 2008; Szmukler 2009; Priebe et al. 2010). Practical considerations also contribute to the controversy (Claassen 2007; Szmukler and Appelbaum 2008; Priebe et al. 2010). Although many clinicians in the UK initially object to them (Claassen 2007; Claassen et al. 2007), those who have used financial incentives in their practice often become convinced of their benefits (Highton-Williamson et al. 2015). The predicted ethical and practical dilemmas (Claassen 2007; Claassen et al. 2007; Szmukler 2009; Priebe et al. 2010) occurred surprisingly infrequently during two pilot studies in Europe (Claassen et al. 2007; Staring et al. 2010), and only in a minority of cases (Highton-Williamson et al. 2015) during the only randomized controlled trial conducted in the UK (Priebe et al. 2013). The intervention group who received a financial incentive in this trial improved their adherence to depot medication significantly, with 28% achieving full adherence. While no difference was found in clinician-reported clinical outcomes, self-reported quality of life improved significantly in the intervention patients (Priebe et al. 2013).

Qualitative studies

There were a small number of qualitative studies of informal coercion within community mental health services identified in this review. Unlike many quantitative papers on informal coercion almost all qualitative studies recruited their own samples of patients. Watts and Priebe (2002) conducted in-depth interviews with 12 patients in one assertive outreach team in London. Early negative (often coercive) experiences at the first episode of psychosis and distrustful and poor therapeutic relationships were the main factors cited for disengagement. Having no choice about seeing clinicians in the community was experienced as coercive. 'Proximal' intervention (e.g. forced medication, physical restraint, involuntary hospitalization, and depot injections) were perceived as more coercive than 'distal' intervention (e.g. feeling pressured to comply with treatment after clinician's help with social welfare benefits). The authors concluded that building trustful and collaborative therapeutic relationships may reduce disengagement and perceived coercion (Watts and Priebe 2002).

Tranulis et al. (2011) interviewed 20 patients with a diagnosis of schizophrenia who were receiving antipsychotic mediation in the community. Patients reported that the personal experience of non-adherence taught them the benefits of adherence. Negative experiences and informal coercion during the first episode were also commonly reported here (Watts and Priebe 2002). Trusting relationships with those employing pressures and pressures from family and clinicians were perceived as necessary for long-term adherence. The personal experience of benefiting from medication seems to be essential for long-term adherence to it (Tranulis et al. 2011).

In focus groups and individual in-depth interviews with staff, patients, and family members from six institutions in the Netherlands, Widdershoven and Berghmans (2007) reported common emotional reactions to pressures such as frustration, powerlessness, and fear. An individual's perception of coercion varied for different forms of treatment pressures and was often not consistent with common assumptions regarding the coerciveness of interventions. For instance, covert pressures such as manipulation may be perceived as more invasive than overt coercion in the form of making a treatment decision for a patient. It appears that some forms of informal coercion may be perceived as more coercive than legal compulsion. On the basis of these empirical data the authors developed quality standards in the use of treatment pressures (Widdershoven and Berghmans 2007). These were: (1) reflecting and talking about emotions should be an important part of interventions containing coercion and pressures; (2) each coercive intervention should be carefully appraised and justified; (3) 'proximal' coercive treatments such as forced medication are perceived as more coercive but patients' perceptions should be always assessed; (4) development of a strong and collaborative therapeutic relationship and communication is essential for preserving and/or rebuilding of trusting relationship (Widdershoven and Berghmans 2007).

A qualitative study involving 32 patients in South London identified a common fear of losing control related to psychosis (Sweeney et al. 2015). Patients also reported fear of detention and involuntary treatment which would delay them seeking the help they needed, as also identified by Van Dorn et al. (2005) in the USA. Staff were perceived to have the power to deny or grant access to services. The basing of treatment decisions on patients' behaviours led to some patients restricting their comments or showing less emotion (Sweeney et al. 2015).

A subgroup of 29 patients in the ULTIMA study were asked about their experiences and perceptions of pressures during in-depth interviews (Canvin et al. 2013). Patients reported a range of pressures from clinicians, family members, friends, professionals, employers, and the police. Many were unsure about their legal status, in common with other studies (Lidz et al. 1995; Høyer et al. 2002). Canvin et al. (2013) suggested a broad definition of treatment pressures. Pressures were grouped as 'pressures for treatment adherence', and 'other aspects of a patient's mental health and wellbeing' ('stay well'). Both types of pressures could be leveraged and non-leveraged. Leveraged pressures should meet three conditions: conditionality, lever, and direct communication. The absence of any of these conditions would categorize the pressure as 'non-leveraged'. This evidence-based definition of leveraged pressures is broader than the common one for leverage (Monahan et al. 2005; Jaeger and Rossler 2010; Burns et al. 2011) and covers a wide range of otherwise 'non-leveraged' (Neale and Rosenheck 2000; Angell 2006; Szmukler and Appelbaum 2008) pressures (Canvin et al. 2013).

In 25 focus groups of patients, clinicians, family carers, and policy makers in England almost all groups identified common themes about the use of financial incentives (Priebe et al. 2010). All feared possible problems such as the use of money for drugs or alcohol, and proposed the need for clear policies for the intervention and its discontinuation. They also believed financial incentives should be used as a 'last resort'. All were concerned about potential negative impacts on adherent patients, the therapeutic relationship, and on patients' attitudes to medication. Concerns over potential coerciveness and the fairness of financial incentives were common (Priebe et al. 2010).

An ethical analysis of Canvin's interviews gave rise to a 'five steps framework for practitioners' to decide on the ethical justification of pressures (Dunn et al. 2014). The first step distinguishes between threats and offers. The second step considers all the possible consequences of pressures. The third step evaluates the possible exploitation of the patient and distinguishes potential benefits to the clinician or the care system. The fourth step requires reflection on the fairness of the offer and justification of the use of health-care resources. The final step establishes whether the voluntariness of the patient's decision would be violated (Dunn et al. 2014).

Sources of informal coercion

With deinstitutionalization and the development of community mental health care the number of professionals involved in each patient's care has expanded. Patients are in contact with a range of other services to assist them to stay well, to minimize risk, and to promote an integrated and meaningful life. To achieve this, a variety of pressures may be employed.

Little is known about who applies pressures as only a handful of studies have investigated the sources. Most housing leverage was applied by landlords (43%) and clinicians (29%), with less by family (11%). Some (9%) was self-imposed by patients who believed they would lose their accommodation if they were non-adherent (Robbins et al. 2009). The analysis of 'general pressures' from the MacArthur study found the major source was mental health clinicians or other medical staff (49%) (Redlich and

Monahan 2006). However, almost a third was imposed by family members (28%), with just 12% and 5–6% by housing officers and legal and social services, respectively. As with housing leverage (Robbins et al. 2009), 10% of 'general pressure' was self-imposed (Redlich and Monahan 2006). These findings of multiple sources including self-imposed pressures are consistent with Canvin et al.'s (2013) qualitative study.

Some authors consider that having multiple social sources of pressure is beneficial (Van Dorn et al. 2006; Canvin et al. 2013). Those who apply the pressures also provide social support. Negative effects of treatment pressures may be reduced by the benefits of social support. However, more research is clearly needed to understand the prevalence and impact of multiple sources of treatment pressures.

Current understanding of informal coercion

Perhaps the most important finding of this review is that informal coercion is widely used in community mental health care. The most researched form of informal coercion is leverage. The 40-plus quantitative empirical papers included here, however, are derived from a limited number of samples and a small number of countries.

Data on the prevalence of informal coercion are still limited. Only a handful of studies in the USA (Elbogen et al. 2003a; Monahan et al. 2005) and in Europe (Jaeger and Rossler 2010; Burns et al. 2011) reported the prevalence of five forms of leverage. The prevalence of other forms of informal coercion and that in other countries with different social welfare, mental health, and legal systems is unknown. Various forms of leverage are often used together (Elbogen et al. 2003a; Appelbaum and Redlich 2006a; Burns et al. 2011) in an attempt to find which is the most effective.

Evidence on the predictors of reported informal coercion is not strong. A history of previous multiple hospitalizations, lower functioning, substance abuse, and severity of mental illness were common predictors for various forms of informal coercion. While informal coercion is routinely used it is still not known whether it is effective. Informal coercion is not legislated for or regulated by any policy. The legality of its use is not always clear.

The generalizability of current evidence is limited. Results vary between different sites such as hospitals, community mental health teams, catchments areas, states, and countries. With the exception of the MacArthur study, participants have been recruited from only one or two sites or service catchment areas. Study samples and sites were usually not selected randomly and different recruitment strategies were used.

There are a number of additional methodological problems with the studies reported. Retrospective, cross-sectional designs and the use of non-concurrent measures have limited the interpretation of causality of associations, potentially masked real undetected associations, and increased the risk of false associations. Results are mostly based on patient self-report, with no confirmation from clinicians or objective measure of treatment pressures. However, patient self-reports were found to correlate highly with researchers' observations (Lidz et al. 1995) and informal coercion is rarely recorded in medical records. Statistical analyses were often made difficult by skewed and problematic variables and the practice of dichotomization was commonly used at the cost of reduced information.

The terminology in this field remains unclear and inconsistent which makes operationalization of measures and comparisons difficult. Terms such as 'mandated community treatment', 'leverage', and 'informal coercion' have been used interchangeably. Broader definitions (Szmukler and Appelbaum 2008; Canvin et al. 2013) have recently been proposed to cover a continuum of various treatment pressures.

Implications and recommendations

Research into informal coercion should include the whole continuum of treatment pressures rather than just leverage. The development of useable research instruments is necessary to make international comparisons possible. Methodologies need to allow international comparisons despite differences in social welfare, legal, and political systems. Future studies should try to include as many different stakeholders (e.g. clinicians, patients, the general public, family members) as possible to capture and better understand their differing experiences. Because perceived and actual coercion do not always match, subjective and objective sources of data are both essential.

Pressures are applied to achieve clinical and social ends and research is needed to test their effectiveness. Identifying the most effective forms of informal coercion and those who may benefit most would inform clinical practice. Identification of the causal impact of informal coercion seems unlikely at present as the random assignment of different forms of informal coercion is enormously difficult.

It is an accepted aim of mental health services to minimize the use of coercion. Pressure to adhere to treatment comes from multiple sources such as family members and housing officers, but clinicians are a major source (Redlich and Monahan 2006; Robbins et al. 2009). The current evidence of widespread informal coercion in community practices needs to be addressed in the training and education of clinicians and requires attention from policy makers. Research evidence should be included in the development of guidelines and safeguards need to be evolved to ensure that pressures are not applied inappropriately or unlawfully.

The evidence suggests that the negative consequences of coercive pressures can be reduced by clinicians' approach to patients. Transparency, encouraging patients to express their views and take some control, listening to the person's suggestions, and striving for collaborative decision-making all help. Full information about both the benefits and risks of treatment and clear enunciation of rights should serve to minimize negative effects on relationships. Greater clarity when pressures are imposed more for the convenience of clinicians or the system would make treatment fairer, more ethical, and probably less coercive (Sjöström 2006; Dunn et al. 2014).

In applying coercive pressures clinicians should be aware of their patients' past experiences of services as these can affect the experience of coercive pressures (Watts and Priebe 2002). Patients and clinicians clearly do not perceive coercive pressures in the same way (Neale and Rosenheck 2000; Szmukler and Appelbaum 2008; Canvin et al. 2013). Canvin et al. (2013) suggest a model of leveraged and non-leveraged pressures that may help clinicians to define pressure more clearly. Clinicians' training should include more teaching of ethics (Lützén 1998) and the five steps framework for practitioners proposed by Dunn et al. (2014) might be a good start. However, an excessively judgemental attitude needs to be avoided and the potential benefits of informal pressures should be weighed against their negative effects.

There is nothing new or unusual about informal coercion in mental health care. What is new is our recognition of its ubiquity. The evidence base is small but growing now that the issue has entered professional consciousness. The challenge ahead will be to develop a vocabulary for discussion that promotes informed clinical debate alongside the evolution of practices that recognize both the potential benefits and potential harms of treatment pressures. This development requires careful ethical analysis and the construction of meaningful measurement scales to inform the debate with high-quality empirical data.

Acknowledgement

I would like to thank Professor Tom Burns for his invaluable assistance in preparing this chapter.

References

Allen M (2003). Waking Rip van Winkle: why developments in the last 20 years should teach the mental health system not to use housing as a tool of coercion. *Sciences and the Law*, **21**:503–521.

Angell B (2006). Measuring strategies used by mental health providers to encourage medication adherence. *Journal of Behavioral Health Services and Research*, **33**:53–72.

Angell B, Martinez NI, Mahoney CA, et al. (2007). Payeeship, financial leverage, and the client–provider relationship. *Psychiatric Services*, **58**:365–372.

Appelbaum PS, Redlich A (2006a). Use of leverage over patients' money to promote adherence to psychiatric treatment. *Journal of Nervous and Mental Disease*, **194**:294–302.

Appelbaum PS, Redlich A (2006b). Impact of decisional capacity on the use of leverage to encourage treatment adherence. *Community Mental Health Journal*, **42**:121–130.

Beauchamp TL, Childress JF (2001). *Principles of biomedical ethics*. New York: Oxford University Press.

Bonnie RJ, Monahan J (2005). From coercion to contract: reframing the debate on mandated community treatment for people with mental disorders. *Law and Human Behavior*, **29**:485–503.

Burns T (2007). Is it acceptable for people to be paid to adhere to medication? Yes. *British Medical Journal*, **335**:232.

Burns T, Yeeles K, Molodynski A, et al. (2011). Pressures to adhere to treatment ('leverage') in English mental healthcare. *British Journal of Psychiatry*, **199**:145–150.

Burns T, Rugkåsa J, Molodynski A, et al. (2013). Community treatment orders for patients with psychosis (OCTET): a randomised controlled trial. *The Lancet*, **381**:1627–1633.

Burton A, Marougka S, Priebe S (2010). Do financial incentives increase treatment adherence in people with severe mental illness? A systematic review. *Epidemiologia e Psichiatria Sociale*, **19**:233–242.

Busch A, Redlich AD (2007). Patients' perception of possible child custody or visitation loss for nonadherence to psychiatric treatment. *Psychiatric Services*, **58**:999–1002.

Canvin K, Rugkåsa J, Sinclair J, et al. (2013). Leverage and other informal pressures in community psychiatry in England. *International Journal of Law and Psychiatry*, **36**:100–106.

Claassen D (2007). Financial incentives for antipsychotic depot medication: ethical issues. *Journal of Medical Ethics*, 33:189–193.

Claassen D, Fakhoury WK, Ford R, et al. (2007). Money for medication: financial incentives to improve medication adherence in assertive outreach. *Psychiatric Bulletin*, 31:4–7.

Curtis LC, Diamond R (1997). Power and coercion in mental health practice. In: *Treatment Compliance and Therapeutic Alliance* (ed. B. Blackwell), pp. 97–122. Amsterdam, NY: Harwood Academic.

Diamond RJ (1995). Coercion in the community: issues for mature treatment systems. *New Directions for Mental Health Services*, 1995(66):3–18.

Draine J, Solomon P (2001). Threats of incarceration in a psychiatric probation and parole service. *American Journal of Orthopsychiatry*, 71:262–267.

Dunn M, Sinclair JM, Canvin KJ, et al. (2014). The use of leverage in community mental health: Ethical guidance for practitioners. *International Journal of Social Psychiatry*, 60:759–765.

Elbogen EB, Swanson JW, Swartz MS (2003a). Psychiatric disability, the use of financial leverage, and perceived coercion in mental health services. *International Journal of Forensic Mental Health*, 2:119–127.

Elbogen EB, Swanson JW, Swartz MS (2003b). Effects of legal mechanisms on perceived coercion and treatment adherence among persons with severe mental illness. *Journal of Nervous and Mental Disease*, 191:629–637.

Elbogen EB, Soriano C, Van Dorn R, et al. (2005). Consumer views of representative payee use of disability funds to leverage treatment adherence. *Psychiatric Services*, 56:45–49.

Gardner W, Hoge SK, Bennett N, et al. (1993). Two scales for measuring patients perceptions for coercion during mental-hospital admission. *Behavioral Sciences and the Law*, 11:307–321.

Godin P (2000). A dirty business: caring for people who are a nuisance or a danger. *Journal of Advanced Nursing*, 32:1396–1402.

Griffin PA, Steadman HJ, Petrila J (2002). The use of criminal charges and sanctions in mental health courts. *Psychiatric Services*, 53:1285–1289.

Hiday VA, Swartz MS, Swanson J, et al. (1997). Patient perceptions of coercion in mental hospital admission. *International Journal of Law and Psychiatry*, 20:227–241.

Highton-Williamson E, Barnicot K, Kareem T, et al. (2015). Offering financial incentives to increase adherence to antipsychotic medication: the clinician experience. *Journal of Clinical Psychopharmacology*, 35:120–127.

Hoge SK, Lidz CW, Eisenberg M, et al. (1997). Perceptions of coercion in the admission of voluntary and involuntary psychiatric patients. *International Journal of Law and Psychiatry*, 20:167–181.

Høyer G, Kjellin L, Engberg M, et al. (2002). Paternalism and autonomy: a presentation of a Nordic study on the use of coercion in the mental health care system. *International Journal of Law and Psychiatry*, 25:93–108.

Jaeger M, Rossler W (2010). Enhancement of outpatient treatment adherence: patients' perceptions of coercion, fairness and effectiveness. *Psychiatry Research*, 180:48–53.

Johansson H, Eklund M (2003). Patients' opinion on what constitutes good psychiatric care. *Scandinavian Journal of Caring Sciences*, 17:339–346.

Kaltiala-Heino R (1996). Involuntary psychiatric treatment. *Nordic Journal of Psychiatry*, 50:27–34.

Katsakou C, Marougka S, Garabette J, et al. (2011). Why do some voluntary patients feel coerced into hospitalisation? A mixed-methods study. *Psychiatry Research*, 187:275–282.

Lakeman R (2000). Negotiating the ethical minefield of psychiatric nursing practice. *Nursing praxis in New Zealand*, **16**:38–48.

Lamberti JS (2007). Understanding and preventing criminal recidivism among adults with psychotic disorders. *Psychiatric Services*, **58**:773–781.

Lidz CW, Hoge SK, Gardner W, et al. (1995). Perceived coercion in mental hospital admission. Pressures and process. *Archives of General Psychiatry*, **52**:1034–1039.

Lidz CW, Mulvey EP, Hoge SK, et al. (1998). Factual sources of psychiatric patients' perceptions of coercion in the hospital admission process. *American Journal of Psychiatry*, **155**:1254–1260.

Lützén K (1998). Subtle coercion in psychiatric practice. *Journal of Psychiatric and Mental Health Nursing*, **5**:101–107.

McNiel DE, Gormley B, Binder RL (2013). Leverage, the treatment relationship, and treatment participation. *Psychiatric Services*, **64**:431–436.

Marson DC, Savage R, Phillips J (2006). Financial capacity in persons with schizophrenia and serious mental illness: clinical and research ethics aspects. *Schizophrenia Bulletin*, **32**:81–91.

Mason T (2000). Managing protest behaviour: from coercion to compassion. *Journal of Psychiatric and Mental Health Nursing*, **7**:269–275.

Monahan J, Hoge SK, Lidz C, et al. (1995). Coercion and commitment—understanding involuntary mental-hospital admission. *International Journal of Law and Psychiatry*, **18**:249–263.

Monahan J, Bonnie RJ, Appelbaum PS, et al. (2001). Mandated community treatment: beyond outpatient commitment. *Psychiatric Services*, **52**:1198–1205.

Monahan J, Redlich AD, Swanson J, et al. (2005). Use of leverage to improve adherence to psychiatric treatment in the community. *Psychiatric Services*, **56**:37–44.

Neale MS, Rosenheck RA (2000). Therapeutic limit setting in an assertive community treatment program. *Psychiatric Services*, **51**:499–505.

Newton-Howes G, Stanley J (2012). Prevalence of perceived coercion among psychiatric patients: literature review and meta-regression modelling. *The Psychiatrist*, **36**:335–340.

Nicholson J (2005). Use of child custody as leverage to improve treatment adherence. *Psychiatric Services*, **56**:357–8 [author reply 358].

Nicholson J, Sweeney EM, Geller JL (1998). Focus on women: mothers with mental illness: I. The competing demands of parenting and living with mental illness. *Psychiatric Services*, **49**:635–642.

Nicholson J, Biebel K, Katz-Leavy J, et al. (2002). The prevalence of parenthood in adults with mental illness: Implications for state and federal policymakers, programs, and providers. In: *Mental Health, United States, 2002* (ed. RW Manderscheid, MJ Henderson), pp. 120–137. Rockville, MD: Substance Abuse and Mental Health Services Administration.

O'Brien AJ, Golding CG (2003). Coercion in mental healthcare: the principle of least coercive care. *Journal of Psychiatric and Mental Health Nursing*, **10**:167–173.

Priebe S, Sinclair J, Burton A, et al. (2010). Acceptability of offering financial incentives to achieve medication adherence in patients with severe mental illness: a focus group study. *Journal of Medical Ethics*, **36**:463–468.

Priebe S, Yeeles K, Bremner S, et al. (2013). Effectiveness of financial incentives to improve adherence to maintenance treatment with antipsychotics: cluster randomised controlled trial. *British Medical Journal*, **347**:f5847.

Redlich AD, Monahan J (2006). General pressures to adhere to psychiatric treatment in the community. *International Journal of Forensic Mental Health*, **5**:125–131.

Redlich AD, Steadman HJ, Robbins PC, et al. (2006). Use of the criminal justice system to leverage mental health treatment: effects on treatment adherence and satisfaction. *Journal of the American Academy of Psychiatry and the Law*, 34:292–299.

Robbins PC, Petrila J, LeMelle S, et al. (2006). The use of housing as leverage to increase adherence to psychiatric treatment in the community. *Administration and Policy in Mental Health*, 33:226–236.

Robbins PC, Callahan L, Monahan J (2009). Perceived coercion to treatment and housing satisfaction in housing-first and supportive housing programs. *Psychiatric Services*, 60:1251–1253.

Rogers A (1993). Coercion and 'voluntary' admission: an examination of psychiatric patient views. *Behavioral Sciences and the Law*, 11:259–267.

Rugkåsa J, Molodynski A, Yeeles K, et al. (2015). Community treatment orders: clinical and social outcomes, and a subgroup analysis from the OCTET RCT. *Acta Psychiatrica Scandinavica*, 131:321–329.

Sjöström S (2006). Invocation of coercion context in compliance communication—power dynamics in psychiatric care. *International Journal of Law and Psychiatry*, 29:36–47.

Staring ABP, Mulder CL, Priebe S (2010). Financial incentives to improve adherence to medication in five patients with schizophrenia in the Netherlands. *Psychopharmacology Bulletin*, 43:5–10.

Susser E, Roche B (1996). 'Coercion' and leverage in clinical outreach. In: *Coercion and aggressive community treatment: a new frontier in mental health law* (ed. D. Dennis and J. Monahan), pp. 73–84. New York: Plenum Press.

Swanson JW, Van Dorn RA, Monahan J, et al. (2006). Violence and leveraged community treatment for persons with mental disorders. *American Journal of Psychiatry*, 163:1404–1411.

Swartz MS, Swanson JW, Wagner HR, et al. (1999a). Can involuntary outpatient commitment reduce hospital recidivism?: Findings from a randomized trial with severely mentally ill individuals. *American Journal of Psychiatry*, 156:1968–1975.

Swartz MS, Hiday VA, Swanson JW, et al. (1999b). Measuring coercion under involuntary outpatient commitment: Initial finding from a randomized controlled trial. In: *Research in community and mental health* (ed. JP Morrissey, J Monahan), pp. 57–80. Stamford, CT: JAI Press.

Swartz MS, Swanson JW, Hannon MJ (2003a). Does fear of coercion keep people away from mental health treatment? Evidence from a survey of persons with schizophrenia and mental health professionals. *Behavioral Sciences and the Law*, 21:459–472.

Swartz MS, Swanson JW, Wagner HR, et al. (2003b). Assessment of four stakeholder groups' preferences concerning outpatient commitment for persons with schizophrenia. *American Journal of Psychiatry*, 160:1139–1146.

Swartz M, Wagner H, Swanson J, et al. (2004). Consumers' perceptions of the fairness and effectiveness of mandated community treatment and related pressures. *Psychiatric Services*, 55:780–785.

Swartz MS, Swanson JW, Kim M, et al. (2006). Use of outpatient commitment or related civil court treatment orders in five U.S. communities. *Psychiatric Services*, 57:343–349.

Sweeney A, Gillard S, Wykes T, et al. (2015). The role of fear in mental health service users' experiences: a qualitative exploration. *Social Psychiatry and Psychiatric Epidemiology*, 50:1079–1087.

Szmukler G (2009). Financial incentives for patients in the treatment of psychosis. *Journal of Medical Ethics*, 35:224–248.

Szmukler G, Appelbaum P (2008). Treatment pressures, leverage, coercion, and compulsion in mental health care. *Journal of Mental Health*, **17**:233–244.

Tranulis C, Goff D, Henderson DC, et al. (2011). Becoming adherent to antipsychotics: a qualitative study of treatment-experienced schizophrenia patients. *Psychiatric Services*, **62**:888–892.

Van Dorn RA, Swartz M, Elbogen EB, et al. (2005). Perceived fairness and effectiveness of leveraged community treatment among public mental health consumers in five U.S. cities. *International Journal of Forensic Mental Health*, **4**:119–133.

Van Dorn RA, Elbogen EB, Redlich AD, et al. (2006). The relationship between mandated community treatment and perceived barriers to care in persons with severe mental illness. *International Journal of Law and Psychiatry*, **29**:495–506.

Watts J, Priebe S (2002). A phenomenological account of users' experiences of assertive community treatment. *Bioethics*, **16**:439–454.

Widdershoven G, Berghmans R (2007). Coercion and pressure in psychiatry: lessons from Ulysses. *Journal of Medical Ethics*, **33**:560–563.

Wong YLI, Lee S, Solomon PL (2010). Structural leverage in housing programs for people with severe mental illness and its relationship to discontinuance of program participation. *American Journal of Psychiatric Rehabilitation*; **13**:276–294.

Chapter 7

Community coercion in mental health: where to for service-user-led research?

Diana Rose

Introduction

There is a dearth of literature reporting user-led research into community coercion. There is one book, Erick Fabris' *Tranquil prisons*, which as the name suggests sees community coercion as being centred on forced medication (Fabris 2011). Writing in Ontario, Canada, Fabris has been coerced himself and has also worked as an advocate. Apart from this, I have had some personal communication with two groups of user/ researchers investigating community coercion from the service user's perspective. One study in London, UK is in its early stages (Evans, pers comm. December 2014) and one in Norway is nearing completion (Loftus, pers comm. March 2015). Finally, Light and colleagues included peer interviewers in their study of service users' experiences of compulsion in Australasia (Light et al. 2014) as did Ridley and colleagues in Scotland (Ridley and Hunter 2013). However, neither of these two investigations distinguished between hospital and community coercion. Since, as far as I can ascertain, the service-user research literature amounts to these five studies, two of which are not even published, I will spend some time sketching what a service-user-led research programme on community coercion might look like. This chapter will not discuss the Convention for the Rights of Persons with Disabilities (CRPD). Whilst highly relevant, it is discussed elsewhere in this volume and, in any case, most of the research and other literature that exists tends towards legalism and abstraction in a way that is not particularly helpful for service users. (This is not to undermine the lively internet and other media presence of service users regarding the CRPD.) Finally, I will also consider a *non*-user-led piece of research that attempted to elicit consumers' views on community coercion to argue that it failed to capture what is important to service users.

Medication

Across the globe, the major ingredient of what is 'compelled' in community coercion is medication. This is uncontroversial for most mental health professionals, whose main worry is about 'adherence' or compliance. Fabris (2011) takes the polar opposite view in seeing medication as more or less poisonous. But let's start with his empirical research.

In Ontario, service users have to 'agree' to being on a community treatment order (CTO) unless they lack capacity, in which case a substitute decision maker (SDM) can be appointed; this can be a relative or the state. Fabris comments that 'agreeing' to be 'compelled' is a contradiction. He decided not to interview people in receipt of CTOs because, despite the fact that he had himself been a service user and coerced, his status as a white, middle-class able-bodied male would introduce a power imbalance into the encounter. He therefore conducted a focus group and individual interviews with a total of ten mental health professionals and collected and analysed his material using institutional ethnography. Following Smith (2005) he adopted the standpoint of con-sumer; thus his own status entered his research in this way. Most of Fabris' participants had been service users and were now working in roles such as peer support workers or advocates. So, whilst not interviewing current service users on CTOs this standpoint was doubly present, and I think this qualifies it to be called user-led research.

Fabris' informants told him that their main task in relation to their service users was to ensure that they took their medication. In many cases this was a daily task that was often resisted. Many of the mental health workers often saw this resistance as entirely reasonable because they witnessed the side effects of neuroleptic medication and could see why their clients found it intolerable. However, they were constrained by law to ensure 'compliance' and this often meant removal to a hospital for forced medica-tion. The participants expressed frustration that the CTO meant they had to focus on medication to the exclusion of other forms of support (but see later). There were also accounts of what this meant for specific groups such as immigrants who could not fulfil their wish to leave Canada because they were committed or women who were forced to live in an abusive relationship.

Fabris' title *Tranquil prisons*, however, leads him to another form of argument about medication altogether, and it is a conceptual one. He argues that neuroleptics, through their effects on different brain structures and pathways, have replaced the walls and restraints of the asylums. Neuroleptics are a neurochemical restraint directly com-parable to physical ones. In addition, they render the recipient docile and compliant and not likely to resist, so that issues such as rights and freedom are of no concern. However, there would appear to be some contradiction here between the resistance to medication described in the empirical research and this argument concerning how neuroleptics render resistance impossible.

To return to the research, interviewees also said that where CTOs did seem accept-able to recipients it may not be the CTO that is key but the access to better services. In Ontario a CTO involves a treatment plan (not always in evidence), so this may give the service user access to, for example, housing and welfare benefits that are not otherwise available. So the key ingredient is not coercion as such but better services. Linked to this, there appear to be inequalities in the Ontario system in access to CTOs with, perhaps surprisingly, middle-class people more likely to be under an order. One possibility is the lobbying activities of relatives' organizations, which are dominated by the middle-class parents of adult children who could use CTOs to 'play the system' and secure a range of services for their relatives.

Fabris' book is avowedly anti-psychiatry and he is aware that his empirical results are not generalizable. However, the book brings together a wide range of literature as well as the interview findings and he is explicit about his standpoint, which is more than can be said about some mainstream research that claims to be value-free and objective. We now turn to some of this.

Consumer satisfaction with compulsory community treatment

There have been many studies of patient experiences with mandated community treatment across the world. Those up to 2007 are summarized by Churchill (2007). In the run-up to the 2007 amendments to the 1983 Mental Health Act for England and Wales, there were studies of patients who the researchers thought were candidates for CTOs (Canvin et al. 2002; Gault 2009). However, none of these were user-led studies and so strictly lie outside the scope of this chapter. What I will do is consider one study, carried out in New Zealand, which considered patients' experiences with CTOs. The work was conducted by Anita Gibbs and colleagues (Gibbs et al. 2005) and two further sub-studies have been published (Gibbs et al. 2004; Gibbs 2010). The work of Gibbs and colleagues was qualitative but with a scale of satisfaction at the end. They paint a rosy picture of satisfaction with CTOs: 'The majority of patients viewed the order as a helpful step towards community stability' (Gibbs et al. 2005, p. 357). However, I would argue that this 'majority' represents a skewed sample. The criteria for the study were those who had been under a CTO, without readmission to hospital, for more than 6 months in the previous 2 years. Half the sample who met these criteria did not participate. Of the 103 eligible patients, 19 were considered (by their psychiatrist) to lack capacity to participate at the outset and were excluded. Of the remaining 84 who were approached, 42 agreed to take part and completed the study, 34 declined to participate, and in 8 cases the research process was unfinished because the patient withdrew, relapsed, or there was a breakdown in communication. In addition, of the 42 service users who completed the research 20 had been discharged from the CTO by the time of the interview, while only 22 remained on it at interview. Finally there is a point about methodology. Although this was purportedly a qualitative study, much of the interpretation represented analysis of a scaled question: 'Overall, do you think the advantages of being on the community treatment order outweigh the disadvantages?'

Now, Gibbs and colleagues removed the 19 patients deemed to lack capacity from their denominator, allowing them to say they had a response rate of 50% rather than 40%. But 'lacking capacity' is more likely to align with disagreeing with one's treatment and treating team and so having negative views. Secondly, there is every reason to suppose that those who declined also had more negative views. Thirdly, nearly half of those interviewed had been discharged from their CTOs so their views may have been coloured by their current freedom. Finally, the reporting of percentages for the final question hardly captures the nuances of views that qualitative research aims to do. That is not to say that some participants were not positive about their legal status. The authors talk about 'voluntary compulsion' just as Fabris did in relation to Ontario's law. There is no doubt that some see it as a safety net. However, this does beg the question of what the key ingredient is here. Is it the formal status or is it access to better support?

Now these objections are basically methodological, and it is true that they apply to all small-scale qualitative research like this. To begin to think about a more substantially user-led programme of research into community coercion we need to go beyond questions of participant characteristics. However, before this it is worth saying a word about the lead author of the Otago studies. Anita Gibbs is a social worker, and in 2001 she wrote a methodological and epistemological position paper on social work research (Gibbs 2001). Here she called for action research and the involvement of service users in social work research, making liberal reference to emerging service-user-led research in social work such as that of Peter Beresford (Beresford and Evans 1999). This work was early in mental health research outside the social work arena. One wonders then about the status of this work in the Otago study, which is not only standard qualitative research but rather poor at that. Interestingly, in her sub-study of women (Gibbs 2010), she is both more flexible about the meanings behind what the women might be saying and concerned about possible skewness of the sample (there were only ten women).

The final study that can be mentioned is the one in Norway, which I have discussed with the service-user researchers there (Loftus, pers comm. March 2015). This is a study of service-user satisfaction with assertive community treatment. Some of the participants were on CTOs and some were not, and the former were more satisfied than the latter. This at first sight seems counter-intuitive from a service-user perspective but it is quite clear that those on CTOs were satisfied because they were in receipt of support that better aligned with their wishes. So once again, the argument must be that the key ingredient is not coercion itself but the services that accompany it. To say it is coercion that is the important thing is obfuscation. Indeed, this leads to the even stronger conclusion that if mental health services were more aligned with the wishes of service users then the need for coercion would greatly reduce. This alignment would include less use of toxic medications.

This is, as far as I can determine, the state of the art in user-led research into community coercion which was the remit for this chapter. So I will spend the second half of this chapter thinking about what a user-led research programme might look like.

A user-led programme for research into community compulsion

Peer interviewers

As already stated, there are two recent studies that employed peer interviewers (Ridley and Hunter 2013; Light et al. 2014). However, in both cases these peers were always accompanied by a professional interviewer and no distinction was drawn between service users detained in hospital and those under forms of community compulsion (or it is difficult to ascertain which form of compulsion applied). For some time now it has been known that peer interviewers gather different information from conventional interviewers (Clark et al. 1999), although the exact contexts are unclear (Gillard et al. 2010a; Rose et al. 2011b). However, there is now consensus, at least amongst service-user researchers, that a user-led programme of research must go beyond having peer interviewers, important though that might be. It must involve or be led by service-user researchers and collaborators from start to finish.

Conceptualizing the research—what is known?

Let us first of all consider what we know about service users' attitudes to coercion—which is not very much because the extant literature takes the perspective of conventional researchers and clinicians and, I would argue, falls at the first hurdle on the question of medication. Most conventional researchers see 'adherence' or compliance as the goal of treatment and as a reason to coerce when this fails. In the literature I have been considering, side effects are seen as just that—secondary. This is not the view of service users, who see side effects as paramount (Crawford et al. 2011; Rose et al. 2014). In addition, most patients under CTOs will be administered depot injections (Patel et al. 2011). Whilst there are service users who prefer depots because they do not have to remember to take oral medication, depots also tend to have a more noxious side-effect profile than oral medication. So when service users express fear of coercion, it is this above all that they are afraid of and indeed it can make them stay away from services. One does not need to be a service user to demonstrate this (Swartz et al. 2003). This is not an argument against medication *tout court* but it is an argument against professionals and conventional researchers who regard adherence as not only unproblematic but the ultimate goal of treatment, coerced if necessary. I am not going as far as Fabris (2011), although I think his book is a welcome antidote.

So let us consider this user-led programme of research in rather a conventional way: management and control; research question; collecting information; analysis and making sense; dissemination.

Management and control

Most service-user researchers do not have financial or administrative control of their projects, although Shaping Our Lives, in the context of social policy, tries to do this (http://www.shapingourlives.org.uk/). Within these constraints, we can have an advisory group and we can employ service-user researchers. The advisory group for this project should have a majority of people who have experienced coercion and a good proportion who have or are experiencing community coercion. A group size of six to eight keeps things manageable. They also need to understand research. It has been argued that the more 'lay' people become 'experts', the less they are valuable as contributors to the research process, and equally the more 'lay' they remain the less they can understand. This has been called the PPI paradox (Ives et al. 2013). Staley (2013) has critiqued this position, drawing mainly on the importance of trained user interviewers in some qualitative research. I would go further and argue that service users involved in research, including on advisory groups, should have research training and strive for a 'double identity', bringing their experience of distress, services, and treatments to bear in advising on and conducting the research (Rose 2014). It is not inconceivable that members of the advisory group adopt other roles as the research proceeds, such as engagement in data interpretation.

The majority of the staff in the project, if not all of them, should be mental health service users and this should be the case for those in supervisory roles too. This is not a pipedream. There is now a robust cadre of mental health service-user researchers, at least in the UK, many of whom have experienced coercion. If a model more crafted to co-production is preferred, this is possible too but the voice of the service user must be paramount (Gillard et al. 2010b).

The research question

The research must be exploratory because little is known from the perspective of the service user. I do not rule out the possibility that we will find what has already been determined by conventional research but counsel keeping an open mind. Exploratory research is usually qualitative research, although it may result subsequently in quantitative measures. I would argue that even the best scales, such as those from the McArthur Foundation (Lidz et al. 1995), are unable fully to capture the experience of coercion. So the research question should be something like: what are service users' experiences of community coercion today: an exploratory study? It should be as general as that so that nothing is ruled out. Such vagueness may trouble those who are used to hypothesis testing but it is usual in more qualitative investigations. For the moment, we must start small, so this project will be confined to one jurisdiction. I won't say which.

Participants

Participants will be in two groups: those currently under a CTO and those discharged in the previous 2 years. It is important to capture the experience of community coercion *in vivo* as well the participants' judgements in hindsight. The study will be advertised at venues that service users choose to frequent, and members of the study team will be available to give more information to anyone interested. This is obviously time-intensive, but it avoids engaging clinicians who might be suspicious of a user-led study and so skew its presentation to service users. The study will also be advertised on social media sites known to the study team (Ennis et al. 2011).

Data collection

First, we must determine a topic guide which could be used both for one-to-one interviews and focus groups. The advisory group has a role here in ensuring everything relevant to community coercion is covered. However, the topic guide must be as open-ended as possible in line with the research question. Potential participants will be given information and consent sheets which will be written in consultation with the advisory group, as often these are very opaque (Rose et al. 2015). Participants will be given a choice of an individual interview or a focus group discussion. For individual interviews, there will be a choice of venue and time; focus groups will be held in community locations. Individual interviewees will be offered breaks and there will be a break for refreshments in the focus groups. Participants will be reimbursed for their time.

The interviewers in the one-to-one interviews will have experienced coercion and there will be two facilitators for the focus groups, one of whom will have experienced coercion and the other who will also be a mental health service-user researcher. We have successfully used this model before in looking at inpatient care (Evans et al. 2012). Although anecdotal, our participants appreciated us sharing our experiences. The aim is to reduce the power differential in the research process (Cornwall and Jewkes 1995), although it has been argued that this is difficult to achieve (Mason and Boutilier 1996). At the same time, comparisons between service-user and clinical interviewers in the context of compulsion have shown that they differ in how they inflect a topic guide in the context of qualitative research (Gillard et al. 2010a). This seems to be less the case with structured, quantitative instruments (Rose et al. 2011b), although surveys can also show a marked difference (Rose et al. 2003).

What do we do with this information?

Many approaches can be used to interpret such data. Some sort of systematic analysis is of course required and the most common way to do this today is through computer software such as NVivo (2010), although other techniques are also available. However, what interests us here is to conduct our interpretations explicitly from the perspective of service users. In case this sounds like 'bias', let it be said that the 'double identity' that researchers who are also service users bring can be argued to result in knowledge that is *more* objective because it combines and synthesizes two sorts of knowledge— experiential and scientific. This has been argued to be the case for feminist studies and research carried out by other marginalized groups, though not yet for mental health service-user researchers (Harding, 1991, Harding, 2004).

I am going to suggest two ways of analysing our data in this community coercion study that follow a model we have used in our team (the Service User Research Enterprise) when researching inpatient detention and compulsion—but this is not the only way of going about things. Steve Gillard and his team have constructed a model of 'co-production' where service users, clinicians, and academics work together to produce knowledge that is more than the sum of its parts. This also enables them to compare the interviews and interpretations of the different groups and show that service-user researchers do indeed bring something special. The first domain to which they applied the co-production model was detention and compulsion in hospital. In both interviews and interpretation the service-user researchers focused more on the emotional aspects of detention and compulsion for service users, whereas psychologists, for example, focused on behaviour and administration (Gillard et al. 2010a,b).

The research proposed here is somewhat different and, as stated earlier, follows on from a project on patients' perspectives on inpatient care, including compulsory inpatient care. This used focus groups, which would be one option for participants in this community coercion study. However, individual interview data are equally applicable, although they lack the collective validation of experience that focus groups can provide. Basically the data are used for two purposes: first, to produce an outcome measure from the perspective of the service user, and second, to conduct an in-depth analysis which will aim to uncover in detail what community coercion means to service users. Returning to earlier parts of this chapter we envisage forced medication to feature strongly and perhaps increased support to be seen as an advantage. A user-led project that has just begun in England has nascent findings in this direction (Evans, pers. comm. December 2014), but our aim here is to be as exploratory as possible as I have said.

Creating a measure and conducting a survey

To create a measure, the focus group data are first of all turned into a draft measure of perceptions of community coercion. This involves mixed methods with Likert scales and open-ended text boxes. This would be done with the assistance of the advisory group. The draft measure is then taken to expert panels of people who have experienced community coercion—one drawn from the focus groups to make sure it captures their views and a new panel to take a fresh look and especially to comment on language and layout. There is then a feasibility phase with the aim of making sure the measure is as easy to complete as possible and with some questions about length, difficulty, and whether any items are distressing. Following this, psychometric testing is undertaken with a special emphasis on test–retest reliability and face and criterion validity. The general model is described by Rose et al. (2011a) and its application to inpatient care including detention and compulsion by Evans et al. (2012).

The final questionnaire is then ready to use as either a self-completed instrument or one that can be completed with an interviewer. We would try to find as many people as possible on CTOs and this would mean a multi-site endeavour. It would be an expensive undertaking, but it would also be possible to make it available on the internet. Although this is an anecdotal view, many people with serious mental health problems seem more comfortable communicating this way, especially in this era of service cutbacks and closure of day centres. The acceptability of electronic communication to people with a diagnosis of psychosis has been investigated by Ennis et al. (2011, 2012).

The immediate response of conventional researchers to this will be that the whole process involves biased and self-selecting samples. This is true. But even the two randomized controlled trials in this area failed in this regard (Churchill 2007). If our method of recruitment and collecting information biases the sample towards those who have more negative views, then perhaps this should be seen as a balance to the skewness introduced by conventional methods. By trying to conduct our study from the explicit perspective of service users, we may shed a different and more balanced light on the experience of community coercion. Of course, we may find exactly what conventional researchers have found, which is a very mixed and muddy picture. But it is incumbent on us to make the effort.

Detailed analysis

The second thing we can do with the information we have collected is an in-depth analysis of the focus group and interview data to capture what may be the complexities and nuances of views of participants as expressed in groups and individual interviews. In our inpatient study we also had the views of nurses and contrasted and compared the two groups (Rose et al. 2015). Here we will only be concerned with service users, partly because this is the main focus but also because community coercion involves a far greater array of staff than does hospital provision.

We will once again engage the assistance of the advisory group in interpreting the focus groups and interviews. It should be pointed out that all qualitative analysis involves interpretation, but that does not mean it is 'subjective'. It should be transparent and reproducible by others, and one way of ensuring this is through reflexivity where analysts constantly interrogate their own interpretive activity (Schwandt et al. 2007).

This should provide us with a picture of how service users experience community coercion that will probably be complex and dense. It comes from the perspective of service users and service-user researchers who are at least explicit about their standpoint. Conventional researchers often are not, believing that what they do is unproblematically objective. But all research has methodological and epistemological underpinnings—we are just more explicit, and are thus also more open to critique. This standpoint and the research that flows from it—sketched here—may or may not produce findings that are radically different from what already exists. But that is what research is for.

Dissemination

The first group of people who need to know the findings of this research are our participants. They have given their time and their stories and we have a moral obligation to tell them what we have done with what they gave us. We will produce an appropriately written report, again in association with our advisory group, and disseminate it widely in both print and electronic form. We will make available the opportunity for meetings for more detailed discussion of the work should anyone want this.

We will disseminate our findings to staff. If we find that service users are unhappy with community coercion, or aspects of it, we will perhaps have to have some difficult conversations. However, I would argue that the research programme sketched above is sufficiently rigorous to count as evidence which, although hard to hear, cannot be ignored.

Finally, this work would join the burgeoning academic literature on community coercion. What place it would find (should anyone be prepared to publish it in the peer-reviewed literature) will depend, I am sure, on the results. It may court controversy if we find that the existing literature does not capture what it is like to be coerced in mental health services. I can anticipate this both from experience and from the position of a researcher. But I may be wrong. It is ultimately service users who will tell us and the research exists to give them voice.

Conclusion

This chapter has moved from a radical alternative to mainstream research (Fabris 2011), through a critique of some conventional qualitative research, a consideration of what is the key ingredient in community coercion, to a proposal for a programme of user-led research. We have seen that there are different perspectives—particularly on forced medication which is a mainstay of community coercion and unquestioned by most mental health professionals—but it is an open question just how far the results of user-led research would depart from what has already been found. What has been found is mixed and the status of user-led research is itself not settled. User-led research in this key area could clarify both uncertainties.

References

Beresford P, Evans C (1999). Research note: research and empowerment. *British Journal of Social Work*, **29**:671–677.

Canvin K, Bartlett A, Pinfold V (2002). A 'bittersweet pill to swallow': learning from mental health service users' responses to compulsory community care in England. *Health and Social Care in the Community*, **10**:361–369.

Churchill R (2007). *International experiences of using community treatment orders.* London: Institute of Psychiatry, Kings College London.

Clark CC, Scott EA, Boydell KM, et al. (1999). Effects of client interviewers on client-reported satisfaction with mental health services. *Psychiatric Services*, **50**:961–963.

Cornwall A, Jewkes R (1995). What is participatory research? *Social Science and Medicine*, **41**:1667–1676.

Crawford MJ, Robotham D, Thana L, et al. (2011). Selecting outcome measures in mental health: the views of service users. *Journal of Mental Health*, **20**:336–346.

Ennis L, Rose D, Callard F, et al. (2011). Rapid progress or lengthy process? Electronic personal health records in mental health. *BMC Psychiatry,* **11**:117.

Ennis L, Rose D, Denis M, et al. (2012). Can't surf, won't surf: the digital divide in mental health. *Journal of Mental Health*, **21**:395–403.

Evans J, Rose D, Flach C, et al. (2012). VOICE: developing a new measure of service users' perceptions of inpatient care, using a participatory methodology. *Journal of Mental Health*, **21**:57–71.

Fabris E (2011). *Tranquil prisons: chemical incarceration under community treatment orders.* Toronto, ON: University of Toronto Press.

Gault I (2009). Service-user and carer perspectives on compliance and compulsory treatment in community mental health services. *Health and Social Care in the Community*, **17**:504–513.

Gibbs A (2001). The changing nature and context of social work research. *British Journal of Social Work*, **31**:687–704.

Gibbs A (2010). Coping with compulsion: women's views of being on a community treatment order. *Australian Social Work*, **63**:223–233.

Gibbs A, Dawson J, Forsyth H, et al. (2004). Maori experience of community treatment orders in Otago, New Zealand. *Australian and New Zealand Journal of Psychiatry*, **38**:830–835.

Gibbs A, Dawson J, Ansley C, et al. (2005). How patients in New Zealand view community treatment orders. *Journal of Mental Health*, **14**:357–368.

Gillard S, Borschmann R, Turner K, et al. (2010a). 'What difference does it make'? Finding evidence of the impact of mental health service user researchers on research into the experiences of detained psychiatric patients. *Health Expectations*, **13**:185–194.

Gillard S, Turner K, Lovell K, et al. (2010b). 'Staying native': coproduction in mental health services research. *International Journal of Public Sector Management*, **23**:567–577.

Harding S (1991). 'Strong objectivity' and socially situated knowledge. In: *Whose science? Whose knowledge?*, pp. 138–163. New York: Cornell University Press.

Harding SG (2004). *The feminist standpoint theory reader: intellectual and political controversies.* New York: Routledge.

Ives J, Damery S, Redwod S (2013). PPI, paradoxes and Plato: who's sailing the ship? *Journal of Medical Ethics*, **39**:181–185.

Lidz CW, Hoge SK, Gardner W, et al. (1995). Perceived coercion in mental hospital admission: pressures and process. *Archives of General Psychiatry*, **52**:1034–1039.

Light EM, Robertson MD, Boyce P, et al. (2014). The lived experience of involuntary community treatment: a qualitative study of mental health consumers and carers. *Australasian Psychiatry*, **22**:345–351.

Mason R, Boutilier M (1996). The challenge of genuine power sharing in participatory research: the gap between theory and practice. *Canadian Journal of Community Mental Health*, **15**:145–152.

NVivo (2010). *NVivo qualitative data analysis software*, version 9. Melbourne: QSR International Pty Ltd.

Patel MX, Matonhodze J, Baig MK, et al. (2011). Increased use of antipsychotic long-acting injections with community treatment orders. *Therapeutic Advances in Psychopharmacology*, **1**:37–45.

Ridley J, Hunter S (2013). Subjective experiences of compulsory treatment from a qualitative study of early implementation of the Mental Health (Care & Treatment) (Scotland) Act 2003. *Health and Social Care in the Community*, **21**:509–518.

Rose D (2014). Patient and public involvement in health research: ethical imperative and/or radical challenge? *Journal of Health Psychology*, **19**:149–158.

Rose D, Fleischmann P, Wykes T, et al. (2003). Patients' perspectives on electroconvulsive therapy: systematic review. *British Medical Journal*, **326**:1363.

Rose D, Evans J, Sweeney A, et al. (2011a). A model for developing outcome measures from the perspectives of mental health service users. *International Review of Psychiatry*, **23**:41–46.

Rose D, Leese M, Oliver D, et al. (2011b). A comparison of participant information elicited by service user and non-service user researchers. *Psychiatric Services*, **62**:210–213.

Rose D, Walke J, Beddoes D et al. (2014). Stratified medicine in psychiatry: what service users, carers and the public think. *Mental Health Today*, May–June:24–27.

Rose D, Evans J, Laker C et al. (2015). Life in acute mental health settings: experiences and perceptions of service users and nurses. *Epidemiology and Psychiatric Sciences*, **24**:90–96.

Schwandt TA, Lincoln YS, Guba EG (2007). Judging interpretations: but is it rigorous? trustworthiness and authenticity in naturalistic evaluation. *New Directions for Evaluation*, 2007(114):11–25.

Smith DE (2005). *Institutional ethnography: a sociology for people.* Lanham, MD: AltaMira Press.

Staley K (2013). There is no paradox with PPI in research. *Journal of Medical Ethics*, **39**:186–187.

Swartz MS, Swanson JW, Hannon MJ (2003). Does fear of coercion keep people away from mental health treatment? Evidence from a survey of persons with schizophrenia and mental health professionals. *Behavioral Sciences and the Law*, **21**:459–472.

Part 3

The experience

Chapter 8

Coercion contexts—how compliance is achieved in interaction

Stefan Sjöström

Introduction

Until the last 50 years or so, psychiatric patients mostly interacted with clinical staff within closed institutions permeated with a paternalistic culture. The transition from hospital-based to community care marked a radical shift in treatment ideologies and the general approach to service users with mental illness. In the community we expect services to have values of participation and respect for autonomy. Staff whom patients meet in the community often have different knowledge and value systems from those primarily trained to function within institutions. Community staff may find the idea of coercing service users into complying with a treatment regime quite troubling. Accordingly, when community treatment orders (CTOs) were to be introduced in Sweden in 2008, representatives of municipal social services expressed concern that their staff would have to start using coercion.

Relatively little is known about the everyday enactment of coercion in community settings. Emerging research suggests that problematic features observed in inpatient settings occur here as well: patients are not always aware of their formal status and may be subject to various kinds of informal coercion (Lambert et al. 2009; Newton-Howes and Mullen 2011; Sjöström 2012; Canvin et al. 2013). A particularly salient phenomenon is how different kinds of 'leverages' (Monahan et al. 2005) or 'influencing behaviors' (Rugkåsa et al. 2014) are brought into play to make patients under a CTO comply with things they would not otherwise have chosen (Szmukler and Appelbaum 2008). This chapter will draw upon my experience gained from a number of studies regarding coercion within Swedish mental health care over the past 20 years, both in hospital and community settings (Sjöström 1997, 2000, 2012; Zetterberg et al. 2014). The Swedish arrangements for community compulsion are similar to those in the USA, Australia, New Zealand, England and Wales, as well as other European countries such as Norway and Finland. For the purpose of discussing the practice of coercion in community settings, they are thus likely to be transferable.

This chapter proposes a theoretical understanding of the micro-level interaction by which community coercion is enacted. A crucial element in analysing human interaction is the context in which it takes place. I will argue that it is meaningful to think about how staff exercise coercion in terms of how they invoke a certain kind of *coercion context* when interacting with people under compulsion in the community.

Coercion context and compliance

The idea of a coercion context was inspired by Glaser and Strauss' 1965 book *Awareness of dying*. Glaser and Strauss undertook clinical observations at a cancer clinic, focusing on how issues regarding the expected death of patients were dealt with. One particular aspect concerned patients' understanding of the uncertainties regarding their chances of survival. Glaser and Strauss coined the concept of an 'awareness context' to capture what participants can know about their circumstances. For their specific purposes, they developed more substantive notions concerning one type of situation—patients at the cancer clinic and their awareness of dying. Analysing interactions between clinical staff and patients, they described four different awareness contexts: closed, suspected, mutual pretence, and open. Closed awareness means that the patient does not know about the terminal diagnosis and suspected awareness means that she or he suspects and tries to verify the truth of the condition. Mutual pretence means that though the patient has knowledge about the diagnosis this is not openly acknowledged in interactions with staff. Open awareness means that everyone including the patient is aware of the diagnosis and can discuss it in an open and honest manner. In their clinical interactions, staff both adapted to and were co-creators of the awareness context surrounding each patient.

Awareness contexts may become quite elaborate in circumstances when they serve an important social function or when there is a certain interactional problem. In the case of the cancer clinic, awareness contexts formed because of the cultural and existential sensitivity of facing death. In analogy to the awareness contexts of dying, I maintain that specific coercion contexts evolve in relation to psychiatric patients under compulsory care. Compulsory care is similarly sensitive in the way it transgresses fundamental values about human rights, autonomy, and expectations that medical staff will respect the patient's stated wishes about treatment. The most significant aspect of awareness of coercion is perhaps that of compliance. After all, compulsory care is fundamentally designed to impose people to accept or do things they oppose or wouldn't otherwise do. Given the sensitivity of forcing adults in our society, there is a need to mitigate coercive acts and—to make them appear acceptable to the unwilling subject—a somewhat paradoxical but nevertheless reasonable approach from the perspective of those who are assigned the difficult task of exercising coercion.

Coercion contexts in hospital settings

In an ethnographic fieldwork extending over 18 months, I followed how hospital staff exerted coercion (Sjöström 1997). The otherwise exceptional social activities of forcing people to comply with strict rules and arduous treatments, to perform body searches, and to restrain and administer injections by physical force tended to become routine matters that occurred on an everyday basis. That is also why there are professional codes of ethics and mechanisms to promote reflection and to help workers cope with the stress and dilemmas involved in such work. For a stranger to the closed psychiatric ward, it is striking how difficult it is to understand which patients are under compulsory care and what actions constitute coercion. One reason for this is the physical layout of the hospital ward, how it is designed to facilitate the monitoring and management of patients, such as locked doors, windows in the doors of patients' rooms, and ready-made beds for restraining patients. In this light, the recurring finding that patients are uncertain about their legal status is not surprising (Lidz et al. 1995; Cascardi and Poythress 1997; Hoge et al. 1997; McKenna et al. 1999; O'Donoghue et al. 2014). Substantial numbers of patients who are not under compulsory legislation in fact believe that they are. Incidentally, the opposite also occurs, with a significant proportion of legally involuntary patients being unaware of their status and rights. In other words, a closed awareness context often seems to be present (Sjöström 2006). But there are other aspects of coercion contexts, such as how the law is written. For example, most mental health legislation allows for voluntary patients to be converted to involuntary status provided that certain legal criteria are met. To the extent that patients are aware of this, they may rightly feel coerced when they comply with treatment recommendations knowing that they otherwise might have their legal status altered. Another aspect of the awareness context of coercion is what kind of powers the law provides to the clinic. Some measures are typically specified in the legislation (e.g. medication, restraint, and containment), but there is considerable leeway for clinicians to specify the actual content of the compulsory regime.

Given how difficult it can be for a patient to understand the legal context, one would expect that the most important factor in patients' perceptions of coercion is what they learn from staff. But this goes far beyond the mandatory information that patients should receive when they are admitted. It is also about what staff convey when a patient sees them interacting with other patients. A patient will draw her own conclusions when she sees a fellow patient being injected under restraint. This may in turn affect her own compliance in accepting the medication recommended to her. The coercion context is also created in mundane interactions that do not immediately relate to coercion. In such events the immediate problem for staff is quite often to manage various situations to maintain order and keep daily activities running efficiently in the ward. For example, staff may allude to a patient's involuntary status when they want her to tend to her personal hygiene (Sjöström 2006).

Drawing from observations of the everyday interactions on psychiatric hospital wards, I would argue that there is a strong strategic element to how hospital staff communicate coercion contexts to patients. Providing patients with sufficient information about the law is not their main priority. Instead they try to solve different kinds of everyday problems in achieving compliance from patients with the strategic invocation of coercion contexts. For example, if a voluntary patient asks a staff member to let her out, the staff member is legally required to simply open the door. However, the staff I followed had developed elaborate 'stalling' techniques to make an unwilling voluntary patient stay at the clinic. The patient may be told to wait until a staff member has completed other chores, or to talk to a nurse and then a doctor before leaving. In doing so, staff members act *as if* the patient does not have the right to leave the premises at her will. Thus, they create an impression—a coercion context—that typically has the effect that the patient will remain at the hospital unless she displays considerable effort in pursuing her wish. If this were taken to its extreme, staff may even break the law by denting fundamental freedoms. Interestingly, even in these cases, they would invoke a coercion context, but in a manner that makes their acts appear legally correct.

Changing conditions for the forming of coercion contexts

What happens to the coercion context when compulsory powers are available in community settings? If coercion is seen as more problematic in the community, how will this affect the creation of coercion contexts? Will they be more open or more closed? Community settings probably allow a wider variety of possible coercive interventions, posing more complex ethical problems (Sjöström et al. 2011; Riley et al. 2014). This will presumably make coercion contexts more complex and multi-faceted than those in closed hospital settings. The day to day social life of the patient becomes more relevant and may be affected on many different levels. Legal compulsion becomes entangled with pressures from the surrounding environment, from family, neighbours, and landlords, to create new types of coercion contexts. Coercion contexts will also be affected by the complexity arising from multiple service providers sharing legal powers. Table 8.1 describes potential differences in the conditions for how coercion contexts develop in hospital versus community settings.

At least some degree of paternalism is inherent in the cultures of hospital and community care alike, although it may have different origins. Hospital wards have a long history of coercion and medical paternalism, whereas the source of paternalism towards people with mental illness in the community stems more from prejudice and stigma in wider society. One consequence of this may be that paternalism in community settings finds other outlets and forms of expression than within institutions. One important difference is the degree to which coercion becomes familiar to staff. Hospital staff face situations where compulsion is involved on an almost daily basis. This makes them more experienced and enables them to develop specific skills in managing the ethical complexities of coercion. It is also more likely that knowledge about coercive practices and legislation is included in their training. However, the daily occurrence of such situations normalizes coercion and can desensitize hospital staff to practices that would be seen as unacceptable in most other settings. The rarity

Table 8.1 Differences in conditions for coercion in hospital versus community settings

Hospital setting	Community setting
Paternalism by psychiatric tradition	Paternalism by cultural stigma
Coercion is commonplace for staff	Coercion is exceptional for staff
Closed, structured setting	Open, limitless setting
Narrow, specialized group of staff	Various staff from different backgrounds
Short-term perspective	Long-term perspective
The patient in her illness	The patient in her ordinary life situation

of coercion in community settings, on the other hand, may make community staff less inclined to invoke formal coercion contexts. The everyday life of inpatients is highly structured compared with community life. This is manifested in terms of space (the limited, structured location where treatment takes place) and time (the strict organization of the day in meal times, the administration of medication, visiting hours, etc.). Life for patients in the community presents much more possibility for variation. Services offered tend to be less structured, and patients have more freedom to engage in a wider range of activities within or outside of what is on offer from service providers. This more multi-faceted context in community settings might provide broader opportunities to extend coercion contexts beyond the law as there are likely to be more leverages available that can be drawn upon. Such extra-legal coercion relies on patients not being fully informed about their legal rights and is an example of a closed coercion context. If those contentions are correct, the risk of breaching legal rights may be higher in community settings. In a hospital ward patients rarely meet staff other than those who more or less exclusively work within those facilities. Community settings offer a wider variety of interactions with different kinds of staff. The narrower composition of staff in the hospital—with more specific experience and training in practising coercion—could theoretically increase the possibility that sufficient knowledge of the law and ethical reflection are brought to bear in the practice of coercion. One might as a result expect more open coercion contexts in the hospital. Temporal perspectives differ between settings and might work to mediate the creation of context. The more extended relations that can develop in community settings may have other effects on the formation of coercion contexts. It seems reasonable that staff–patient relations will become more personal, which could open the way for more informal pressures on patients, perhaps alongside a greater reluctance to impose formal coercion. The final distinction regards the extent to which the patient is seen as a whole person or not. The specialized, shorter-term focus on illness within institutions may increase the probability that patients are objectified and depersonalized. One might argue that reducing a person to symptoms and a diagnosis would also lessen the concerns with human rights issues and thus an increased tendency to invoke coercion contexts. This may be less likely in open community settings. On the other hand, knowing a patient well for a long time in community settings could promote a paternalism that nourishes informal coercion.

Coercion contexts in the community

Researching the use of compulsion in the community is particularly challenging. It is difficult to pinpoint the practice to a specific location or a specific instance. Requirements to take medication or not to drink alcohol are realized in any place where the patient happens to be. The enactment of compulsion cannot be observed in the same relatively straightforward way as coercion inside institutions. How, for example, do we capture the coercive nature of a lone person taking medicine in their home? To a large extent, researchers have to rely on participants' descriptions of events and their own opinions about them.

Before looking closer at some examples of how coercion contexts unfold in practice, I will provide a brief background view of community compulsion in Sweden.

Compulsory community care can be initiated when a patient under compulsory care at a hospital is discharged. The treating psychiatrist then applies to an administrative court for a CTO. In 99% of cases (Zetterberg et al. 2014) the court approves the application and states so-called *special provisions* that the patient must abide to (e.g. taking medication, living in a designated place, abstaining from alcohol, staying in touch with outpatient psychiatric services). The care of the patient is managed collaboratively between a hospital clinic and a municipal social service organization, with the latter more involved in day-to-day interactions such as home support. Some staff within social services may serve functions closely related to the special provisions dictated by the court, such as giving medication. Although Swedish law does not allow for forced medication in the community, social services staff do monitor that patients act in accordance with the legal requirements. For the patient who is interacting with a wide array of helpers, it may be difficult to understand each party's role in enforcing compulsory care. Notably, Swedish legislation does not give service providers any powers to actually make patients follow their special provisions. The law does not provide any sanctions such as forcing non-compliant patients to return to hospital. Quite understandably, this is a source of confusion and misunderstanding for patients and service providers alike. Similar concerns have been raised in other jurisdictions such as in New York State (Swartz et al. 2009).

A recurring theme in the interviews I have carried out with CTO patients (Sjöström 2012) was their uncertainty regarding their legal status and what it really meant. This cannot be attributed to lack of the capability to understand information. Most interviewees were perfectly capable of having nuanced discussions, and several kept the written decisions of the administrative court issuing the CTO. Some of this uncertainty relates to the legislation itself. When asked about the consequences of departing from special provisions, almost all interviewees replied that they would risk being returned to the hospital. This authority does not exist, as outlined above. Very few patients knew what their special provisions were or had even heard of the notion. Despite this, most had an idea of certain things that they were obliged to do as a result of their legal status. This status set a coercion context which made patients understand that they had to follow some sort of regime. However, the specific contents of that regime or the consequences of not abiding to it were mostly unclear to patients. Some patients made distinctions about how strictly different provisions were upheld, with some provisions appearing 'softer'. Regularly taking medication and keeping appointments with their doctor were generally taken seriously, whereas some had a more flexible approach to other provisions. For example, they chose to skip mandatory undertakings at an activity centre or allowed themselves a drink on a Friday evening. They reported that they could do so without this being raised as a violation of their special provisions. A conclusion from these findings is that responsible clinicians may fail to provide sufficient information to patients about their legal status, what special provisions they are subjected to, and the consequences of failure to comply. This is likely to do with a wish to ensure flexibility in invoking a coercion context. Given the lack of teeth in CTO regulations, psychiatrists may be concerned about their usefulness if patients are aware they can ignore them. This appears to be one reason why the coercion context surrounding special provisions is so vague.

In a similar way to that described earlier in relation to institutions, the everyday practice of community compulsion has established coercion contexts in the community that extend what the law prescribes. Particularly in supported housing, patients often believed that trivial rules about domestic chores and weekly routines were part of the provisions. Some patients expressed strong frustration over rules that interfered with features of life that were fundamental to them: one man described that he was not allowed to have a dog in his apartment and a 25-year-old man complained that the staff had banned his girlfriend from sleeping over in his apartment. From the point of view of the nursing staff, providing a coercion context where house rules are presented as legally binding could serve to facilitate the efficient running of a supported housing facility. It is unclear to what extent staff deliberately reinforce such beliefs, and it is clear that coercion contexts do not always result from conscious actions on behalf of staff. The combination of vague statutes and complex service provision in community mental health is likely to increase the risk that the coercion context is expanded. A contributing factor could be the fact that some patients live in housing conditions that closely resemble hospital wards. These facilities have a similar structure, with the staff office in the centre, shared spaces for watching television, playing games, and having meals, and corridors where each client had her own apartment (quite often with the doors open). It was in such settings that I observed the most examples of informal coercion. This resemblance to the traditional, paternalistic institution is likely to reinforce coercion contexts in which clients are generally expected to do what staff tell them to.

Coercion contexts without coercive legislation

It appears that the introduction of powers to compel in the community has opened up new modes of informal coercion. One question that arises is: how did staff handle similar issues before CTOs existed? First of all, one should note that Swedish legislation prior to the introduction of CTOs, like that of many other countries, did have mechanisms that allowed for extending coercive powers into the community over long periods of time. In the Swedish case 'long-term leave' was used to accomplish some of the things that CTOs do today. To provide some insight into how staff solved everyday problems without creating a coercion context related to CTOs, I will turn to a few examples from ethnographic fieldwork I conducted some 8 years prior to their introduction. For about a year I followed a group of people with severe mental illness who all lived in the same neighbourhood. They lived in their own apartments, but with varying degrees of support from staff, usually on a daily basis. All of them had been permanently discharged from hospital care.

Clear-cut situations that required coercive measures were rare. Several clients had their medicines in a cabinet in the apartment to which only staff had the keys. Once or twice a day, staff opened the cabinet for the patients to take their medicines. This offered an opportunity for staff to monitor that patients took their medicines in a way similar to when they were in hospital. This arrangement required that the client agreed to have such a cabinet in the apartment. If agreement is sought in the context of being offered an apartment, it may be difficult for a patient to reject it. One woman lived under heavy surveillance due to the risk she posed of setting fire to the building. Her contract for an apartment came with the requirement that she agreed to have two staff members with her in the apartment at all times. Sometimes residents would refuse to open their apartment door when staff paid a visit. This created a problem for staff, since they had a responsibility to support and monitor patients. In rare and extreme situations, staff could actually call the police to assist in entering the apartment and bring the person to hospital for assessment for inpatient compulsory care. On other rare occasions, staff simply gave up and accepted that they could not check on the client for the time being. In general, however, they managed to somehow persuade the client to open the door. Occasionally staff would point out to the resident that they might call the police. Even when they refrained from doing so, residents would still be aware of that possibility. Staff were thus able to create a coercion context to manage the problem of patients who would not let them into their homes.

Dimensions, conditions, and implications of coercion contexts

Rugkåsa et al. (2014) highlight the need for micro-level analysis of clinical encounters relating to coercion in community care. I would like to add that it is necessary to ground such analysis in substantive theory (cf. Glaser and Strauss 2009), which applies concepts that are general enough to manage the diversity among national settings but specific enough to capture the essential and unique features of compulsory community care. A starting point for such theorizing must be the fuzziness of CTOs, which can be conceptualized in terms of how they are used *spatially* and *temporally*. The notion of coercion contexts is helpful in analysing how CTOs are enacted in everyday situations. In the asymmetrical relationship between staff and patient, the former wields more power in defining the coercion context. The invocation of coercion context is often a means to achieve compliance. It may be helpful to think of such contexts in terms of three dimensions that refer to their reality, their source of powers, and the patient's awareness (as illustrated in Table 8.2).

Reality of the context

There are components in the coercion context that are external to the participants. In addition to having temporal and/or spatial features, such factors can be material

Table 8.2 Dimensions of coercion contexts

Reality of the context	Inherent Material, formal, personal, social status	versus	Constructed Interaction, negotiation Partly conditioned by inherent context
Source of powers	Formal Legal and other regulations	versus	Informal Leverage, pressures, threats
Patient's knowledge	Open About: legal status and rights, provisions, sanctions	versus	Closed (Patient unaware of those)

(the layout of housing facilities, having a medicine cabinet in the apartment), formal (how the law is written, regulations pertaining to medical care, social services, housing, etc.), organizational (responsibilities of and coordination between different service providers), personal (staff qualifications, the patient's condition and capacities) or social (the patient's dependence on staff, pressures from family and neighbours). These components are inherent in the situation and 'set the stage'. There are other components that do not exist in themselves and are constructed in the interaction between staff and patients. One example of this is the portrayal of certain arrangements as part of the conditions of a CTO. In such interactions, inherent components of the coercion context become building blocks for construction of the coercion context. The meanings and consequences of these components are not fixed, and this is where strategic communication can have an impact on patients' understanding of the coercion context. Going back to the example of the medicine cabinets, the existence of a cabinet in an apartment will condition the negotiations between the parties about how to administer medicines. Nevertheless, the inherent context does not decide the outcome, and it is perfectly possible for the parties to define the medicine cabinet as part of the patient's private sphere that the staff would not interfere with.

Source of powers

The relationship between staff and patients is inherently imbalanced in terms of power. Formal rules can impinge on the constructed coercion context, such as when staff explain that patients have to abide by certain restrictions because of their legal status The coercion context in relation to a CTO can be seen as formal regardless of whether the participants have a correct understanding of the law or not. An informal coercion context is present when there is a sense that the patient has to accept something she is against, but without anyone explicitly invoking the law. This is where leverage and patients' general dependence on staff may come in to effect. A patient may accept having a locked medicine cabinet in her home rather than making time-consuming trips to the pharmacy to fetch the medicines by herself. Informal coercion can also consist of threats of sanctions, such as imposing coercive legislation or filing criminal charges. One alternative described in the literature is to simply envisage or predict unwanted consequences for the non-compliant patient. This kind of informal coercion has been discussed in relation to the assertive community services that have emerged in many countries over recent decades (Davidson and Campbell 2007). Informal coercion is not limited to relationships between staff and patients; a number of studies have highlighted the role of families, friends, employers, and wider social networks.

Patient's knowledge

As with the awareness context in relation to dying described by Glaser and Strauss (1965), coercion contexts can be open or closed. A minimum requirement for a coercion context to be open is for patients to be aware of their legal status. In a truly open context the patient would also be aware of the specific meaning of the law, what treatment measures she has to comply with, and what will happen if she does not. Moreover an open coercion context would entail knowledge of rights to legal counsel and appeal. A closed context can be either inherent or constructed, or indeed contain elements of both. An example of the former is how the Swedish legislation is written in a way that gives the misleading impression that non-compliance will lead to readmission to hospital. The primary source of closed coercion contexts appears to be constructed by strategic withholding of information on behalf of staff, in combination with their lack of knowledge. Staff may also want to downplay the reality of coercion when talking to patients to avoid stigmatizing them and reminding them of the power imbalances in their relationship.

Conclusions

We currently have limited knowledge about how coercion contexts are affected when compulsory care enters community settings. At this early juncture, it seems that coercion contexts may be more informal and closed for service recipients in the community. It is probable that coercive powers are extended to new and more personal domains of people's lives. From an ethical point of view, all this raises serious concerns, as the effect of coercion in the community reaches further into someone's natural living circumstances and interferes more profoundly with identity. In this chapter I have attempted to demonstrate the relevance of the concept of coercion context. Thinking in terms of the dimensions of coercion contexts may help us to understand more about the delicate workings of compulsory care, as well as informal coercion and leverage. This may aid the development of concrete research questions and guide the analysis of empirical data. For policy makers, it may provide insight into the gaps between law, policy, and practice. This may in turn enable care providers, legislators, and policy makers to fill some of these gaps and limit the ongoing expansion of community coercion. Increased attention on how coercion contexts are formed may enable service providers in the community to be more mindful of their interactions with patients.

References

Canvin K, Rugkåsa J, Sinclair J, et al. (2013). Leverage and other informal pressures in community psychiatry in England. *International Journal of Law and Psychiatry*, **36**:100–106.

Cascardi M, Poythress NG (1997). Correlates of perceived coercion during psychiatric hospital admission. *International Journal of Law and Psychiatry*, **20**:445–458.

Davidson G, Campbell J (2007). An examination of the use of coercion by assertive outreach and community mental health teams in Northern Ireland. *British Journal of Social Work*, **37**:537–555.

Glaser B, Strauss A (1965). *Awareness of dying*. Chicago: Aldine.

Glaser B, Strauss A (2009). *The discovery of grounded theory: strategies for qualitative research*. Piscataway, NJ: Aldine Transaction.

Hoge SK, Lidz CW, Eisenberg M, et al. (1997). Perceptions of coercion in the admission of voluntary and involuntary psychiatric patients. *International Journal of Law and Psychiatry*, **20**:167–181.

Lambert TJ, Singh BS, Patel MX (2009). Community treatment orders and antipsychotic long-acting injections. *British Journal of Psychiatry*, **195**:S57–S62.

Lidz CW, Hoge SK, Gardner W (1995). Perceived coercion in mental hospital admission. *Archives of General Psychiatry*, **52**:1034–1039.

McKenna BG, Simpson AIF, Laidlaw TM (1999). Patient perception of coercion on admission to acute psychiatric services; the New Zealand experience. *International Journal of Law and Psychiatry*, **22**:143–153.

Monahan J, Redlich AD, Swanson J, et al. (2005). Use of leverage to improve adherence to psychiatric treatment in the community. *Psychiatric Services*, **56**:37–44.

Newton-Howes G, Mullen R (2011). Coercion in psychiatric care: systematic review of correlates and themes. *Psychiatric Services*, **62**:465–470.

O'Donoghue B, Roche E, Shannon S, et al. (2014). Perceived coercion in voluntary hospital admission. *Psychiatry Research*, **215**:120–126.

Riley H, Høyer G, Lorem GF (2014). 'When coercion moves into your home'—a qualitative study of patient experiences with outpatient commitment in Norway. *Health and Social Care in the Community*, **22**:506–514.

Rugkåsa J, Canvin K, Sinclair J, et al. (2014). Trust, deals and authority: community mental health professionals' experiences of influencing reluctant patients. *Community Mental Health Journal*, **50**:886–895.

Sjöström S (1997). *Party or patient? Discursive practices relating to coercion in psychiatric and legal settings*. Umeå: Boréa Bokförlag.

Sjöström S (2000). Hemligt och hemlikt. Professionella samtal i bostaden. *Kulturella Perspektiv*, **9**:66–72. [Secret and homelike. Professional discourse in home settings. *Swedish Journal of Ethnology*]

Sjöström S (2006). Invocation of coercion context in compliance communication—power dynamics in psychiatric care. *International Journal of Law and Psychiatry*, **29**:36–47.

Sjöström S (2012). *Det diffusa tvånget. Patienters upplevelser av tvångsvård.* Stockholm: Socialstyrelsen. [*Fuzzy coercion. Patient perceptions of coercive care.* The Swedish National Board of Health and Welfare]

Sjöström S, Zetterberg L, Markström U (2011). Why community compulsion became the solution. Reforming mental health law in Sweden. *International Journal of Law and Psychiatry*, **34**:419–428.

Swartz M, Swanson J, Steadman HJ, et al. (2009). *New York State assisted outpatient treatment program evaluation*. Durham, NC: Duke University School of Medicine.

Szmukler G, Appelbaum PS (2008). Treatment pressures, leverage, coercion, and compulsion in mental health care. *Journal of Mental Health*, **17**:233–244.

Zetterberg L, Sjöström S, Markström U (2014). The compliant court—procedural fairness and social control in compulsory community care. *International Journal of Law and Psychiatry*, **37**:543–550.

Chapter 9

Patient experiences and perceptions of coercion: universal meaning, individual experiences?

Krysia Canvin

Introduction

This chapter presents a synthesis of major research themes and findings on patients' subjective experiences and perceptions of coercion in community psychiatry. It is specifically concerned with *patient-reported* experiences of community coercion rather than those reported by clinicians or observed by researchers. Studies of patient perspectives on health and illness have produced major methodological and substantive insights, and the field of psychiatric coercion is no exception. The MacArthur Coercion Study, conducted in the USA in the 1990s, made two important observations that would alter the study of coercion from that point onwards. The MacArthur team found that legal status—whether a patient is voluntarily or involuntarily admitted to hospital—is only a 'blunt' measure of experienced coercion during hospital admission:

> A significant minority of legally 'voluntary' patients experience coercion, and a significant minority of legally 'involuntary' patients believe that they freely chose to be hospitalised.

> Monahan et al. (1999)

The same research programme produced the MacArthur Perceived Coercion Scale (Gardner et al. 1993), a validated instrument that has been adopted for use in many studies. Additionally, the MacArthur Study found that patients who perceived that their admission to hospital was characterized by 'procedural justice' perceived less coercion than patients who reported that they had no 'voice' in the proceedings and were not respected (Lidz et al. 2000). These findings clearly indicate that patients' *subjective* experiences and perceptions of inpatient and community coercion matter for a range of outcomes, including patients' behaviours (Rhodes 2000; Swartz et al. 2003c, 2004; Szmukler and Appelbaum 2008). The bulk of the literature to date on patients' perspectives on coercion derives from studies of involuntary hospital admission and inpatient experiences.

Deinstitutionalization, however, has led to the increasing, perhaps inevitable, use of coercion in community settings and the subsequent introduction of legal frameworks to support its use (see Chapters 2 and 3). Such developments have demanded that researchers turn their attention to the community, and as a consequence there is small but growing literature.

Coercion is widely regarded as a slippery concept (e.g. Newton-Howes and Mullen 2011), although few concerns have been expressed in the literature about how to operationalize it in research with patients. The generic term coercion is used extensively throughout the psychiatric literature to refer to a range of practices, both legal and extra-legal, yet is little used by patients. Which practices amount to coercion—and according to what criteria—is the focus of ongoing debate and is far from clear (see Wertheimer 1987; Dunn et al. 2012). In this chapter I use the term community coercion as a catch-all, but adopt specific terms such as community treatment order, outpatient commitment, leverage, and so on, when reporting findings from particular studies. While it is my intention to focus on what coercion means to patients, it is important to point out that the experiences and perceptions reported in the literature are subject to researchers' (who may also be clinicians) interpretations and priorities. As such they constitute *representations* of patients' perspectives.

The literature reviewed for the purposes of this chapter was extracted from a search for articles on patients' experiences of coercion in the community over the 20-year period from 1994 to 2014. A variety of alternative terms for 'coercion' were specified (i.e. commitment, involuntary, compulsion/compulsory, persuasion/persuasive, leverage, threat, force, Mental Health Act). The search yielded a total of 215 papers and was supplemented with papers from my own archive, hand-searching of reference lists, and some additional internet searches. Nevertheless, it does not purport to be exhaustive. In this review I focus on *psychiatric* interventions in response to adult mental illness, and for the purposes of simplicity I exclude those related to incapacity, eating disorders, and dementia. Nor do I include forensic, substance misuse, or child and adolescent services. For reasons of space, I will not address the literature on patients' perceptions and experiences of specific aspects of mental health services (e.g. treatments) as coercive (as opposed to those that are coercive by design).

The literature to date is almost exclusively from developed, industrialized countries in the West and there is an urgent need for this gap to be filled. Although the existing literature does encompass a variety of legal and socio-cultural settings, spanning the USA, Europe, and Australasia and includes a few studies that pay special attention to the experiences of minority ethnic groups (e.g. Gibbs et al. 2004; Newton-Howes et al. 2013; Mfoafo-M'Carthy 2014), this should not be considered as even approaching what is required to achieve a truly global picture of patients' perspectives on coercion.

This chapter will focus on studies of patients' perceptions and experiences of coercion, that is, legislation, programmes, and services that are commonly described as and agreed to be of a coercive nature. Examples studied by the literature include: community treatment orders (CTOs), or their equivalent, supervised discharge orders, guardianship orders, drug treatment and testing orders (DTTO), jail diversion, co-occurring disorders treatment programmes, and use of the Mental Health Act in general. 'Informal' coercion refers to 'non-legislative' or 'extra-legal' coercion and includes studies of assertive community treatment (ACT), leverage, and other 'treatment pressures'. In some studies informal coercion is used synonymously with the term 'leverage', although recent work in this area argues that leverage is not necessarily 'coercive' (Dunn et al. 2012) and that non-legislative coercion—or pressure—may be leveraged or non-leveraged (Canvin et al. 2013). The range of informal practices that might be employed in an attempt to influence patients' behaviours is expansive (see Rugkåsa et al. 2014 for a summary). Only those practices specifically identified in the literature as informal coercion, pressure, or leverage are included in this review.

Patient perceptions of community coercion: universal meaning?

Four concepts are repeatedly used to characterize patients' perceptions of coercion: interventions (what they perceive is done to them), obligations (what they perceive they must do), threats (what they perceive might be done to them), and safety (what they perceive they might gain). In particular, obligation and threat are unwaveringly presented as synonymous with coercion. The universality of these four components is implied by the absence of counter-narratives: if there are patients who do not perceive coercion to comprise these components, then the literature to date does not report their views.

Coercion as intervention

The literature depicts coercion in terms of patients enduring a series of interventions: taking medication or other treatment, seeing the mental health team, being supervised or subjected to 'compliance monitoring' (Ridley and Hunter 2013). This is coercion at its most basic and practical level.

Coercion as obligation

For the most part, depictions of coercion as intervention are presented as perceived obligations. For example, patients are cited as describing 'having to' comply with treatment or 'having to' see the psychiatrist. The literature presents patients' perceptions of a range of obligations from the general and all-encompassing, such as following legal requirements, rules, and regulations, to the specific, such as ceasing alcohol use and self-harm. Some studies also report patients' perceptions of less tangible obligations such as having to 'play the game', 'stay in the good books of the doctor' (Brophy and Ring 2004), 'do as they say', and 'live up to their expectations' (Riley et al. 2014). Many patients are reported to perceive coercion as draconian (Ridley and Hunter 2013), professionals as 'authoritarian' (Gibbs et al. 2005, p. 363), and life as having 'more discipline' and being 'more regimented' (Canvin et al. 2002, p. 364).

Coercion as threat

Throughout the literature, there are countless examples of how living with coercion means living with the (perceived) omnipresent threat of hospitalization. Other (perceived) sanctions are mentioned too, including being reprimanded by the doctor (Canvin et al. 2002), getting into trouble (Castille et al. 2011), losing custody of a child (Canvin et al. 2013; Mfoafo-M'Carthy 2014), losing a driving licence (Schwartz et al.

Table 9.1 Patient conceptualization of coercion

Conceptualization	Illustrative interview extracts from the international literature	
	Formal coercion	**Informal coercion**
Intervention	'I must do as they say, go to the doctor to get an injection, go to a psychiatrist to talk, go to a psychiatric nurse to talk' 'There was a time they rang every day, (…) the medicine people come here every morning' (Riley et al. 2014, pp. 510–11; outpatient commitment, Norway)	'They come to your house' 'They mess with your money' (Appelbaum and Le Melle 2008, p.462; assertive community treatment, New York, USA)
Obligation	'Just basically restricting because I've got to keep to rules and regulations under it (…) I normally like to do things at my leisure (…) I don't like the emotional threat of 'you'll be re-called into hospital' if you don't' (Ridley and Hunter 2013, pp. 7–8; CTO, Scotland)	'Just trying to work out how I can stop them seeing me now. I don't have a choice, they just come. They don't listen sometimes. They'll change some appointments but they won't change them all' (Watts and Priebe 2002, p. 449; ACT, England)
Threat	'It were just threatening if I had missed a day or something like that, they would, um, hospitalize me again' (Castille et al. 2011, p. 258; assisted outpatient treatment, New York, USA)	'The other slight pressure that was put on me was people saying things like, 'Well of course if you're going to be self-harming you won't be allowed to have your daughter with you'. (…) This open threat really' (Canvin et al. 2013, p. 3; leverage, England)
Safety	'I accept now that it is best for me and best for my family (…) it protects me and it protects other people' (Gibbs 2010, p. 229; CTO, New Zealand)	'Once you get to know the team, you realize that it really works. It works in the way that you have a sense of safety in that … well, it's not just that one time in the week … because if you need more help, the door is open …' (Thøgersen et al. 2010, p. 43; ACT, Denmark)

2010), police involvement (Brophy and Ring 2004), and the use of force (Gibbs et al. 2004, p. 833, 2005; Riley et al. 2014). The threat component of community coercion is described by Castille et al. (2011) as its 'punitive hand'; indeed, elsewhere patients are reported as experiencing community coercion as punitive in itself (Brophy and Ring 2004) or as punishment for wrongdoing (Canvin et al. 2002).

Coercion as safety

Alongside these negative aspects of coercion, the literature presents a more positive connotation: coercion as safety. Patients are said to perceive community coercion as a 'safety net' or 'safeguard', 'security' and 'protection', not just for themselves but sometimes also for their whole family and other people (Gibbs et al. 2005; Gibbs 2010). Swartz et al. (2003b) asked patients to complete a preference-ordering task, and found that they placed 'being safe' higher than 'staying out of hospital' and 'being free to participate in treatment or not'. They concluded that this meant that participants were 'willing to accept the coerciveness of outpatient commitment to gain improved outcomes'. As this finding suggests, the fact that coercion holds some positive meaning for patients is used by some in an attempt to justify the use of coercion or suggest that patients are willing to tolerate its negative aspects in order to achieve safety (or other benefits). This portrayal of the patient perspective is problematic and I return to this later.

This four-component conceptualization of coercion is common to representations of patients' perceptions of both formal and informal community coercion (see Table 9.1). The apparent absence of difference in perception between the two serves to reinforce the findings of the MacArthur studies that patients' legal status has little consequence for patient perceptions of coercion.

Although all patients have the potential to experience an intervention as coercive (Newton-Howes and Mullen 2011), some do not. Despite the implied universality of the *meaning* of coercion to patients, it is worth noting that what exactly patients consider to *constitute* coercion can and does vary. Based on patients' accounts that appear in the literature and my own encounters with patients, those who report coercion do so in terms of the universal components I have described, but not all patients who experience these components consider themselves as having experienced coercion. To add to the complexity, patients have different views about what constitutes an intervention, what they are (and are not) obliged to do, what words or actions denote a threat, and under what circumstances coercion amounts to safety.

Variations in patients' experiences of community coercion: individual experiences?

When it comes to presenting patients' experiences of coercion, the literature revolves around five themes. The first theme compares hospital and community coercion while the remainder focus on the various potential implications of coercion for self-determination, 'normality', care and services, and wellness. Similar to the universal components already described, these themes are common to characterizations of patients' experiences of coercion across the literature. Here, however, counter-narratives are abundant both within and across studies. Patients are reported to experience community coercion as both enhancing and restricting their self-determination, as enabling and preventing a return to 'normality', as providing access to or causing the loss of housing, and as facilitating or undermining their wellness. In some cases, individual patients have been reported to hold seemingly inconsistent views (Canvin et al. 2005). Much of the variation, however, is obscured by the way in which research findings are usually reported as themes, majority experiences or attitudes, and/or associations between variables. The use of the somewhat reductionist categories of benefits and disadvantages compounds this. One example is the categorization of patients' simultaneous expressions of positive and negative views of coercion as 'ambivalence' (e.g. Gibbs 2010). I will return to this issue later.

Hospital versus community coercion

The literature often represents formal community-based coercion—meaning CTOs or their equivalent—as a preferable alternative to hospitalization for patients (e.g. Stroud et al. 2013). Patients are quoted as making statements such as: 'anywhere but in hospital' (Crawford et al. 2004). Riley et al. (2014) describe one patient as preferring outpatient commitment to hospitalization even though she disagreed with her treatment, and other studies report how patients state a preference for taking (unwanted) medication over the risk of being (involuntarily) hospitalized (O'Reilly et al. 2006; Canvin et al. 2014). Studies of patients' attitudes (as opposed to experiences) have found that patients express a preference for treatment at home both retrospectively (following treatment in hospital) (O'Donoghue et al. 2010) and regarding future compulsory treatment (Crawford et al. 2004). Crawford et al. (2004) documented the reasons for this preference as including a dislike of hospitals, familiarity with home, the upheaval of hospital admission and discharge, and the belief that home treatment offered greater freedom and independence. Reasons reported by other studies include feeling 'freer' in the community to 'being away from everybody' (Canvin et al. 2014) and because being in the community meant 'clearer agreements and regular people. It's not just suddenly changing doctors, or changing what's going to happen' (Riley et al. 2014, p. 510).

Although few studies include a counter-narrative to this preference, they do exist: some patients do not prefer community coercion to hospitalization. In their study of patient attitudes, O'Donoghue et al. (2010) found that 59% of participants thought that people should be admitted to hospital if they were going to be administered medication without consent. Such preferences are based on patients' beliefs about hospital and home: patients reported to prefer hospital care thought they would receive more support in hospital than at home: 'I needed to be watched and encouraged' (Crawford et al. 2004). Other patients regarded home to be a private and safe place, unsuitable for professionals to visit (Crawford et al. 2004; Canvin et al. 2005).

Implications for self-determination

Community coercion is portrayed as having a pivotal role in patients' self-determination, capable of enhancing or impairing it. Several studies report that patients perceive coercion in the community as affording greater freedom, free time, and autonomy compared with being in hospital (Canvin et al. 2002, 2014), especially when patients were living in their own accommodation (Riley et al. 2014). Swartz et al.'s (2003b) finding that patients ranked 'staying out of the hospital' higher than 'being free to participate in treatment or not' as an area of concern suggests that it is the avoidance of hospital rather than achieving freedom per se that is a priority to patients. The authors concluded that patients would therefore be prepared to have their freedom in the community curtailed if that meant being able to avoid hospital. Others highlight the negative impact that CTOs have on patients' sense of liberty and freedom of action, such as having to organize their daily lives around visits to/from the mental health team and/or medication (Newton-Howes 2013; Riley et al. 2014). We can see illustrations of this impact in patient narratives in which they compare, for example, CTOs with prison (Canvin et al. 2002, 2014; Gibbs et al. 2005) or with community-based criminal justice sentences (Brophy and Ring 2004). One patient is reported as describing being on a CTO as like 'being in jail without any walls' (Brophy and Ring 2004, p. 165), while another is reported as saying she 'felt as if I was in prison but outside' (Gibbs 2010, p. 228). Given that a significant proportion of psychiatric patients will have encountered the criminal justice system it is unsurprising that such comparisons emerge.

The literature also reports patients' experiences of how coercion impacts on feelings of empowerment (Canvin et al. 2002; Gault 2009; Castille et al. 2011). In one study patients on CTOs reported feeling in control of themselves and able to make their own decisions (Gibbs 2010). Galon and Wineman (2011) found that patients subject to outpatient commitment felt significantly more empowered than those receiving ACT or usual care. Elsewhere, patients have been reported as saying that coercion in the community gave them more choice, influence, and responsibility than being in hospital (Canvin et al. 2002; Riley et al. 2014) and that going on a CTO was their choice (Jobling 2014). Others, including Gibbs et al. (2005, 2010) and Schwartz et al. (2010), discuss how CTOs can also be perceived as taking away patients' power: 'The psychiatrist who took my driver's licence away, I think he had too much power, he didn't know me.' (Schwartz et al. 2010).

The relationship between empowerment and community coercion remains far from clear, however, as suggested by Galon and Wineman's (2011) finding that coercion/negative pressure was unrelated to empowerment.

Implications for 'normality'

The implications of community coercion for patients' perceptions of 'normality' are similarly indisputable, but are again varied. Patients reportedly describe community coercion as providing employment prospects, a 'better' future (Canvin et al. 2005; Schwartz et al. 2010), and an opportunity to live a fulfilling life (Canvin et al. 2002). The structure and routine associated with some forms of community coercion kept some patients occupied and gave them something to get up for (Canvin et al. 2005). In the words of one patient: '[The] CTO makes sure I'm not lazy' (Mfoafo-M'Carthy 2014, p. 5). On the other hand, patients have also been reported as describing how community coercion interferes with various aspects of 'everyday life' and 'normality' (Brophy and Ring 2004; Ridley and Hunter 2013; Canvin et al. 2014; Jobling 2014). This is illustrated by the following extract:

> Right now all I need is a job, a possible [*sic.*] go to church, and a job, and live a normal life and they don't, they say, 'Well, you're taking medication, you're doing much better, don't go too fast, go slow'.

> Castille et al. (2011, p. 261)

The literature also reports how patients describe the way in which the combination of appointments, medication, and care in the home require everyday activities to be planned, reported, and adapted (Riley et al. 2014). Such restrictions can make it difficult to get or maintain employment, limit the type of work patients are able to do (Schwartz et al. 2010), and restrict social and leisure activities (including taking holidays) (Riley et al. 2014).

Another way in which patients subject to community coercion reportedly perceive normality to be suspended is through the stigma that they feel. Some patients are said to feel 'locked' into the patient identity (Gibbs 2010; Riley et al. 2014), which, in the words of one patient, stopped her from 'getting on with my life like a normal person would get on with their life' (Jobling 2014, p. 61). Others are reported as feeling as though they have lost a 'credible' identity (Gault 2009) and are like second-class citizens (Mfoafo-M'Carthy 2014). Accordingly, patients are said to feel isolated, treated as outsiders (Gibbs 2010; Schwartz et al. 2010), and feared and judged (Schwartz et al. 2010). These kinds of feelings reportedly lead some to express concerns about not being able to look after children or work, or worry that their employer would find out about the order (Brophy and Ring 2004; Gibbs 2010). Moreover, Brophy and Ring (2004) describe patients who believed that the stigma of CTOs was *worse* than that associated with mental illness per se.

Implications for (better) care and services

It is often reported that patients consider being subject to community coercion as being associated with improved access to a range of mental health and related social welfare services, such as housing provision. For example, patients reportedly say that they received increased support and attention from a range of professionals (Canvin et al. 2005; Schwartz et al. 2010) and that community coercion meant having someone to talk to (O'Reilly et al. 2006). Many (though not all) are reported as perceiving increased monitoring or supervision as *better* care (Canvin et al. 2002; Gault 2009). Studies report how the presence of ongoing supervision or being kept 'in the system' (Ridley and Hunter 2013) following discharge from hospital was understood as better than being 'just dumped out in the community to get on with it' (Canvin et al. 2005, p. 459). Others report that patients perceived that community coercion meant they could access care when they needed it and that it was much quicker to do so (Gibbs 2010): one patient is reported as saying 'you don't have to go via the emergency service, you just go straight in' (Riley et al. 2014, p. 510). Similarly, there is evidence of an associated perception of services as more responsive (Brophy and Ring 2004). This takes two forms: perceiving that someone will come if called (Gault 2009) and that they will be taken seriously, listened to, and involved in decision-making about their care (Castille et al. 2011; Riley et al. 2014). Riley et al. (2014) report that patients on CTOs perceived themselves as having more influence and being subject to less coercion than when they were in hospital. Similarly, Castille et al. (2011) found that patients perceived services as empowering rather than coercive where they experienced help with negotiating the system and their concerns and goals were listened to and facilitated. Given this, it is less surprising that several studies report that patients perceive good-quality relationships with mental health professionals involved in their coercive care. For example, Jobling (2014) describes collaborative relationships between professionals and patients, mutual positive regard, trust, and a common sense of purpose. Riley et al. (2014) report stable relationships with 'regular people' which made their lives more predictable and O'Reilly et al. (2006) describe ambivalent (but not negative) relationships.

Another positive aspect of community coercion presented by the literature is patients' attainment of housing and associated benefits, such as freedom and increased predictability (Riley et al. 2014). In some jurisdictions, housing and outpatient commitment have an interdependent relationship. For example, in Norway, housing is a precondition for outpatient commitment. In New York outpatient commitment is a precondition for housing or makes patients a priority for housing placements (Castille et al. 2011). Patients are reported as placing great emphasis on the importance of receiving help with finding housing (Castille et al. 2011; Riley et al. 2014). Perhaps as a consequence, many of the patients in Castille et al.'s (2011) study who perceived that they accessed housing as a result of community coercion reportedly did not perceive that they had experienced coercion.

Running parallel to these positive narratives about care is a less positive narrative about the over-reliance of community coercion on medication. In the words of one patient: 'I was given drugs instead of support … I needed support'! (Gibbs 2010, p. 228). Ridley and Hunter (2013) report that the one-dimensional focus on medication led some patients in their study to perceive the Scottish CTO as a 'medication order'. Such perceptions reportedly lead patients to express disappointment that they did not receive a holistic care package (Brophy and Ring 2004; Gibbs 2010; Ridley and Hunter 2013) and to express a desire for 'someone who would really listen' (Brophy and Ring 2004, p. 166). Moreover, Swartz et al. (2003a) present evidence to support the argument that both mandated and informal community coercion act as a *barrier* to care and treatment. Roughly a third (36.4%) of subjects with schizophrenia spectrum disorders reported one or more barriers to care related to mandated treatment: delay in treatment seeking for fear of involuntary hospitalization was the most frequently cited, followed by fear of being forced to take medications or other treatment and fear of trouble with the law (Swartz et al. 2003a).

Implications for wellness

As I have already described, according to the literature, coercion can also mean safety to patients. Some patients perceive community coercion quite literally as a life saver, protecting them from self-harm and suicide (Canvin et al. 2005; Gibbs et al. 2005; Gibbs 2010). Less dramatically, patients also reportedly perceive community coercion as an opportunity to get well and 'stay well' (Canvin et al. 2013), protecting them from relapse and hospitalization.

In contrast to positive depictions of community coercion, Swartz et al. (2003c) found that the majority of patients in their study *did not* perceive outpatient commitment to be personally beneficial. Most had a negative view both at the beginning of the study and 1 year later, with the number expressing positive views declining over this period (Swartz et al. 2003c). This view was associated with the view that outpatient commitment was ineffective, or because they did not acknowledge their own need for treatment, or both. Patients who experienced a positive outcome (i.e. stayed out hospital, avoided violence, achieved an above average Global Assessment of Functioning score) under outpatient commitment were twice as likely as those with negative outcomes to convert from a negative attitude at the start of the study to a positive one at the end. This effect was only true of patients who experienced outpatient commitment and not the control group. Swartz et al. (2003c) conclude that their findings do not support Stone's (1975) 'thank-you' theory because of the 'modest rates of endorsement' and because patients ultimately did not want outpatient commitment because they perceived it to be ineffective or believed future treatment was unnecessary. In a later study, Swartz et al. (2004) examined whether patients subject to treatment mandates endorsed their effectiveness. They found that higher levels of *perceived* coercion amongst patients were associated with significantly lower perceived effectiveness scores, although actual numbers of mandated treatments were not.

When it comes to patients' quality of life scores, the quantitative evidence regarding the benefits of coercion is mixed. Two studies have shown that patients' perception of coercion/negative pressure are not related to quality of life (Galon and Wineman 2011; Newton-Howes 2013), while two others produced conflicting results. Phelan et al. (2010) detected an insignificant increase in quality of life scores amongst patients on assisted outpatient treatment, while Castille et al. (2011) found that the higher coercion score, the lower the quality of life score.

Despite the consistency of themes throughout two decades of community coercion research, representations of patients' individual experiences repeatedly demonstrate that there is no single experience of coercion in the community. In general, the literature makes little acknowledgement of the extent of variation and sheds little light on why it might be so. The only exception is the suggestion that (as with inpatient coercion) it is not whether a patient is coerced in the community but how they are coerced and whether they perceive procedural justice that matters. Galon and Wineman (2011) found that patients who reported higher levels of procedural justice (defined as the 'client's belief that others are acting out of genuine concern, that they are treated with respect, and that they are afforded the opportunity to tell their side of the story') tended to perceive lower levels of coercion/negative pressure, while Swartz et al. (2004) found that the higher perceived coercion scores were associated with lower perceived fairness. Swartz et al. also found that the number of reported episodes of coercion (mandated treatment) was not significantly associated with their perceived fairness. Galon and Wineman (2011) also found that patients subject to outpatient commitment (but not ACT) experienced higher levels of perceived coercion and also perceived less procedural justice than the treatment as usual group.

Representations of community coercion: positive, negative, and ambivalent patients

The justifiability of coercion is a central concern in psychiatry (see Chapter 14) and the literature often turns to patient experience to inform the debate. What emerges is a body of contradictory evidence, as I described. It is essential that the literature represents the full range of patient experiences and views rather than majority views or consensus. People with mental illness are individuals with unique histories, experiences, and aspirations: psychiatric services are only one aspect of their lives. It is increasingly recognized that there is no single 'patient perspective', although it is not that long since patient perspectives held little value. The patient voice, however, has long been synonymous with a critique of the mental health system and its techniques. Such a limited portrayal does an enormous disservice to patients and their experiences. To see variety amongst patients' views on coercion is therefore useful for researchers, clinicians, service providers, and policy makers.

Unfortunately, the literature generally offers a rather limited dichotomous categorization of patients' experiences of community coercion. Patients whose views do not fall neatly into the positive/negative binary, such as those who reflect that coercion might bring advantages as well as disadvantages, are designated as 'ambivalent'. This limited categorization underplays the diversity and nuance in patients' experiences and is a disservice to those who participated.

Another problem is the disproportionate weight given to positive experiences of coercion. A case in point is the work of Gibbs et al. (2006), who report the frequency of patients' experiences. They state that 19% of participants expressed 'wholly favourable' experiences of CTOs and 46% were 'generally favourable but noted disadvantages'. A naïve interpretation of this type of reporting could assume that there are more patients with something positive to say about community coercion than with negative views, but making quantified claims based on purposive, not randomized samples, lacks meaning.

Based on the most robust evidence available to date, we know that formal community coercion (i.e. the CTO) does not lead to improvements for patients across a range of outcome measures (see Chapters 4 and 5; Churchill et al. 2007; Burns et al. 2013; Maughan et al. 2014; Rugkåsa et al. 2015). Despite this, some argue that the evidence provided by quasi-experimental and naturalistic studies (i.e. excluding the most recent randomized controlled trial by Burns et al. 2013) is 'definitive enough' (Swanson and Swartz 2014, p. 3). Stroud and colleagues assert that the findings from their qualitative study with 72 participants (a combination of patients, professionals, and nearest relatives) suggest that CTOs 'can be effective for the "right" service user with certain needs and perceptions' (Stroud et al. 2015, p. 4). Others acknowledge the weakness of the quantitative evidence but point to the qualitative evidence as showing the benefits of CTOs (e.g. Lally 2013). It is beyond the remit of this chapter to review the defence by Burns and colleagues of their randomized controlled trial and its results, which is detailed elsewhere (see Chapter 5).

Throughout the literature there is evidence of patients' perceptions being used to support the argument that community coercion offers safety and improved access to better services (though the latter is contested). Stroud and colleagues found that CTOs 'enabled an increase in support' (Stroud et al. 2015, p. 4), while Mfoafo-M'Carthy asserts the significance of his finding that 'participants in this study believed CTOs enabled them to access treatment resources which otherwise would not have been available to them' (Mfoafo-M'Carthy 2014, p. 9). What is of particular interest here is how the literature presents the meeting of patients' basic needs as a *benefit of community coercion*, which seems inherently questionable. Stroud et al. (2015) do question the impact on patients who are not subject to CTOs, but only given the 'constrained resources' available. Patients should expect to feel safe or able to acquire adequate support or accommodation without having to be subjected to coercion, not least because tying together services and coercion could create a 'perverse incentive' to employ coercion where it is otherwise considered unnecessary (Canvin et al. 2014). To present patients' surmising of the upside of coercion as positive is equally perverse. The presentation of benefit in this way raises the question of whether patients subject to formal community coercion are more likely to access and/or receive better services (objectively measured) compared with patients who are not. Burns et al. (2013) found no difference between the number of clinical contacts experienced by patients subject to CTOs and their control group in England. Such questions, however, must take into account the jurisdiction in which they are asked. In many parts of the USA it is common practice to link treatment with the provision of services such as housing, whereas this is largely unnecessary in Europe where citizens enjoy unconditional welfare rights in many countries (Burns et al. 2011; Canvin et al. 2013).

It is therefore inappropriate that patients' positive views should be used as a basis for justifying coercive interventions. Although Stone's (1975) 'thank-you theory' provides a rationale for involuntary inpatient treatment, Swartz et al. (2003c) found no evidence to support it in the context of community coercion. Patients' positive views have been cited as providing support for the use of CTOs (e.g. see O'Reilly et al. 2006; Stroud et al. 2015). These views fit with Wertheimer's (1987) definition of coercion, in which only interventions that result in a patient being worse off amount to a coercive threat, meaning that any patient able to identify gains from their experience of coercion might be deemed not to have experienced coercion at all. Sen's argument—that to focus on the 'desire fulfilment' of a 'deprived person' is misleading in an assessment of well-being because they may have become accustomed to their deprivation (Sen 1992)—seems applicable here. Yet discussions of benefit seem irrelevant to deciding whether a patient has been coerced or not. This is especially the case given that patients see safety as one of the defining features of coercion, that the same features can be experienced as positive by some patients but as negative by others, and that most patients have mixed views and experiences. The extent of such variation is often obscured by the dichotomous presentation of patients' views. Community coercion then is perhaps best conceptualized as, in the words of one patient, 'a bittersweet pill' (Canvin et al. 2002).

Where do we go from here?

Together, the literature provides a rich and varied, though as yet incomplete, understanding of what it is to experience coercion as a community psychiatry patient. One conspicuous gap in the current literature is an understanding of why patients' perceptions and experiences differ. We do not fully understand why one person would perceive home visits as coercive while another would not, for example. Nor do we fully understand why one patient would experience a CTO as an opportunity to get better and live a 'normal' life while another would experience it as reinforcing their patient identity and preventing them from working.

There are many possible explanations, but one way forward might be to get to grips with the context within which coercion takes place. This is important, as one of the defining changes in the delivery of mental health care in recent years has been its mass relocation from hospital to community settings. On the face of it, however, context seems to hold little promise. Variations in patients' (reported) experiences do not appear to be related to differences between teams, services, or legal jurisdictions. Most studies include patients from the same team and/or service who report different experiences, and there are no apparent differences between experiences reported by studies conducted in different jurisdictions, despite the differences in legislation and operation (see Dawson 2005). Whether these variations are attributable to such differences in context, we simply do not know.

One argument for turning to context to improve our understanding of patients' experiences can be found in the work of Stefan Sjöström (2006; see Chapter 8). Sjöström argues that context determines whether patients perceive coercion, where context refers to patients' past experiences of mental health care and coercion as well as the physical setting in which care is received. In order to understand more about patients' experiences, then, we need to know more about the contexts within which they occur. There is a need to examine the coerciveness of particular mental health-care providers, from the regional policy-making level, to the local team-implementation level, to the individual clinician level. Are some providers more coercive than others? Do patients' perceptions of coercion vary across providers? Thinking more broadly, there is a need to develop cross-country comparative work. In particular, we need to look beyond the USA, Europe, and Australasia. How do differences in culture, mental health-care funding, and availability of services and treatment impact on the use of coercion? How do different cultures, policies, and legal frameworks impact on patients' perceptions and experiences of coercion? Another question relating to context that is as yet underexplored is whether and to what extent patients' experiences and perceptions of coercion change over time. Can we identify turning points (Denzin 1989) in patients' accounts and, if so, under what circumstances did they occur? Finally, what role is played by changes in patients' personal circumstances, their relationships and living arrangements, their responsibilities and expectations? If we seek answers to these questions we can begin to incorporate more nuance and complexity into our representations of patients' experiences of community coercion.

References

Appelbaum PS, Le Melle S (2008). Techniques used by assertive community treatment (ACT) teams to encourage adherence: patient and staff perceptions. *Community Mental Health Journal*, **44**:459–464. [Focus groups with 21 patients in New York, USA.]

Brophy L, Ring D (2004). The efficacy of involuntary treatment in the community: consumer and service provider perspectives. *Social Work in Mental Health*, **2**:157–174. [Focus groups with 30 consumers in Victoria, Australia.]

Burns T, Yeeles K, Molodynski A, et al. (2011). Pressures to adhere to treatment ('leverage') in English mental healthcare. *British Journal of Psychiatry*, **199**:145–150. [Structured interviews with 417 mental health service users including substance misuse, England.]

Burns T, Rugkåsa J, Molodynksi A, et al. and the OCTET Team (2013). Community Treatment Orders for patients with psychosis: a randomised controlled trial (OCTET). *The Lancet*, **381**:1627–1633.

Canvin K, Bartlett A, Pinfold V (2002). A 'bittersweet pill to swallow': learning from mental health service users' responses to compulsory community care. *Health and Social Care in the Community*, **10**:361–369. [In-depth interviews with hypothetical questions with 20 service users on supervised discharge or guardianship in England.]

Canvin K, Bartlett A, Pinfold V (2005). Acceptability of compulsory powers in the community: the ethical considerations of mental health service users on supervised discharge and guardianship. *Journal of Medical Ethics*, **31**:457–462. [In-depth interviews with hypothetical questions with 20 service users on supervised discharge or guardianship in England.]

Canvin K, Rugkåsa J, Sinclair J, et al. (2013). Leverage and other informal pressures in community psychiatry in England. *International Journal of Psychiatry and Law*, **36**:100–106. [Qualitative interviews with 29 service users in England.]

Canvin K, Rugkåsa J, Sinclair J, et al. (2014). Patient, psychiatrist and family carer experiences of community treatment orders: qualitative study. *Social Psychiatry and Psychiatric Epidemiology*, **49**:1873–1882. [Qualitative interviews with 26 mental health service users on CTOs in England.]

Castille D, Muenzenmaier K, Link B (2011). Coercion—point, perception, process. In: *Coercive treatment in psychiatry: clinical, legal and ethical aspects* (ed. T Kallert, J Mezzich, J Monahan), pp. 245–268. Chichester: John Wiley and Sons. [Mixed methods study with 184 service users (including 20 qualitative interviews) in New York, USA.]

Churchill R, Owen G, Singh S, et al. (2007). *International experiences of using community treatment orders*. London: Institute of Psychiatry.

Crawford M, Gibbon R, Ellis E, et al. (2004). In hospital, at home, or not at all. A cross-sectional survey of patient preferences for receipt of compulsory treatment. *Psychiatric Bulletin*, **28**:360–363. [Cross-sectional survey with 109 patients discharged from two in-patient units in West London, England.]

Dawson J (2005). *Community treatment orders: international comparisons*. Dunedin: Otago University Print.

Denzin NK (1989). *Interpretive biography*. Newbury Park, CA: Sage.

Dunn M, Maughan D, Hope T, et al. (2012). Threats and offers in community mental health care. *Journal of Medical Ethics*, **38**:204–209.

Galon P, Wineman NM (2011). Quasi-experimental comparison of coercive interventions on client outcomes in individuals with severe and persistent mental illness. *Archives of Psychiatric Nursing*, **25**:404–418. [Quasi-experimental research had a 2 × 2 factorial design. Compares outpatient commitment (OPC) and assertive community treatment (ACT) with 180 service users in Ohio, USA.]

Gardner W, Hoge S, Bennett N, et al. (1993). Two scales for measuring patients' perceptions of coercion during hospital admission. *Behavioral Sciences and the Law*, **20**:307–321.

Gault I (2009). Service-user and carer perspectives on compliance and compulsory treatment in community mental health services. *Health and Social Care in the Community*, **17**:504–513. [Qualitative interviews with 11 service users in England.]

Gibbs A (2010). Coping with compulsion: women's views of being on a community treatment order. *Australian Social Work*, **63**:223–233. [Qualitative interviews with ten women with experience of CTO in Otago, New Zealand.]

Gibbs A, Dawson J, Forsyth H, et al. (2004). Maori experience of community treatment in Otago, New Zealand. *Australian and New Zealand Journal of Psychiatry*, 38:830–835. [Qualitative interviews with eight Maori patients with experience of CTOs in Otago, New Zealand.]

Gibbs A, Dawson J, Ansley C, et al. (2005). How patients in New Zealand view community treatment orders. *Journal of Mental Health*, 14:357–368. [Qualitative interviews with 42 patients on CTO in Otago, New Zealand.]

Gibbs A, Dawson J, Mullen R (2006). Community treatment orders for people with serious mental illness: a New Zealand study. *British Journal of Social Work*, 36:1085–1100. [Qualitative interviews with 42 patients on CTO in Otago, New Zealand.]

Jobling H (2014). Using ethnography to explore causality in mental health policy and practice. *Qualitative Social Work*, 13:49–68. [Ethnography including interviews with 18 mental health service users in England.]

Lally J (2013). Liberty or dignity: community treatment orders and rights. *Irish Journal of Psychological Medicine*, 30:141–149.

Lidz C, Mulvey E, Hoge S, et al. (2000). Sources of coercive behaviors in psychiatric admissions. *Acta Psychiatrica Scandinavica*, 101:73–79.

Maughan D, Molodynski A, Rugkåsa J, et al. (2014). A systematic review of the effect of community treatment orders on service use. *Social Psychiatry and Psychiatric Epidemiology*, 49:651–663.

Mfoafo-M'Carthy M (2014). Community treatment orders and the experiences of ethnic minority individuals diagnosed with serious mental illness in the Canadian mental health system. *International Journal for Equity in Health*, 13:69. [Qualitative interviews with 24 patients with an ethnic minority background and experience of community treatment orders in Toronto, Canada.]

Monahan J, Lidz C, Hoge S, et al. (1999). Coercion in the provision of mental health services: the MacArthur studies. In: *Research in community and mental health, Vol. 10: Coercion in mental health services—international perspectives* (ed. J Morrissey, J Monahan), pp. 13–30. Stamford, CT: JAI Press.

Newton-Howes G (2013). A factor analysis of patients' views of compulsory community treatment orders: the factors associated with detention. *Psychiatry, Psychology and Law*, 20:519–526. [Questionnaires completed by 79 patients in New Zealand.]

Newton-Howes G, Mullen R (2011). Coercion in psychiatric care: systematic review of correlates and themes. *Psychiatric Services*, 62:465–470.

Newton-Howes G, Lacey C, Banks D (2013). Community treatment orders: the experiences of non-Maori and Maori within mainstream and Maori mental health services. *Social Psychiatry and Psychiatric Epidemiology*, 49:267–273.

O'Donoghue B, Lyne J, Hill M, et al. (2010). Patient attitudes towards compulsory community treatment orders and advance directives. *Irish Journal of Psychological Medicine*, 27:66–71. [Structured interviews with 67 service users 1 year post-discharge from psychiatric hospital in Ireland.]

O'Reilly RL, Keegan DL, Corring D, et al. (2006). A qualitative analysis of the use of community treatment orders in Saskatchewan. *International Journal of Law and Psychiatry*, 29:516–524. [In-depth interviews with patient with experience of CTO in Saskatchewan, Canada.]

Phelan JC, Sinkewicz M, Castille DM, et al. (2010). Effectiveness and outcomes of assisted outpatient treatment in New York State. *Psychiatric Services*, 61:137–143. [Interviews with

184 mental health service users mandated to OPC or recently discharged from psychiatric hospitals in New York State, USA.]

Rhodes M (2000). The nature of coercion. *Journal of Value Inquiry*, **34**:369–381.

Ridley J, Hunter S (2013). Subjective experiences of compulsory treatment from a qualitative study of early implementation of the Mental Health (Care & Treatment) (Scotland) Act 2003. *Health and Social Care in the Community*, **21**:509–518. [Semi-structured interviews by peer and professional interviewers with 49 mental health service users with experience of CTO in Scotland.]

Riley H, Høyer G, Lorem G (2014). When coercion moves into your home'—a qualitative study of patient experiences with outpatient commitment in Norway. *Health and Social Care in the Community*, **22**:506–514. [In-depth interviews with 11 patients subject to outpatient commitment in Norway.]

Rugkåsa J, Canvin K, Sinclair J, et al. (2014). Trust, deals and authority: community mental health professionals' experiences of influencing reluctant patients. *Community Mental Health Journal*, **50**:886–895.

Rugkåsa J, Molodynski A, Yeeles K, et al., the OCTET Group (2015). Community treatment orders: clinical and social outcomes, and a subgroup analysis from the OCTET RCT. *Acta Psychiatrica Scandinavica*, **131**:321–329.

Schwartz K, O'Brian AM, Morel V, et al. (2010). Community treatment orders: the service user speaks. exploring the lived experience of community treatment orders. *International Journal of Psychosocial Rehabilitation*, **15**:39–50. [Qualitative interviews with 6 service users on CTO in Ontario, Canada.]

Sen A (1992). *Inequality reexamined*. Oxford: Clarendon.

Stone A (1975). *Mental health and law: a system in transition*. Rockville, MD: NIMH Center for Studies of Crime and Delinquency.

Stroud J, Doughty K, Banks L (2013). *An exploration of service user and practitioner experiences of community treatment orders*. Executive Summary of Research. University of Brighton. [Qualitative interviews with 21 service users in Sussex, England.]

Stroud J, Banks L, Doughty K (2015). Community treatment orders: learning from experiences of service users, practitioners and nearest relatives. *Journal of Mental Health*, **24**:88–92. [Qualitative interviews with 21 service users in Sussex, England.]

Swanson JW, Swartz MS (2014). Why the evidence for outpatient commitment is good enough. *Psychiatric Services*, **65**:808–811.

Swartz MS, Swanson JW, Hannon MJ (2003a). Does fear of coercion keep people away from mental health treatment? Evidence from a survey of persons with schizophrenia and mental health professionals. *Behavioral Sciences and the Law*, **21**:459–472. [Survey of 104 individuals with schizophrenia spectrum conditions in Piedmont, North Carolina, USA.]

Swartz M, Swanson J, Wagner H, et al. (2003b). Assessment of four stakeholder groups' preferences concerning outpatient commitment for persons with schizophrenia. *American Journal of Psychiatry*, **160**:1139–1146. [Rated vignettes, compares views of four groups including persons in treatment for schizophrenia and related disorders in North Carolina, USA.]

Swartz M, Swanson J, Monahan J (2003c). Endorsement of personal benefit of outpatient commitment among persons with severe mental illness. *Psychology, Public Policy, and Law*, **9**(1/2):70–93. [North Carolina, USA.]

Swartz M, Wagner H, Swanson J, et al. (2004). Consumers' perceptions of the fairness and effectiveness of mandated community treatment and related pressures. *Psychiatric Services*,

55:780–785. [Structured interviews with 104 consumers treated for schizophrenia or similar in the USA.]

Szmukler G, Appelbaum P (2008). Treatment pressures, leverage, coercion and compulsion in mental health care. *Journal of Mental Health*, **17**:233–244.

Thøgersen M, Morthorst B, Nordentoft M (2010). Perceptions of coercion in the community: a qualitative study of patients in a Danish assertive community treatment team. *Psychiatric Quarterly*, **81**:35–47. [In-depth interviews with six patients in Danish assertive community teams.]

Watts J, Priebe S (2002). A phenomenological account of users' experiences of assertive community treatment. *Bioethics*, **16**:439–454.

Wertheimer A (1987). *Coercion*. Princeton, NJ: Princeton University Press.

Chapter 10

Family carers and coercion in the community

Jorun Rugkåsa

Caring is embedded in relationships of obligation such as marriage, parenthood, or kinship, in which people feel responsible for spouses, children, or parents and obliged to give care. These are not voluntary relationships, and these feelings of obligation have consequences for their lives.

Twigg and Atkin (1994, p. 10)

Introduction

Family members have always cared for those who are ill. In the absence of welfare states or health service systems, members of the family might be the sole source of help for many people with severe mental illness in many parts of the world. In the West, various studies indicate that around half of patients with severe and enduring mental illness live with their families (Hallam 2007; Fleury et al. 2008; Hughes et al. 2011) who are involved in helping and supporting them in different ways and to varying degrees. As the opening quote indicates, family caregiving forms part of normative cultural expectations and has emotional and social consequences. Chapters 15–20 illustrate how family life across the world constitutes part of the context within which people with mental illness can experience being influenced and pressured. Families also often have a role in the delivery of community-based services, including coercive interventions, and, as described later, their role in this regard is increasingly written into mental health policy and law.

The purpose of this chapter is to outline current knowledge about the role of the family in coercive practices in the community. Despite a substantive body of research on the experience of caring for an adult family member with severe mental illness, there is a remarkable lack of studies that specifically investigate how family members exert influence in ways that may be described as *informal coercion* (see Chapter 1) when they help a relative with medication, finances, housing, social activities, and so forth. While there are some studies of family involvement in assertive community services and in formal community coercion (such as the use of community treatment orders, CTOs) this is also limited (Kallert 2008). A literature search performed for the purposes of writing this chapter (using Ovid, Web of Science, MEDLINE, Sociological Abstract, Embase, and CINAHL) identified only a very small number of studies on formal or informal coercion, so I also draw on the more general literature on family caregivers in mental health which indirectly comment on these issues. I place particular emphasis on carers' own experiences (as opposed to how patients or health professionals perceive interventions by family members) and I investigate three dimensions of relevance to coercive practices. First, carers' interactions with the family member who is unwell; second, their involvement in community treatment; and third, the role attributed to family carers in welfare states. Throughout I comment on how family carers may be both at the giving and the receiving end of community coercion. In common with what is observed in other chapters of this volume, there is an almost complete lack of published research from outside Europe, North America, and Australasia.

I will refer to *family care* as help and support given beyond what is considered normal reciprocity among adults in a given cultural context (Twigg and Atkin 1994) and to *family carers* as those providing such support. As the topic of this chapter is coercion, it focuses attention on difficult aspects of family relationships. It is important to keep in mind that family carers—and those they care for—also describe affectionate and loving relationships even if these relationships at times are difficult to manage or be part of. The variation in the experiences of family carers is vast and impossible to do justice to in one chapter. Instead, I aim to extract some general themes of what is currently known that is of relevance to future research and clinical practice.

Family carers' interactions with an unwell relative

Family care as part of family life

Care situations often emerge gradually, sometimes over many years. Family members might observe uncharacteristic behaviours in their relative over time: people talking to themselves, becoming withdrawn, hearing voices, or displaying aggressive or suicidal behaviour. At the milder end of the spectrum, these symptoms are often understood as normal teenage behaviour or interpreted in the light of other culturally available explanations in an attempt to normalize that which can be frightening or hard understand (Johl et al. 2014; Rossen et al. 2014). Symptoms often become increasingly pronounced until the person eventually has a psychotic episode or it is otherwise clear that their problems are due to mental illness. Despite early signs, family members often experience the eventual diagnosis as a shock.

Emerging as it does within the context of families, the role of family carer is embedded in family life. For carers this does not represent a new relationship, but a continuation of enduring and consequential bonds (Johl et al. 2014) that touches on love, compassion, and identity as well as frustrations, sadness, and anger. During the initial period, the carer typically gradually takes on new tasks or responsibilities to help their relative. What mental health carers often describe as the dominant feature of their caregiving, however, is the emotional support involved in sharing one's life (Weimand et al. 2013). As we shall see, family carers' interactions with patients are shaped by different cultural models of what mental illness is and how it should be treated, and of family obligations. The role of family carer is thus simultaneously cultural, social, and deeply personal (Rugkåsa 2015).

Potentially coercive aspects of family care

The tasks that family carers do to support their ill relative may serve different functions. According to Keady and Nolan (2003) they may be:

- anticipatory,
- instrumental,
- preventative,
- supervisory,
- proactive, or
- preservative.

Many of these tasks may directly or indirectly influence or coerce the patient, or at least be perceived to do so. It is important to keep in mind, though, that attempts to influence each other occur in *all* families. We all 'try to shape each other's behaviour by suggesting, nagging, threatening, arguing, criticising, playing on feeling of obligation and guilt' (Greenley 1986, p. 25, quoted in Solomon 1996, p. 140). Given the ubiquitous presence of such social control mechanisms, it may be difficult to isolate dynamics that are specifically or directly related to mental illness. This may partly explain the lack of research on potentially coercive aspects of family care. From the more general literature on the experiences of family mental health caregiving, three broad interrelated themes of what family members perceive to be key tasks and which may include a coercive element can be identified.

Maintenance of 'normality' and autonomy

The overarching aim for many family carers is to create a stable environment which can protect the patient's 'normality' and autonomy as well as promote their wellbeing. Family carers often see it as their task to contribute to a positive social environment, meaningful activities, and the patient's sense of belonging (Monteiro et al. 2006; Villatoro and Aneshensel 2014). Substantial encouragement or pressure may be needed when the patient lacks motivation to engage socially (Rugkåsa 2015).

Sometimes family carers are intimately involved in many areas of patients' lives in ways they would not be with other relatives, such as looking after finances or medication. Conflicts between patients and their families often stem from disagreement about what is legitimate influencing behaviour within families and what constitutes a coercive action. Many family carers struggle to find a balance between too much involvement, which can undermine autonomy, and too little involvement, which can place patients in vulnerable positions that also, in turn, affect autonomy (Weimand et al. 2013; Rugkåsa 2015). Finding the optimal forms of influence that preserve autonomy and wellbeing while also being acceptable to all parties remains a challenge for many, particularly when situations fluctuate with the illness.

Control as protection

Family carers are frequently those who most closely observe such fluctuations and they are often affected when patients relapse (Lefley 1997). During these periods their unwell relative may reject support, neglect themselves, or even put themselves and others at risk. Agreed arrangements, deals, or boundaries might be broken, and family carers may need to deal with strained relationships, bad financial decisions, or huge credit card bills (Lefley 1997). In some cases violence or the threat of violence to themselves or other loved ones may be a real worry. To prevent or ease such situations, family carers may try to apply different forms of control (Saunders 2003). In practical terms, this could be ensuring that the patient eats and sleeps well and manages everyday tasks, accompanying them to make sure they keep medical appointments, or staying with them around the clock when they are upset, hallucinating, or suicidal. Some are involved in money management or in other ways set boundaries to help the patient maintain as much stability as possible.

Medication adherence is a common area of conflict between family carers and patients. They may disagree about the role that antipsychotics can play in remaining well and in control. Many carers routinely remind their relatives to take their medication (Gibbs et al. 2006). Some collect it at the pharmacy, administer it to the patient, or bring them to outpatient clinics to receive depot injections (Gibbs et al. 2004). To avoid upsetting the patient or risk damage to their relationship, some carers hide their communication with medical professionals, sometimes resorting to 'white lies' (Weimand et al. 2013). In other cases family carers tailor or limit the information they give about treatment or side effects to increase the likelihood of patients accepting it (Weimand et al. 2013). While some carers are concerned about unpleasant side effects of psychiatric medication or may doubt their utility, others have considerable faith in them. Some believe medicines could justifiably be smuggled into food or drinks to ensure they are taken (Hallam, 2007). In some countries, such surreptitious treatment by carers is reported as fairly routine and supervised by psychiatrists (Shah and Basu 2010).

Families often find effective ways of interacting with their relative during psychotic episodes, which in many cases may prevent the need for coercive service involvement. In acute situations when there is risk to health or safety, some 'try everything' to influence treatment adherence, including making implicit or explicit threats of contacting the police or the hospital (Solomon 1996; Mullen et al. 2006). Most mental health laws have provision for family to apply for legal compulsion. Initiating involuntary interventions is described by carers as a last resort, done in desperation as it is humiliating and painful for all concerned. Even so, involuntary treatment can represent an essential 'safety net' (Lefley 1997) or respite (Hallam 2007) for carers.

Severe mental illness is stigmatizing across cultural traditions, and legal compulsion (whether in hospital or the community) particularly so. Stigma and its consequences vary and are closely linked with cultural understandings of the aetiology and manifestation of mental illness. Stigmatization may affect the entire household or extended family and can impact on individual and family status, honour, employment opportunities, or marriage prospects (Shefer et al. 2013; Connor et al. 2014). Family carers therefore often experience a need to protect the patient, themselves, and sometimes the whole family from these effects and this may add pressure to the patient and to other family members alike. For example, there may be strong pressure to maintain secrecy about mental illness (Shefer et al. 2013), and this can lead to a high degree of social isolation (Connor et al. 2014; Johl et al. 2014; Rossen et al. 2014). Some may change or carefully frame what they say to others to make situations more socially acceptable, such as focusing on the physical aspects of the illness or saying that their relative has depression instead of schizophrenia (Monteiro et al. 2006). Some only accept home-based services to avoid disclosure.

Influence on help-seeking

Both an initial normalization of signs and symptoms and subsequent interventions by family to protect against stigma may delay presentation to services (Villatoro and Aneshensel 2014). A wide range of other social and cultural factors may also shape how families influence help-seeking (Wynaden et al. 2005). For example, those who understand mental illness as chemical imbalances in the brain and hold a strong belief in pharmaceutical solutions to redress these may influence or pressure patients to seek medical advice as soon as a problem is identified. If, however, mental illness is understood as spiritual or social imbalances resulting from witchcraft, spirit possessions, or misconduct by the patient or her ancestors, addressing symptoms with psychiatric medication may not take highest priority (Monteiro et al. 2006). While medication is often considered complementary to other forms of addressing the issues at stake, those who do not share Western perceptions of mental illness may not direct their relative towards medical services at all (Lavender et al. 2006). Other cultural factors can also affect help-seeking, such as the common portrayal in the media of overly coercive psychiatric services with excessive medication, straitjackets, or other forms of constraint (Monteiro et al. 2006). Familial pressure may thus lead away from as well as towards different forms of treatment, and the family's role in help-seeking can be a consequence of wider cultural influence as well as individual preference (Villatoro and Aneshensel 2014).

Potential for coercive practices to damage family relationships

Many family carers express that they do not wish to attach conditions to the support they offer their relative. This would constitute a breach of family values of unconditional support and can also damage trust and undermine the relationship (Canvin et al. 2014; Rugkåsa 2015). Carers may, however, face competing demands, such as when repeated relapses create chaotic circumstances for other family members for whom they also hold responsibility (Lefley 1997; Weimand et al. 2013): should one continue to expose everyone to a problematic situation or would it be better to impose some limits or conditions on the patient or even evict (and possibly alienate) them? Involuntary admissions or community compulsion may be safeguards in such situations, but if initiated by carers this may also endanger relationships (Shefer et al. 2013; Rugkåsa 2015). With today's service emphasis on short admissions, family carers may also find that an admitted patient is discharged within days, still symptomatic but with added feelings of anger and alienation (Lefley 1997). Also, if a family carer's approach to services does not lead to hospitalization, this has in some cases been found to increase the risk of violence (Hallam 2007). Indeed, one study reported that when an assault on a carer has occurred, attempts to place limits on their unwell relative have frequently preceded it (Straznickas 1993, quoted in Lefley 1997). Being involved in interventions that the patient objects to can damage or have detrimental effects on family relationships (Mullen et al. 2006). To reduce such risks to relationships and people, family carers often avoid confrontation or criticism and try to calm and sooth patients rather than imposing limits (Lefley 1997) and to conduct any monitoring as discreetly as possible (Weimand et al. 2013). When considering using informal coercion or initiating legal compulsion carers need to weigh up a range of issues: 'they must balance the indignity to their loved one against his or her own self-destructive behaviour, threats to themselves and others, and the very real possibility that their relative will be arrested, severely neglect himself or herself, or even die on the streets' (Lefley 1997, p.9).

The burden of family care

The effects of family caregiving are well documented. Sleep disturbance, fatigue, ill-health, absence of reward, guilt, loneliness, family conflict, isolation, stigma, and loss of income or opportunities for paid work have all been reported (Saunders 2003; Jones 2004; Werner et al. 2010; Johl et al. 2014). Some live with fear that patients will threaten or carry out physical abuse during bad phases, and some have reported going to extreme measures such as barricading their bedroom door to feel safe at night (Hallam 2007). There is an extensive international literature on the 'burden' of family caregiving based on research instruments developed to measure and compare it, some of which are designed for specific cultural contexts or care situations.[1]

While providing important data on the extent of the consequences of family caregiving, these pre-defined measures may fail to detect how carers themselves perceive their situation (Wynaden 2007). For example, patients' lack of motivation, poor sleep, and diet have, maybe surprisingly, been identified by some carers as more disruptive than their violence, drug, or alcohol use (Saunders 2003). Qualitative work has found that the emotional impact of a temporary or permanent change to social relationships is particularly hard to deal with (Johl et al. 2014; Rugkåsa 2015), such as when an equal relationship between two adults changes into one more like that of parent and child (Perry 2002). Similarly, broken expectations for the future may be a burden, such as knowing that a loved one will never be able to marry or have a family of their own (Adamson and Donovan 2005; Ahmed and Jones 2010).

Despite the widespread use of instruments measuring caregiving burden, there are almost no studies that measure the impact on carers when a family member is treated under community compulsion. The North Carolina RCT (see Chapter 5) is an exception as it did investigate carer strain. It found no difference between those caring for someone under a CTO and those caring for a voluntary patient. When analysing

---

[1] Examples include the Family Burden Interview Schedule (Pai and Kapur 1981), the Threshold Parental Burden Questionnaire (Cook and Pickett 1988), the Role Overload Scale (Pearlin et al. 1990), and the Caregiver Burden Scale (Montgomery 2002).

non-randomized samples (including patients with a history of violence who were all on CTOs), a significant difference was found (Groff et al. 2004), but this might reflect the effect of violent behaviour or selection bias and not the CTO itself. A Swedish controlled before and after study failed to find any difference in family burden between those caring for someone admitted voluntarily or involuntarily (Östman and Hansson 2000), and another Swedish study did not find any association between caregiver burden and violence (Kjellin and Östman 2005). Small cross-sectional studies in the UK and Australia also found no association between compulsory treatment and caregiving burden (Boydell et al. 2014; Vine and Komiti 2015), but carers of those under compulsion identified more problems with services (Boydell et al. 2014).

Family carers' involvement in coercive community treatment

The role of family carers in health-care systems

The deinstitutionalization of mental health services in many countries has shifted a significant proportion of the day-to-day care of patients onto their families. This policy move is thus to some extent premised on unpaid work, mostly by women, in their own homes (Reay-Young 2001) and relies on cultural obligations for family members to look after one another (Adamson and Donovan 2005; Johl et al. 2014). The way in which the family is portrayed in psychiatric theory and practice has also changed from a potential part of the problem to a definite part of the solution. Today, ideas linking family dysfunction and mental illness (Laing and Esterson 1964; Lidz et al. 1965) are less prominent even if links between *expressed emotion* in families and mental illness remains a topic of research (Healey et al. 2006). Expressed emotion is also identified as a potential source of informal coercion by the family (Mullen et al. 2006). Today there is more focus on families' role in treatment (such as through family interventions), as partners in service delivery, or on their home as a locus for community care. A changed relationship between family carers and health professionals is reflected in public policy in many countries, with it encouraging or even requiring family involvement (Brand 2001; Mullen et al. 2006; Hallam 2007). There are studies reporting associations between family involvement and improved patient engagement (Weine et al. 2005; Fischer et al. 2008) and professionals are now explicitly encouraged to view family caregivers as integral to health-care systems, to involve them in service delivery, and to recognize their *carer expertise* (Department of Health 2008a).

In many cases this works well, with a real partnership between family carers and health professionals (Weimand et al. 2011). A fairly substantial literature, however, demonstrates the difficulties in achieving this (Eassom et al. 2014) and mental health carers in many countries are often very dissatisfied with how they are involved. Their role remains ill-defined and family carers often feel marginalized and undervalued, or that their views and experience go unrecognized despite their intimate knowledge of a patient's circumstances and changing needs (Brand 2001; Rapaport et al. 2006; Jankovic et al. 2011; Simmons et al. 2011; Outram et al. 2015). Disagreements between families and professionals are not uncommon (Macpherson et al. 2008), and carers report that the 'shared' nature of decision making is inadequate, sometimes to the extent that it may leave patients at risk (Colombo 2008). A great deal of conflict relates to patients' rights to confidentiality and carers' wishes be involved and to help (Gibbs et al. 2004). Accusations have been made that professionals hide behind confidentiality issues as a means of marginalizing carers (Rapaport et al. 2006; Hallam 2007). When patient capacity fluctuates, these issues become even more complex, and the community context can sometimes add to this. For example, a Scottish mother of a patient on a CTO found it frustrating that despite being her son's day-to-day carer she was not informed about treatment activities that happened in her own living room (Ridley et al. 2010).

The ways in which family members are involved in services vary in different parts of the world. The prioritization of patient autonomy in Western health care is not necessarily shared by other traditions, where collective family goals are given more emphasis (Shah and Basu 2010). To have someone other than the patient making decisions is, for example, 'part and parcel of the illness experience in India, one that carries important symbolic implications with regard to one's place in society and one's spiritual well-being' (Nunley 1988, p. 325). From such a perspective, a devaluation of family is perceived as a potentially negative effect of the Western mental health system. In many parts of India it is required that a family member resides with a hospitalized patient and this is perceived to provide for better overall care. Family carers make sure the patient remains in the hospital, they cook for them, and assist with personal hygiene. They are a key source of information for clinicians. Families are also closely involved in outpatient care, often ensuring that patients take their medication (Kar and Tiwari 2014), and in systems where medical records are not in regular use, psychiatrists often depend on a patient's family to obtain information about them. Nunley's (1988) study from India suggested that, confidentiality is less of a concern there than in many Western coutries, in particular regarding intrafamilial information. Similar practices with extensive family involvement and control have been observed in settings as diverse as Papa New Guinea, Cameroon, and Japan (Nunley 1988). In South Korea, patients' families have an even stronger position in that they not only have the right to request an involuntary hospitalization, they also have the authority to determine it (Lee and Park 2014). It has been suggested that the prevailing notion within Western psychiatry of autonomous individuals (as opposed to autonomous families) has prevented the discipline from gaining a firm foothold in cultural traditions where familial interdependence is a strongly held value (Nunley 1988).

Carer experience with coercive community interventions

In general, family carers seem to welcome the development of community-based services (the findings of one Korean study being an exception; Lee and Park 2014) that involves more assertive delivery models and increased use of outpatient compulsion if this means improved services for patients. They particularly want to find ways to prevent patients from fully relapsing before services intervene (Lefley 1997; Ridley et al. 2010). A handful of studies that describe carers' experiences of assertive services and of formal compulsion in the community (CTOs) identify overall support, but also a range of difficulties in implementation.

Informal practices: assertive community treatment

Community service models, such as assertive community treatment (ACT) involve active intervention and monitoring of patients' adherence and functioning in the community, and many of the related activities take place in the patient's home environment. Originally, the ACT model was directed towards patients with no family or little contact with them. This may partly explain the limited research on family caregiving and ACT (Weimand et al. 2014). Variations of the ACT model (e.g. family-assisted ACT) involve patients' families performing many of the monitoring task such as ensuring medication is taken. These also seek to modify behaviour vis-à-vis the patient that is perceived to prevent recovery and includes, among other things, structured educational sessions for the family (McFarlane et al. 1992). Studies have shown that this approach improves patient outcomes (Petersen et al. 2005), for example in terms of employment (McFarlane et al. 1996).

In general, family caregivers seem to value the ACT approach. A UK study found that it was experienced as helpful to patients as well as being less imposing and more attuned to family needs than standard services (Hughes et al. 2011). A small study in Norway reported mixed experiences of carer involvement, but carers still found ACT to be superior in that regard compared with other services (Weimand et al. 2014). Many caregivers seem to find the authoritative role of the ACT team helpful even if their relative does not like it. This is partly because the authority of staff means family carers do not need to risk damaging family relationships by setting or enforcing limits when there is a need to control medication adherence or financial or other behaviour (Hughes et al. 2011). The taking on of some of these responsibilities by staff may explain why the ACT approach has been found to reduce carer burden and stress (Jeppesen et al. 2005; Hughes et al. 2011). Family carers also perceive that ACT leads to clinical improvement in patients, increased independence, and more participation in meaningful activities (Gault 2009; Hughes et al. 2011; Weimand et al. 2014). ACT has not been found to improve carers' knowledge of mental illness (Jeppesen et al. 2005).

Formal community coercion: CTOs

A role for family carers in the planning and execution of formal community coercion is usually written into mental health legislation, often in their capacity of 'nearest relative'.[2] The implementation of the law is thus premised on the participation of family in the coercion of patients. For example, the code of practice accompanying the CTO legislation for England and Wales specifies their role in supervising patients:

> Particular attention should be paid to carers and relatives when they raise a concern that the patient is not complying with the conditions or that the patient's mental health appears to be deteriorating. The team responsible for the patient needs to give due weight to those concerns and any requests made by the carers or relatives in deciding what action to take. Carers and relatives are typically in much more frequent contact with the patient than

---

[2] Various terms are used in legal frameworks (e.g. nearest relative, next of kin, named person) to identify a person with specified rights to make decisions in relation to patient care, including in some instances proxy decisions when the patient lacks capacity.

professionals, even under well-run care plans. Their concerns may prompt a review of how [the CTO] is working for that patient and whether the criteria for recall to hospital might be met. The managers of responsible hospitals should ensure that local protocols are in place to cover how concerns raised should be addressed and taken forward.

Department of Health (2008b, paragraph 25.46)

While family carers in general seem to support the intentions behind CTOs, the literature on their experiences of them shows a mixed picture. For some, the specific role allocated to them in the administration of the CTO has led to increased involvement and influence over decisions (Hallam 2007; Ridley et al. 2010; Stroud et al. 2015). Many see their involvement as potentially contributing to how CTOs may work, particularly through providing everyone involved with the right information at the right time. Some find that their views are taken more seriously, and that help during crises is more forthcoming (Mullen et al. 2006; Ridley et al. 2010; Stroud et al. 2015). The existence of an order is thought to direct attention to the duty of the services to provide care (Gibbs et al. 2006; Ridley et al. 2010) and to intervene earlier when someone relapses, serving as a safety net (Canvin et al. 2014; Stroud et al. 2015). This is not a universal experience, however, as some family carers find that rapid readmission means CTO patients actually receive less therapeutic attention which, in turn, can increase the demand on their family (Hallam 2007). Also, demands on beds mean patients can be discharged onto CTOs prematurely with the expectations that the family is ready and able to look after them (Lefley 1997; Hallam 2007). Such gaps between theory and practice, resulting in the responsibility for patients remaining with carers (Ridley et al. 2010) has raised concern that CTOs in some cases mean family carers become de facto responsible for the administration of involuntary treatment (Mullen et al. 2006).

Studies in New Zealand and the UK report that many family carers have not been consulted or involved in the CTO process in the ways required by law (Gibbs et al. 2004; Owens and Brophy 2013). Many carers describe a lack of adequate consultation, that their views are ignored, and/or that they are not given adequate information (Gibbs et al. 2006; Hallam, 2007; Ridley et al. 2010; Canvin et al. 2014). Some find it unreasonable to expect that they should remember details about how the legislation works (Hallam 2007). A lack of understanding of legal regimes has been observed, (Canvin et al. 2014; Stroud et al. 2015) which also has implications for how carers are involved.

While being a 'nearest relative' can increase involvement, patients may exercise their right to revoke such a role. Carers have reported that their involvement as a result depends on them agreeing with the patient's judgements (Ridley et al. 2010). Conversely, refusing to take on this role may equally harm the relationship (Hallam 2007). In both events, carers are prevented from letting their view have an impact on decisions.

While some family carers monitor compliance with medication and other CTO conditions and communicate closely with the team about the need for recall to hospital (Stroud et al. 2015), others express relief that responsibility for medication is taken from them (Gibbs et al. 2006; Mullen et al. 2006; Hallam 2007) so that they can focus on being a mother or a father (Canvin et al. 2014). Knowing that a CTO is in place provides some with a sense of security, reduced stress, and increased stability (Ridley et al. 2010) even if it does not necessarily lead to a better relationship with the patient. Indeed some say that their involvement with the order has an adverse effect on family relationships (Mullen et al. 2006). As such, involvement with legal coercion can sometimes place family members in adversarial positions vis-à-vis each other (Lefley 1997; Kallert 2008).

In general, family carers seem to find CTOs useful insofar as they improve treatment adherence. Many of them perceive CTOs to have this effect (Mullen et al. 2006; Canvin et al. 2014; Vine and Komiti 2015) and they explain this as being due to patients' respect for the law and/or the threat of readmission (Mullen et al. 2006; Canvin et al. 2014; Stroud et al. 2015). Medication adherence is commonly viewed by carers as the key justification for the order. A number of studies report that carers are concerned that this focus on medication is too narrow and that CTOs fail to help people more widely, to live better lives, or to recover (Gibbs et al. 2004; Canvin et al. 2014). Family carers in Australia, for example, found that a CTO did not improve access to case management or accommodation (Hallam 2007). When discussing whether they think CTOs work, many carers seem to struggle to distinguish the effect of the coercion from that of the service model (often ACT). Some UK carers raised the concern that perhaps CTOs were not needed because intensive services could achieve the same on their own in terms of patient engagement and adherence (Gault 2009; Canvin et al. 2014).

It has been suggested that it is possible to reduce the use of formal coercion (particularly hospital detention) by increasing the involvement of family carers (Clarke 2010), especially during discharge planning (Gibbs et al. 2004; Nurjannah et al. 2014), which is what many carers ask for (Wilkinson and McAndrew 2008; Ridley et al. 2010; Outram et al. 2015). This would depend on family carers having the information and skills to deal with mental illness. There is, however, considerable unmet need with regard to providing family carers with the support or information they need (Rapaport et al. 2006).

Services pressurizing carers—carers pressurizing services

Some studies indicate that services or interventions which seek to influence patients in effect also pressurize or leverage their families. For example in the USA, avoidance of jail for some patients who instead come on a CTO is sometimes contingent on their relatives participating in family therapy (Lefley 1997). It may be difficult for carers to decline this due to the consequences for the patient. Other examples, reported from the UK, include how services rely on family carers to gain access to patients who do not wish to see clinicians. A patient may be more likely to pick up the phone or open the door if approached by a family member, and family may even be able to trespass in ways professionals cannot (Rugkåsa 2015). While serving as an access point may be important so that the patient is seen by clinicians, being seen to be in 'cahoots' with health professionals may be risky for carers. Some experience that professionals are keen for them to sign papers initiating involuntary treatment because it makes the process easier. In such situations, family carers who are eager for their relative to get treatment may experience little choice despite the potential for damage to relationships.

As mentioned, the influence that family carers experience in interactions with services varies greatly. In the study from India referred to earlier, the patient's family could to a large extent decide which clinical recommendations were put into practice. Families in many contexts thus retain considerable power (Nunley 1988). Such gate-keeping functions are also reported elsewhere, as we saw earlier regarding help-seeking. Concern has been raised that the recent Mental Health Care Bill in India could, by increasing the remit for community compulsion, decrease caregivers' trust in services and trigger them to increasingly divert patients to traditional healers (Kar and Tiwari 2014).

A few studies show that family carers may attempt to influence or leverage services when it is difficult to obtain assistance for a patient. Some carers even make threats (e.g. to involve the media) or make formal complaints in order for the patient to get help or to be taken seriously. Some say they resort to deceit in order to ensure patients get the treatment they need (Hallam 2007). It has been anecdotally reported from Philadelphia, USA, that some family carers in a desperate attempt to get treatment for their relative obtain a restraining order though the court to bar them from the family home. Violation of the order can then lead to arrest and detention in jail where the patient receives treatment (Solomon 1996).

Some family carers experience that they are pushed out or allowed less involvement during crises, which is precisely when they perhaps feel an extra urgency about being involved (Cleary et al. 2006). During such periods, however, patients sometimes distance themselves from their family and may inform health professionals that they do not wish family carers to be present or informed. How to integrate carer involvement and patient confidentiality is a recognized problem, and carers commonly express that health professionals lack the willingness to find ways around these issues (Rugkåsa 2015). A review of policies in England about how to involve carers when patients withhold consent for their involvement found that of 56 policies and 35 supporting documents, only one in five specifically addressed information-sharing and only one in 20 gave practical advice (Slade et al. 2007). So despite the current policy drive towards carer involvement, local practice seems to remain guarded. From a carer's perspective, this may be experienced as a coercive intervention in family life.

While many carers feel forced out of involvement, it is important to note that some family carers also want to be *less* involved in the care of their relative, especially with regard to the monitoring of medication. They may, however, fear that the available services are insufficient for it to be safe for them to take a step back (Rugkåsa 2015). Some, particularly where community services are limited, therefore do more than they feel is right, or that they have the resources to, because of a lack of alternatives: 'families feel coerced by a system that offers inadequate resources and makes it difficult to save persons during a critical period when they are perceived as incapable of saving themselves' (Lefley 1997, p. 9).

Family cares and the welfare state

From relative to 'carer'

Labelling the assistance that family members provide for one another as 'care' and those performing it as 'carers' is a relatively new development within welfare states and is mostly lacking in countries where this contribution is less formalized. The UK provides an example of a particularly pronounced politicization or professionalization of caregiving within families. The carer role was first recognized in law in The Carers (Recognition and Services) Act 1995 which ensured carers the right to an assessment of their support needs. The Carers and Disabled Children Act 2000 then placed a duty on local authorities to inform carers of this right and introduced an additional right to a written plan for how to meet assessed need. A national carers' strategy (Department of Health 2008a) set out the direction for carer involvement and highlighted the importance of recognizing carers' expertise across health and social services. In a number of countries, eligible family carers are entitled to financial compensation, a process that has been described as a 'commodification of care' (Ungerson 1997). This manifests differently across welfare states. In Scandinavia, where carers' contribution is considered work, payment can be substantial, whereas in Britain, where care primarily is considered a family responsibility, payment is modest or even symbolic (Knijn and Kremer 1997). By offering payment, family care is portrayed as somehow conducted on behalf of the state. Family obligations are thus linked to citizenship. In this way, modern welfare states have used legal and policy frameworks to convert aspects of the traditional roles of mothers, fathers, sisters, or other relatives into the role of 'carer' with specified rights and obligations attached. This can be seen as a form of reciprocal transaction with the state, one that can be said to be voluntary only to a limited extent (Rugkåsa 2015). It seems, therefore, that 'the very acceptance of the label of carer represents a transition in one's status vis-à-vis the state' (Keywood 2003, p. 356).

Despite these policy developments of state support, few UK carers receive what they are entitled to (Rapaport et al. 2006; Milne and Larkin 2015). This is a particular issue for mental health carers, even if many of them do not qualify for statutory support because the care they provide is not constant but fluctuates with the illness. Many also remain unaware of their rights (Wilkinson and McAndrew 2008) or do not recognize or adopt the title of carer but see themselves primarily as mothers, sisters, husband, or wives (Ridley et al. 2010; Johl et al. 2014; Milne and Larkin 2015). To the extent that they exist, support services to family carers are in general delivered by the voluntary sector and are therefore organizationally divorced from services to patients (Rapaport et al. 2006). This may represent a missed opportunity to provide comprehensive services for families affected by mental illness.

Competing roles: family carers and mental health legislation

Carer involvement is, as already mentioned, written into the laws governing coerced treatment both in hospital and in the community. Three partly overlapping roles for carers in the administration of such law have been identified (Keywood 2003). First, carers act as 'gatekeepers' in that they often monitor patients and decide when professional intervention (including coercion) is required. Second, carers serve as a 'proxy' for patients without capacity. Third, carers are portrayed as 'advocates' working in partnership with professionals and in the interests of patients by representing their wishes. As we have seen throughout this chapter, there is potential for these three roles to conflict with each other and with other roles that family carers have and value. For example, the role of a gatekeeper initiating compulsion may conflict with the role of 'mother' and may damage family relationships. The role of 'proxy', often as a 'nearest relative' may in practice only be possible if the family carer supports the patient's views, which may exclude the input of the 'expert carer' which is also envisaged to be essential for the delivery of community care. Being an effective 'advocate' depends on the carer having considerable knowledge and voice. While some want this, others find it unreasonable that they should be the ones to ensure that legal regimes are used optimally. A general lack of information, sometimes impeded by issues of confidentiality, can also prevent effective family advocacy.

Future areas for research

For family carers, the wellbeing of the patient and the family unit is their highest priority, even if it comes at a considerable cost. The nature of the tasks they do shows how their role may add pressure to the patient, but also how caregiving is understood as inseparable from wider family life. These tasks revolve around safety, control, reputation management, and keeping families together, as well as improving the health and quality of life and increasing the autonomy of the patient. These concerns display a strong sense of interconnectedness between caregiver and care recipient underpinned by fundamental relationships of obligation and emotion.

Family carers want good services for their relatives. As we have seen, carers are in different ways involved in the limit setting and coercion of patients by services in the community setting. Both assertive outreach services and CTOs are usually valued by family carers if it means patients get good services. There seems, however, to be a long way to go before services interact with family carers in a way that both parties experience as useful and respectful.

The way in which family carers are involved in pressurizing or coercing patients, either as part of family life or via their involvement with services, varies between and within societies. Future comparative analysis might shed new light on the role of carers in the interaction between informal and formal community coercion. The current evidence regarding the role of family carers in community coercive treatment is scarce, and the scope and quality of existing studies vary greatly. We particularly need further research from countries where formal health services or mental health legislation is lacking or in development.

The very limited literature on family carers and community coercion to date tends to focus either on (1) family interactions or the burden on family carers, (2) the (often difficult) interactions with health professionals, or (3) the role of the family carer as expressed in policy and law. In this chapter I have tried to shed light on how these three dimensions to the caregiving role may mutually influence one another so that carers engage in processes where they simultaneously may coerce others and be coerced themselves. These interactions are in turn connected to cultural, social, and personal features of care situations. Further research is needed to obtain a fuller understanding of the role of families in community coercion. In the meantime, family carers everywhere will continue to look after some of the most vulnerable among us.

References

Adamson J, Donovan J (2005). 'Normal disruption': South Asian and African/Caribbean relatives caring for an older family member in the UK. *Social Science and Medicine*, 60:37–48.

Ahmed N, Jones IR (2010). 'Habitus and bureaucratic routines', cultural and structural factors in the experience of informal care. *Current Sociology*, 56:57–76.

Boydell J, Onwumere J, Dutta R, et al. (2014). Caregiving in first-episode psychosis: social characteristics associated with perceived 'burden' and associations with compulsory treatment. *Early Intervention in Psychiatry*, 8:122–129.

Brand U (2001). European perspectives: a carer's view. *Acta Psychiatrica Scandinavica*, 104:96–101.

Canvin K, Rugkåsa J, Sinclair J, et al. (2014). Patient, psychiatrist and family carer experiences of community treatment orders: qualitative study. *Social Psychiatry and Psychiatric Epidemiology*, 49:1873–1882.

Clarke L (2010). Prevention of coercion in public mental health with family group conferencing. *Journal of Psychiatric and Mental Health Nursing*, 17:846–848.

Cleary M, Freeman A, Walter G (2006). Carer participation in mental health service delivery. *International Journal of Mental Health Nursing*, 15:189–194.

Colombo A (2008). Models of mental disorder: how philosophy and the social sciences can illuminate psychiatric ethics. In: *Empirical ethics in psychiatry* (ed. G Widdershoven, J McMillan, T Hope, et al.), pp. 69–94. Oxford: Oxford University Press.

Connor C, Greenfield S, Lester H, et al. (2014). Seeking help for first-episode psychosis: a family narrative. *Early Intervention in Psychiatry*. doi: 10.1111/eip.12177

Cook JA, Pickett SA (1988). Feelings of burden and criticalness among parents residing with chronically mentally ill offspring. *Journal of Applied Social Science*, 12:79–107.

Department of Health (2008a). *Caring at the heart of 21st century families and communities: a caring system on your side, a life of your own*. London: Department of Health.

Department of Health (2008b). *Code of Practice: Mental Health Act 1983*. London: Stationery Office.

Eassom E, Giacco D, Dirik A, et al. (2014). Implementing family involvement in the treatment of patients with psychosis: a systematic review of facilitating and hindering factors. *BMJ Open*, 4(10):e006108.

Fischer EP, McSweeney JC, Pyne JM, et al. (2008). Influence of family involvement and substance use on sustained utilization of services for schizophrenia. *Psychiatric Services*, 59:902–908.

Fleury MJ, Grenier G, Caron J, et al. (2008). Patients' report of help provided by relatives and services to meet their needs. *Community Mental Health Journal*, 44:271–281.

Gault I (2009). Service-user and carer perspectives on compliance and compulsory treatment in community mental health services. *Health and Social Care in the Community*, 17:504–513.

Gibbs A, Dawson J, Forsyth H, et al (2004). Maori experience of community treatment orders in Otago, New Zealand. *Australian and New Zealand Journal of Psychiatry*, 38:830–835.

Gibbs A, Dawson J, Mullen R (2006). Community treatment orders for people with serious mental illness: a New Zealand study. *British Journal of Social Work*, 36:1085–1100.

Groff A, Burns B, Swanson J, et al. (2004). Caregiving for persons with mental illness: the impact of outpatient commitment on caregiving strain. *Journal of Nervous and Mental Disease*, 192:554–562.

Hallam L (2007). How involuntary commitment impacts on the burden of care of the family. *International Journal of Mental Health Nursing*, **16**:247–256.

Healey F, Tan VL, Chong SA (2006). Cross-cultural validation of expressed emotion in caregivers of Chinese patients with first episode psychosis in Singapore: a qualitative study. *International Journal of Social Psychiatry*, **52**:199–213.

Hughes H, Meddings S, Vandrevala T, et al. (2011). Carers' experiences of assertive outreach services: an exploratory study. *Journal of Mental Health*, **20**:70–78.

Jankovic J, Yeeles K, Katsakou C, et al. (2011). Family caregivers' experiences of involuntary psychiatric hospital admissions of their relatives—a qualitative study. *PloS One*, **6**:e25425.

Jeppesen P, Petersen L, Thorup A, et al. (2005). Integrated treatment of first-episode psychosis: effect of treatment on family burden. *British Journal of Psychiatry*, **187**(Suppl.):s85–s90.

Johl N, Patterson T, Pearson L (2014). What do we know about the attitudes, experiences and needs of Black and minority ethnic carers of people with dementia in the United Kingdom? A systematic review of empirical research findings. *Dementia*, doi: 10.1177/1471301214534424.

Jones DW (2004). Families and serious mental illness: working with loss and ambivalence. *British Journal of Social Work*, **34**:361–387.

Kallert TW (2008). Coercion in psychiatry. *Current Opinion in Psychiatry*, **21**:485–489.

Kar SK, Tiwari R (2014). Impact of Mental Health Care Bill on caregivers of mentally ill: boon or bane. *Asian Journal of Psychiatry*, **12**:3–6.

Keady J, Nolan M (2003). The dynamics of dementia: working together, working separately or working alone? In: *The dynamics of dementia: working together, working separately or working alone?* (ed. M Nolan, U Lundh, G Grant, et al.), pp. 15–32. Maidenhead: Open University Press.

Keywood K (2003). Gatekeepers, proxies, advocates? The evolving role of carers under mental health and mental incapacity law reforms. *Family Law*, **24**:355–368.

Kjellin L, Östman M (2005). Relatives of psychiatric inpatients—do physical violence and suicide attempts of patients influence family burden and participation in care? *Nordic Journal of Psychiatry*, **59**:7–11.

Knijn T, Kremer M (1997). Gender and the caring dimension of welfare states: towards inclusive citizenship. *Social Politics*, **4**:328–361.

Laing RD, Esterson A (1964). *Sanity, madness and the family*. London: Penguin.

Lavender H, Khondoker AH, Jones R (2006). Understandings of depression: an interview study of Yoruba, Bangladeshi and White British people. *Family Practice*, **23**:651–658.

Lee MS, Park JI (2014). Caregivers' acceptance of alternatives to long-term psychiatric hospitalization; lessons and debates from the South Korean situation. *International Journal of Mental Health Systems*, **8**(1):4.

Lefley HP (1997). Mandatory treatment from the family's perspective. *New Directions for Mental Health Services*, **1997**(75):7–16.

Lidz T, Fleck S, Cornelison A (1965). *Schizophrenia and the family*. Boston, MA: International Universities Press.

McFarlane WR, Dushay RA, Stastny P, et al. (1996). A comparison of two levels of family-aided assertive community treatment. *Psychiatric Services*, **47**:744–750.

McFarlane WR, Stastny P, Deakins S (1992). Family-aided assertive community treatment: a comprehensive rehabilitation and intensive case management approach for persons with schizophrenic disorders. *New Directions for Mental Health Services*, **1992**(53):43–54.

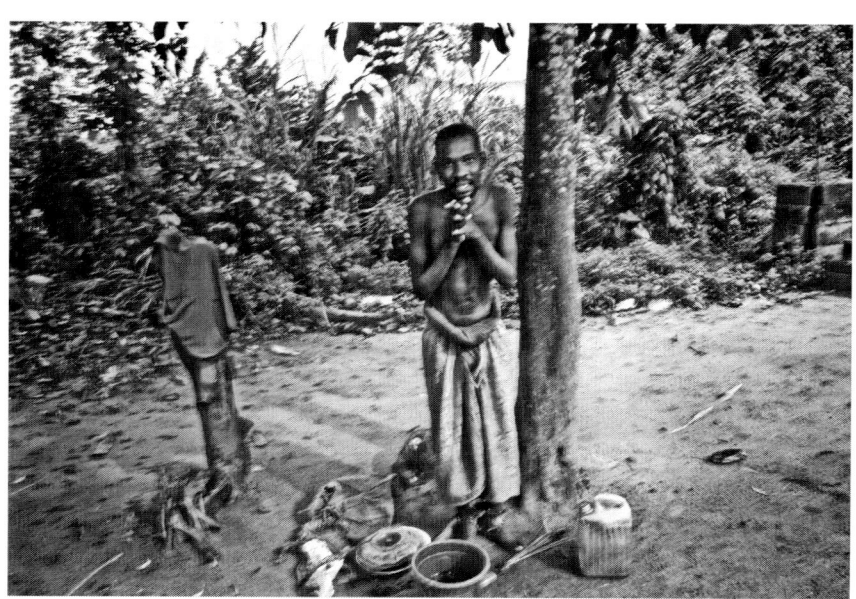

Figure 19.1 A native doctor claims to heal mental illness through the power of prayer and traditional herbal medicines. While receiving treatment, which can sometimes take months, his patients are chained to trees in his courtyard. They are not given shelter or protection from the elements. They are visibly terrified of the doctor. Away from the doctor the patients beg the photographer for food. They say they are only fed once a day, sometimes only once every 3 days. One cries and says how cold he gets and that he is attacked by mosquitoes every night. His body is covered in bites. He says they are sometimes beaten for no reason and if a piece of fruit falls from the tree and they try to eat it they are beaten. In regions where both fortune and sickness are attributed to the spirit world, mental illness is considered a curse. Spiritual remedies are often sought, and chains regularly used as restraints. The Niger Delta, Nigeria. October 2012. Photo Robin Hammond/Panos.

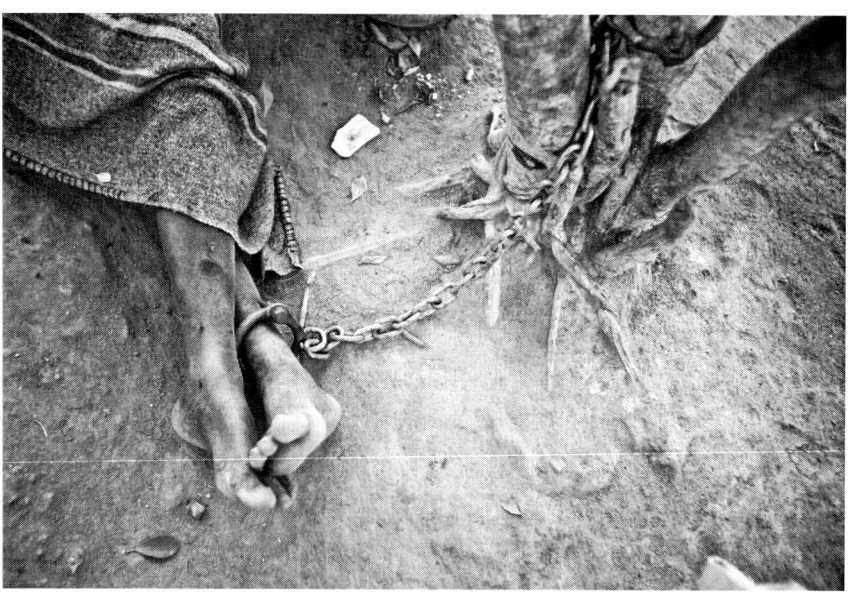

Figure 19.2 Men and women with mental illness and/or intellectual disability are shackled and locked away in Juba Central Prison for years on end. The new nation of South Sudan faces a tremendous challenge to build a modern country capable of caring for all of its citizens. Juba, Sudan. January 2011. Photo Robin Hammond/Panos.

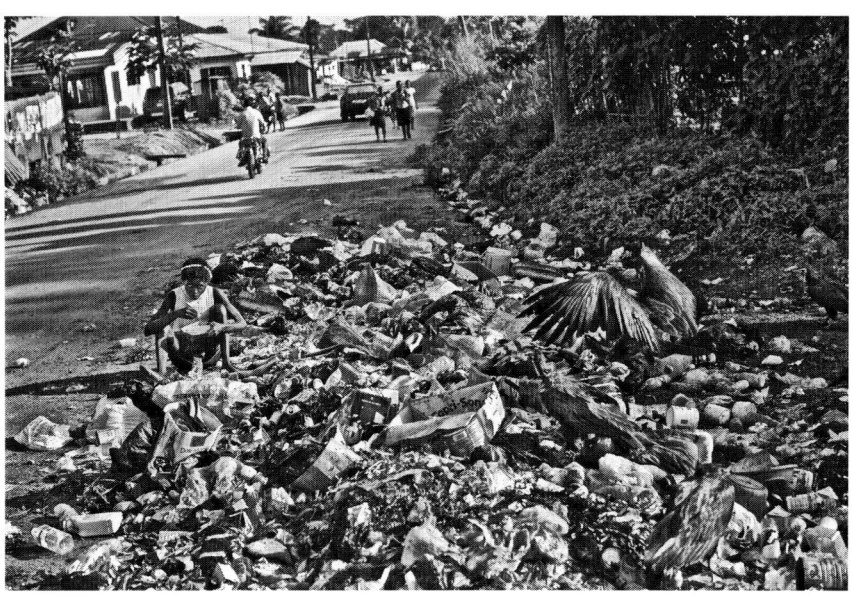
Figure 21.1 Mental health is not a priority to the state government of the Niger Delta. Many people with mental illness and/or intellectual disability are abandoned to the streets where they wander searching for food and shelter. The Niger Delta, Nigeria. October 2012. Photo Robin Hammond/Panos.

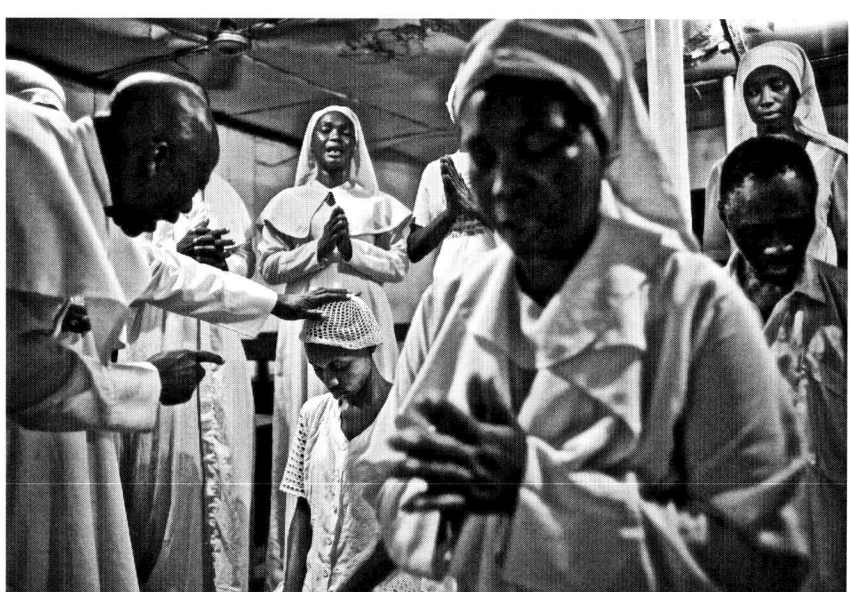

Figure 21.2 Christ's Universal Spiritual Hospital claims, through the power of prayer, to be able to heal mental illness. In a society that cannot trust government organizations, churches have become a sanctuary from the perceived wickedness and greed of the modern culture. In regions where both fortune and sickness are attributed to the spirit world, mental illness is considered a curse. Spiritual remedies are often sought. The Niger Delta, Nigeria. October 2012. Photo Robin Hammond/Panos.

Macpherson R, Collins-Atkins C, Gregory N, et al. (2008). The relationships between user, carer and staff perceptions of need in an assertive outreach team. *Journal of Mental Health*, 17:452–461.

Milne A, Larkin M (2015). Knowledge generation about care-giving in the UK: a critical review of research paradigms. *Health and Social Care in the Community*, 23:4–13.

Monteiro VB, dos Santos JQ, Martin D (2006). Patients' relatives delayed help seeking after a first psychotic episode. *Revista Brasileira de Psiquiatria*, 28:104–110.

Montgomery RJV (2002). *Using and interpreting the Montgomery Borgatta Caregiving Burden Scale*. Available at: http://www4.uwm.edu/hbssw/PDF/Burden%20Scale.pdf (accessed 27 March 2015).

Mullen R, Gibbs A, Dawson J (2006). Family perspective on community treatment orders: a New Zealand study. *International Journal of Social Psychiatry*, 52:469–478.

Nunley M (1988). The involvement of families in Indian psychiatry. *Culture, Medicine and Psychiatry*, 22:317–353.

Nurjannah I, Mills J, Usher K, et al. (2014). Discharge planning in mental health care: an integrative review of the literature. *Journal of Clinical Nursing*, 23:1175–1185.

Östman M, Hansson L (2000). Comparisons between parent, spouses, and grown-up children of voluntary and compulsory admitted psychiatric patients. *Nordic Journal of Psychiatry*, 51:31–36.

Outram S, Harris G, Kelly B, et al. (2015). 'We didn't have a clue': family caregivers' experiences of the communication of a diagnosis of schizophrenia. *International Journal of Social Psychiatry*, 61:10–16.

Owens N, Brophy L (2013). Revocation of community treatment orders in a mental health service network. *Australasian Psychiatry*, 21:46–50.

Pai S, Kapur RL (1981). The burden on the family of a psychiatric patient: development of an interview schedule. *British Journal of Psychiatry*, 138:332–335.

Pearlin LI, Mullan JT, Semple SJ, et al. (1990). Caregiving and the stress process: An overview of concepts and their measures. *Gerontologist*, 30:583–594.

Perry J (2002). Wives giving care to husbands with Alzheimer's disease: a process of interpretive caring. *Research in Nursing and Health*, 25:307–316.

Petersen L, Jeppesen P, Thorup A, et al. (2005). A randomised multicentre trial of integrated versus standard treatment for patients with a first episode of psychotic illness. *British Medical Journal*, 331:602.

Rapaport J, Bellringer S, Pinfold V, et al. (2006). Carers and confidentiality in mental health care: considering the role of the carer's assessment: a study of service users', carers' and practitioners' views. *Health and Social Care in the Community*, 14:357–365.

Reay-Young R (2001). Support groups for relatives of people living with a serious mental illness: an overview. *International Journal of Psychosocial Rehabilitation*, 5:147–168.

Ridley J, Hunter S, Rosengard A (2010). Partners in care?: views and experiences of carers from a cohort study of the early implementation of the Mental Health (Care & Treatment) (Scotland) Act 2003. *Health and Social Care in the Community*, 18:474–482.

Rossen C, Stenager E, Bruun N (2014). The experiences of being close relative and informal carers of mentally ill Iraqi refugees: a qualitative study. *International Journal of Culture and Mental Health*, 7:452–463.

Rugkåsa J (2015). *Care and culture. Care relations from the perspectives of mental health caregivers in ethnic minority families*. Cambridge: Cambridge Scholars Publishing.

Saunders JC (2003). Families living with severe mental illness: a literature review. *Issues in Mental Health Nursing*, 24:175–198.

Shah R, Basu D (2010). Coercion in psychiatric care: global and Indian perspective. *Indian Journal of Psychiatry*, **52**:203–206.

Shefer G, Rose D, Nellums L, et al. (2013). 'Our community is the worst': the influence of cultural beliefs on stigma, relationships with family and help-seeking in three ethnic communities in London. *International Journal of Social Psychiatry*, **59**:535–544.

Simmons MB, Hetrick SE, Jorm AF (2011). Experiences of treatment decision making for young people diagnosed with depressive disorders: a qualitative study in primary care and specialist mental health settings. *BMC Psychiatry*, **11**:194.

Slade M, Pinfold V, Rapaport J, et al. (2007). Best practice when service users do not consent to sharing information with carers. National multimethod study. *British Journal of Psychiatry*, **190**:148–155.

Solomon P (1996). Research on the coercion of persons with severe mental illness. In: *Coercion and aggressive community treatment* (ed. D Dennis, J Monahan), pp. 129–145. New York: Springer.

Stroud J, Banks L, Doughty K (2015). Community treatment orders: learning from experiences of service users, practitioners and nearest relatives. *Journal of Mental Health*, **24**:88–92.

Twigg J, Atkin K (1994). *Carers perceived. Policy and practice in informal care.* Buckingham: Open University Press.

Ungerson C (1997). Social policy and the commodification of care. *Social Politics*, **4**:362–381.

Villatoro AP, Aneshensel CS (2014). Family Influences on the Use of Mental Health Services among African Americans. *Journal of Health and Social Behavior*, **55**:161–180.

Vine R, Komiti A (2015). Carer experience of community treatment orders: implications for rights based/recovery-oriented mental health legislation. *Australasian Psychiatry*, **23**:154–157.

Weimand BM, Hedelin B, Hall-Lord ML, et al. (2011). 'Left alone with straining but inescapable responsibilities:' relatives' experiences with mental health services. *Issues in Mental Health Nursing*, **32**:703–710.

Weimand BM, Hall-Lord ML, Sallstrom C, et al. (2013). Life-sharing experiences of relatives of persons with severe mental illness—a phenomenographic study. *Scandinavian Journal of Caring Sciences*, **27**:99–107.

Weimand BM, Israel P, Ruud T (2014). *Pårørende og ACT-team [Caregivers and ACT teams]*. Oslo: Akershus Universitetssykehus and Landsforeningen for Pårørende innen Psykisk Helse.

Weine S, Ukshini S, Griffith J, et al. (2005). A family approach to severe mental illness in post-war Kosovo. *Psychiatry: Interpersonal and Biological Processes*, **68**:17–27.

Werner P, Goldstein D, Buchbinder E (2010). Subjective experience of family stigma as reported by children of Alzheimer's disease patients. *Qualitative Health Research*, **20**:159–169.

Wilkinson C, McAndrew S (2008). 'I'm not an outsider, I'm his mother'! A phenomenological enquiry into carer experiences of exclusion from acute psychiatric settings. *International Journal of Mental Health Nursing*, **17**:392–401.

Wynaden D (2007). The experience of caring for a person with a mental illness: a grounded theory study. *International Journal of Mental Health* Nursing, **16**:381–389.

Wynaden D, Chapman R, Orb A, et al. (2005). Factors that influence Asian communities' access to mental health care. *International Journal of Mental Health* Nursing, **14**:88–95.

Chapter 11

Clinician attitudes, experiences, and use of coercion

Beth Angell

Introduction

It is essential to consider and understand the perspectives of psychiatric providers (e.g. psychiatrists, psychologists, social workers, caseworkers/keyworkers) on coercion, given their prominent role in implementing treatment mandates and in carrying out practices aimed at promoting treatment adherence in the community. This chapter describes the results of research using the direct reports of mental health providers across two broad areas:

(1) practices and strategies providers report using in promoting compliance or adherence;

(2) practitioner views about the utility, effectiveness, and ethics of such practices.

In addition, provider perspectives will be characterized across the different types of treatment contexts in which they have been studied.

Clinical work in the involuntary context is a longstanding concern in many fields of practice, including forensics and social work (Rooney 2013). Although at one time involuntary treatment was characterized narrowly as legally mandated treatment (in either an inpatient or outpatient setting), the conceptualization of coercion has broadened considerably to include a range of formal and informal mechanisms. Monahan et al. (2001) were among the first to parse the different forms of legal and bureaucratic leverage available for promoting compliance with community mental health treatment, including civil commitment (variously called outpatient commitment or community treatment orders), commitment via the criminal justice system for those who have committed minor offences or criminal acts, and bureaucratic pressures achieved by contingently withholding an individual's resources and entitlements, such as housing, custody of children, or employment or disability benefits. In addition, scholarship has illuminated various ways that informal pressures may be applied to induce compliance (Angell et al. 2006; Szmukler and Appelbaum 2008). For example, practitioners may attempt to persuade their patients, reward them with food, cigarettes, or verbal praise, or threaten to terminate the treatment relationship if compliance expectations are not met. This chapter, in keeping with a broad conceptualization of coercion, includes all of the above mechanisms and practices. While it draws from research conducted around the world, it is important to note that such research has been conducted mainly in Western countries. As a result less is known about these issues in developing nations.

Legally mandated community treatment

Involuntary community treatment refers to treatment mandated under a civil commitment order. In the USA these arrangements are commonly termed involuntary outpatient commitment (IOC) or assisted outpatient treatment (AOT); in the UK and Australasia, they are referred to as community treatment orders (CTOs). CTOs are becoming more prevalent in many countries, though their effectiveness is a subject of intense debate (Maughan et al. 2014; Morrissey et al. 2014; Swanson and Swartz 2014). Studies focusing on providers' perspectives on CTOs fall into two general categories: (1) large-scale surveys of providers to ascertain their opinions about the utility and favourability of CTOs and their perceptions of the barriers and challenges to their use; and (2) smaller-scale qualitative studies of how providers use and implement CTOs, typically within the context of one region or practice context.

Surveys of providers

Surveys of provider groups are typically designed to inform local debates about the potential effectiveness and likelihood that CTO mechanisms will be used. Some such studies were conducted prior to the introduction of legislation, such as the 2007 amendments to the Mental Health Act (England and Wales), which followed nearly 10 years of debate over draft legislation (Churchill et al. 2007), or following the passage of legislation such as the Mental Health and Compulsory Assessment and Treatment Act of 1992 in New Zealand. Other studies were undertaken after the passage of legislation and were designed to evaluate its effectiveness or effects on stakeholder groups.

During the lead-up to the 2007 changes in the Mental Health Act for England and Wales, Pinfold et al. (2002) surveyed 579 mental health professionals to examine the attitudes of providers toward supervised discharge orders and guardianship, both of which were components of the 1995 amendments to the Mental Health Act that preceded the later addition of CTOs. They found that practitioners generally favoured guardianship over CTOs, but endorsed neither wholeheartedly because of the limitations on power to enforce the order and, particularly, the limits on requiring patients to take medication.

Following the introduction of CTOs in the 2007 amendments, Manning et al. (2011) conducted a national survey of 714 psychiatrists in England and Wales, finding that a slight majority (60%) preferred having CTOs to not having them. These clinicians cited important benefits (promoting adherence, protecting patients from negative outcomes of relapse, and ensuring engagement with services), but also barriers such as administrative burden, unavailability of certain service options (supported housing, depot forms of some medications), and difficulty enforcing adherence to medication, which is a permissible statutory component of CTOs but which cannot be administered forcibly. Coyle et al. (2013) extended the Manning study by replicating it with 288 professionals, including a broader range of team leaders, nurses, and social workers in addition to psychiatrists. Again, they found that more than half the sample endorsed the use of CTOs and believed that their benefits outweighed the possible harms of increased perceived coercion; however, professional differences were observed, with psychiatrists endorsing CTOs more strongly than other professional groups, particularly nurses.

In the USA, IOC (as CTOs are typically called) has been introduced in a more gradual manner, as different states have introduced IOC laws at different times (and a few states do not currently have such legislation). Swartz et al. (2003) surveyed 85 mental health professionals working in a region of North Carolina in which IOC was already well established, as well as a companion sample of mental health patients, about their perceptions of whether legal and coercive pressures made people more likely to stay in treatment and the degree to which respondents perceived that mandates would deter people from seeking help in the future. They found that the majority (78%) of providers endorsed the helpfulness of mandated treatment in keeping people in treatment and disagreed (81%) that there would be harmful effects on help-seeking, but found, in contrast, that patients were less sanguine about the benefits and absence of harms. Following the passage of the Baker Act, which introduced IOC in Florida in 2005, Christy et al. (2009) conducted an online survey of 498 clinicians, the majority of whom were working in positions that could hypothetically involve working with IOC. Most participants agreed with the philosophy behind IOC, but reported significant barriers to its use, including underfunding of the services to be rendered under the order, insufficiency of treatment resources, difficulty persuading outpatient mental health providers to accept court-ordered cases, the time demands associated with negotiating court orders, and anticipated problems enforcing the order if patients failed to comply. Thus, research in the USA suggests that clinicians find IOC helpful in principle, but features of the national debate regarding the need to allocate sufficient resources for the provision of services (Swanson and Swartz, 2014) are reflected in the experiences of professionals as well.

Canadian provinces have likewise introduced CTOs at different times, and studies of professional attitudes have been conducted as part of efforts to evaluate their effectiveness. Saskatchewan introduced CTOs in 1995, and initially they were used sparingly. In response, O'Reilly et al. (2000) administered a survey to all licensed psychiatrists in the province, about half of whom had used a CTO with at least one patient. Psychiatrists who had not used CTOs reported that they had not done so because their patients did not meet the criteria, because they lacked information about how to use them, and because they believed that enforcement powers were inadequate. Overall, reported satisfaction with the policy was moderate. In Ontario, CTOs were featured in changes to Mental Health Legislation Bill 68 in 2000, and a legislatively mandated evaluation was recently completed (RA Malatest and Associates Ltd 2012). Their comprehensive evaluation included group and individual interviews with case managers, psychiatrists, and other service providers as well as an online survey of 411 stakeholders, of which providers were the largest group. Providers reported that they believed CTOs to be effective in providing a good quality of life, wellbeing, adherence, stability, reduced hospitalizations, connections in the community, physical health, and re-engagement in work and school. However, they noted that these benefits often took longer than the typical length of a CTO (6 months), consistent with the outcomes of IOC evaluations performed in the USA (Swartz et al. 1999, 2010). Concerns and perceived barriers to the use of CTOs included perceptions that CTOs diverted resources from voluntary patients, the administrative burden of petitioning and renewing CTOs, availability of community resources, and screening requirements that excluded patients who would benefit from CTOs such as recently released prisoners with mental illness. As in other studies, clinicians complained about the limited ability to enforce commitments if patients did not fear or respect the order. Finally, providers raised concerns about the effectiveness of CTOs in serving rural, Francophone, and aboriginal communities, due to cultural differences in beliefs about mental illness and mental wellness among con-sumers and their family members in these communities.

CTOs were introduced in New Zealand in 1992, and several studies undertook to examine provider responses. An early study (Currier et al. 1997) surveyed 232 psy-chiatrists registered with the Medical Council of New Zealand to determine the rates of CTO use as well as perceptions of their utility. Results indicated significant dis-satisfaction with the law, with some reporting that it placed patients at risk by releas-ing them into the community, a perception that judges varied in their interpretation of legal standards, and a majority indicating that the Act required major revision. Dawson and Romans (2001) surveyed 55 psychiatrists, representing 14% of qualified psychiatrists in New Zealand. Respondents indicated that the benefit of CTOs relative to its harms (primarily coercion) was moderate (1.9 on a four-point scale). In a later study, Romans et al. (2004) surveyed 202 psychiatrists and 82 mental health profes-sionals in Otago, using a similar methodology to subsequent studies in the UK (e.g. Manning et al. 2011; Coyle et al. 2013). In their survey, the majority of respondents reported that they felt it was better to work in a system with CTOs than without, and that the benefits of CTOs outweighed the harms. Concerns cited included insufficient treatment and community resources (e.g. housing, certain therapies, depot forms of some medications), problems in enforcing the order, and some moderate concerns about damage to the therapeutic alliance. A subsequent New Zealand study (Gibbs et al. 2006) likewise found that providers with experience of using CTOs were largely favourable toward the orders, perceiving that they provided an opportunity to help patients become stabilized so that they would be able to move onto other life goals. Because of these positive effects, concerns the participants revealed about CTOs per-tained to dilemmas about the length of time for which CTOs should be maintained in order to avoid disruption of positive gains.

Qualitative studies and small-scale surveys

Whereas the aim of large-scale quantitative surveys is to determine general profes-sional opinion about CTOs, smaller-scale studies using qualitative (and sometimes survey) methods generally seek information regarding specific issues and challenges in using CTOs. Scheid-Cook (1993) conducted an early study of participant construc-tions of CTOs in the USA, focusing on the state of North Carolina, an early adopter. Clinicians in that study saw CTOs as helpful tools because they provided a source of leverage over patients, but they also complained that this leverage was somewhat symbolic as there were no 'teeth' or tangible ways to enforce the order if the patient did not need to be rehospitalized. In a strikingly similar fashion, Rawala and Gupta (2014) examined the views of assertive outreach providers in one London programme; these providers described that leverage—the 'power of recall'—was most central to the effectiveness of CTOs, but that effectiveness was diminished if the patient did not believe in the potential threat of recall. Mullen et al. (2006) elicited the views of psychiatrists in New Zealand regarding their experiences of CTOs, and found that in contrast to the foregoing studies, the capacity to recall patients to hospital was quite feasible, and although not used prolifically was seen as a useful option for patients who did not take the order seriously. Another recent study, conducted within the context of the OCTET Trial (Canvin et al. 2014), illustrated how clinicians instituted workarounds when recall procedures proved to be cumbersome. Some psychiatrists in that study reported that they wrote the CTO using broad provisions that made it easier to implement and enforce without the need for frequent changes in response to patient status and personnel changes. Their orders typically stipulated medication adherence and contact with the treatment team, and they relied on the hypothetical power or 'legal clout' to motivate patient compliance with the order as uncertainty about the limits of the recall procedure was expressed by both patients and psychiatrists.

Additional qualitative studies of providers of assertive community treatment (ACT) suggest ways in which clinicians deploy commitment orders in the context of their broader efforts to promote adherence, and how they respond to the enforcement challenges highlighted in nearly every survey discussed above. Angell et al. (2006), in a study that identified adherence-promoting strategies in ACT practice, found that when patients were under a CTO or guardianship order, clinicians perceived that they had greater discretion to use more forceful and directive strategies to enforce the order, even if these powers were not specifically entailed in the legal statute. For the psychiatrists in a New Zealand study, the broad power to use the CTO to control a wide range of behaviour was seen as both an advantage and an ethical grey area (Mullen et al. 2006). Brodwin (2012), in a study of the use of outpatient commitment within an ACT programme, examined how clinicians avoid the difficult task of enforcing commitments via formal legal proceedings by building an 'assemblage' of compliance. The coercive logic of ACT, he argued, begins with the signing of an informed consent for treatment (which warns patients that if they do not comply with treatment recommendations, the team may pursue involuntary treatment) and pressuring patients to take medication by altering its form (e.g. liquid instead of a pill) and verbally insisting that they ingest the medication under watchful supervision. In a countervailing strategy, he describes that when ACT teams wish to pursue enforcement of commitment, they must cease their efforts to pressure compliance and, instead, watchfully document non-compliance and decompensation in hope of satisfying legal criteria for a more stringent legal order in the brief period between substantial deterioration and eventual harm to self or other.

Criminal justice leverage

An alternative form of legally mandated treatment occurs when treatment is ordered by the court as a condition of release from jail or prison, as a diversion from being prosecuted for a criminal offence, or as an alternative to serving time in prison for an adjudicated offence (Monahan et al. 2001). In the USA these arrangements may be designated through community supervision (probation and parole) or mental health courts. If compliance with the court order is not met, the patient may (in theory) be remanded to prison. Across all types of criminal justice leverage, the order for treatment specifies a plan of care to which the patient is accountable and the entities (correctional officers, judges, treatment providers) to which he or she is expected to report in order to monitor compliance. Research on the provider perspective in the context of criminal justice leverage has tended to focus either on criminal justice personnel (most often probation officers) or mental health providers (typically case managers).

Research focusing on the perspectives of criminal justice personnel most often hones in on the unique features of specialty corrections, particularly specialized probation. Specialized probation officers carry a 'smaller-than-usual' caseload of probationers who have serious mental illness and they are provided with training in behavioural health management (Epperson et al. 2014). Studies of practice patterns show that, compared with usual probation, specialized parole agencies tend to eschew punitive practices such as surveillance and sanctions, relying instead on problem-solving techniques and linkage to community resources (Skeem et al. 2006). In addition, specialized officers tend to allocate time during supervision meetings to the discussion of mental health needs and to rely on positive inducements and only a sparing use of sanctions and threats of reincarceration (Eno Louden et al. 2012; Epperson et al. 2014). They use relational strategies in order to build trust and increase the probationer's motivation and capacity for self-regulation (Epperson et al. 2014). These patterns are at odds with an earlier investigation by Solomon and Draine (1995) highlighting punitive practices used in specialized probation and parole, which yielded the unintended consequence of increasing reincarceration among people with mental illness. A recent quasi-experimental evaluation of specialized probation showed that the officers did not specifically avoid the use of sanctions for order violations but that, overall, probationers receiving specialized probation services showed lower rates of reincarceration and spent less time in jail than their regular probation counterparts (Wolff et al. 2014). Taken together, these results suggest that a gradual infusion of therapeutic jurisprudence principles has shaped the evolution of specialized correctional services over time.

Because treatment orders administered through the criminal justice system entail the use of mental health treatment as a component of the order, mental health professionals who serve patients involved in the justice system must achieve some degree of collaboration with criminal justice authorities in monitoring compliance with the order. As Wilson and Draine (2006) describe, the levels of collaboration range from highly integrated (e.g. a team in which mental health professionals and correctional staff work side by side) to more limited alliances that involve coordination of monitoring activities. Research on the provider perspective in this area highlights the potential for role conflict among mental health professionals, who may be professionally socialized to advocate for clients rather than collude with a punitive system. Brodwin (2014), for example, describes in an ethnographic vignette the experiences of an ACT team when one of their patients receives a mental health probation order to avoid incarceration for drug and prostitution charges. The ACT workers, unused to working in such a context, exhibited profound ambivalence about their new role in monitoring and reporting compliance and non-compliance, particularly given that their longstanding relationship with the patient was premised on principles of trust and advocacy. On the other hand, the arrangement into which the team entered was aimed at avoiding a negative outcome for the patient (i.e. incarceration). As a result they struggled intensely with everyday decisions of whether to report infractions or to leverage compliance from the patient in order to avoid the need to report her behaviour to authorities. Studies of mental health programmes which are designed to work with a population involved in the criminal justice system suggest that providers working within a dual system are typically more savvy and less conflicted about these roles, and acquire ways to balance the 'care' and 'control' functions entailed within them (Angell et al. 2014).

Bureaucratic leverage

Monahan (2001), arguing for an expanded consideration of the varieties of mandated treatment, drew a distinction between court-ordered treatment through the civil commitment system and varieties of leverage that occur through bureaucratic channels. As such, bureaucratic leverage through systems such as housing, employer assistance programmes, child custody systems, and money management authorities occupy a middle ground between legally coerced treatment and purely informal methods of persuasion and pressure. Of these bureaucratic mechanisms, housing and money have received the most empirical attention.

Housing leverage occurs when the conditions of receiving housing through a supported housing programme, group home, or housing voucher require the tenant to adhere to particular rules, such as taking medication, attending treatment, or abstaining from consuming alcohol or drugs. In a landmark study of the prevalence of different types of adherence pressures reported by people receiving mental health treatment in five US cities, Monahan et al. (2005) found that between 23% and 40% of participants (depending on the city) had experienced housing leverage at some point in the past. This result was replicated in a similar study subsequently conducted in the UK (Burns et al. 2011). In a recent study comparing the practices of housing providers, Henwood et al. (2011) found that the tendency to use the threat of eviction to enforce treatment adherence or other behavioural goals was more commonly reported among providers working in a traditional treatment-first housing model, where tenants are expected to earn the right to move into gradually more independent housing based on the accomplishment of programme goals. Providers in a housing-first model, however, tended to eschew such practices, instead using the 'gift' of housing as a way of building trust with the patient, so that it was easier to help him or her build motivation to adhere in order to meet his or her own goals.

Financial leverage occurs when an appointed money manager (appointed legally, through the representative payee system, or informally, as the chosen money manager) makes the disbursement of the funds belonging to the person with mental illness contingent upon adherence behaviour. In the USA it is quite common for adults with serious mental illness to have a payee appointed to manage their funds, and mental health agencies and family members commonly perform the payee role (Dixon et al. 1999; Elbogen et al. 2003; Moser and Bond 2009). In either case, maintenance of control over patient funds makes it possible to withhold the funds contingently. Such practices are common in programmes that withhold a daily allowance, for example, until patients take their medications or come to treatment appointments. In the USA, a five-site study showed that between 7% and 19% of a sample of adults with mental illness reported ever experiencing financial leverage, and the prevalence was greater among those for whom a payee managed their money (15–31%, depending on the city). In contrast, such practices are reported far less frequently in the UK, where professional money management is less commonly used (Burns et al. 2011).

Studies conducted from the provider perspective have examined self-reports of using money as a form of contingent withholding. Angell (2005) administered a scale measuring practices aimed at increasing medication adherence to a sample of ACT providers and a sample of staff at a community mental health centre ($n = 55$), in which the staff were asked to rate the frequency of the practices in relation to a particular patient. For contingent withholding of funds or cigarettes, ACT providers reported using the strategy more frequently than did the mental health centre staff (14% versus 4%). In a similar study, Moser and Bond (2011) surveyed 122 ACT providers in one US state regarding a range of limit-setting practices. A relatively small number of providers reported that they would explicitly withhold resources (such as cigarettes or a daily money allowance) from patients for not taking their medications (18% reported occasionally doing this, while only 4% did so often or always). However, more than half of the providers reported making sure that the patient had taken the medication dose before undertaking an activity such as providing them with money or taking them shopping. This suggests that the practice of financial leverage may be implied rather than spelled out as a quid pro quo, and may account for the disparity in provider reports of the practice compared with the relatively more common patient reports of experiencing financial leverage.

Several qualitative studies of ACT and case management providers shed light on how expectations of treatment adherence and their connection to the patient's access to his or her funds are conveyed to patients in subtle ways. Angell et al. (2006), in an intensive study of two ACT teams, found that providers conveyed unspoken expectations of adherence by arranging daily delivery of medication and money to the patient's home. This arrangement, while presented as a convenience to the patient, represented the baseline arrangement from which a gradual transition to independent control of medications and money would occur when the patient was judged to be insightful and capable of managing these tasks. Brodwin (2012), in an in-depth ethnographic study of a single ACT programme, honed in on the logic underpinning the institutionalized representative payeeship system, highlighting the ways that this logic justifies the removal of rights of the patient and the discretionary disbursement or withholding of funds as a strategy for managing adherence. He argues that having an appointed payee establishes two categories of dependence for the patient— an inability to provide for oneself, and in interpersonal dependency wherein clients 'are vulnerable to their case managers who can release or withhold money in order to influence behavior. According to the logic of this system, the relationship of dependency is demanded by and uniquely appropriate to the client's baseline biology' (Brodwin 2012, p. 120). Brodwin also notes, as Angell et al. (2006) did, that this dependence becomes viewed as the default condition from which the patient must prove fitness to exit and become an independent custodian of their own money and administrator of their own medication. While these arrangements are perceived by providers as an important tool for promoting adherence, they are not without challenges. In a survey of providers, Dixon et al. (1999) found that about a fifth of the respondents reported that being a payee for a patient has negative effects on the therapeutic relationship, a finding echoed in a quantitative study which showed that patients who reported experiencing financial leverage had more conflicted relationships with their case managers than those not experiencing leverage (Angell et al. 2007). Ethnographic studies (Floersch 2002; Brodwin 2012) also depict the money management relationship between patients and staff as highly contentious, fraught with conflict over everyday decisions about how much money to disburse and in what form, about the possible purchase of illicit drugs instead of food, and often assuming the dominant focus of clinical encounters. Concerns about minimizing the negative effects of money management have led to the development of manualized money management programmes that clarify lines of authority and minimize the effects of implicit linking of money to adherence (e.g. Serowik et al. 2013).

Informal coercion

While research on formal coercion has had most attention, scholars have also looked at the ways that providers may pressurize patients to adhere to treatment or conform to behavioural expectations through more subtle and informal methods (Angell et al. 2006; Szmukler and Appelbaum 2008). Awareness of the potential for informal coercion was heightened by a series of commentaries on one particular type of treatment, ACT (Diamond, 1996; Gomory, 1999; Fisher & Ahearn, 2000). Treatment teams based on the principles of ACT, such as assertive outreach in the UK and related, yet less intensive, models such as intensive case management, are common vehicles for organizing the treatment of people with mental illness who are considered the most difficult to treat due to revolving-door hospitalization and inconsistent adherence to treatment. Such programmes are considered highly effective in reducing hospitalization, and some studies show that they effect modest improvements in symptoms, quality of life, and reduction of family burden (Bond et al. 2001). However, debate about whether ACT achieves these effects through excessive paternalism and control has prompted a proliferation of studies in both the USA and the UK.

Studies of therapeutic limit setting

Michael Neale and Robert Rosenheck were among the first to study informal coercion as self-reported by mental health professionals (Neale and Rosenheck 2000; Rosenheck and Neale 2004). They developed a quantitative measure [the Therapeutic Limit Setting (TLS) Scale] which asked providers to rate the frequency with which they employed an array of 'therapeutic limit setting' behaviours that ranged from verbal persuasion to the pursuit of involuntary detention in a hospital. The researchers then administered the measure to a large sample of case managers working with clients with serious mental illness in the Veterans Affairs health system in the USA, and further refined the scale to several components: verbal guidance, money management, contingent withholding, enforced hospitalization, and invocation of institutional authorities. Findings revealed that low-coercion strategies such as verbal guidance were used far more frequently than more forceful strategies, and that the more forceful strategies were more likely to be used when the client had a history of arrest or substance abuse, when the client was being seen more frequently, and when the alliance between client and case manager was poor. In the follow-up report (Rosenheck and Neale 2004), the authors analysed the effects of limit setting by examining whether the limit-setting measure predicted outcomes 6 months later. Contrary to expectation, they found that clients who received the most limit setting had the poorest outcomes on most indicators, such as symptoms, functioning, quality of life, and violence, suggesting that limit setting was not only ineffective, but possibly harmful. Because of its cross-sectional design, however, the authors had difficulty establishing the directionality of effects, but they note that the results are potentially troubling with respect to the potential for the use of limit setting to have unintended negative consequences.

In another study using the TLS Scale, Davidson and Campbell (2007) surveyed 60 keyworkers (case managers) in ACT teams and standard community mental health teams in Northern Ireland. They found a significant effect for type of programme, with community mental health team staff reporting a higher use of TLS than ACT teams. Both teams, however, increased use of TLS over time, and all keyworkers reported using at least one of the strategies at all three points in time. More recently, Manuel et al. (2014) adapted the TLS Scale to encompass additional limit setting behaviours and modified the items to target average behaviour rather than behaviour related to a given client, as was the measurement strategy in the original scale. Again, they found that verbal guidance and positive inducements were most frequently employed, though more directive strategies such as conditional involvement and reporting behaviour to authorities were used occasionally. These more directive strategies were more likely, in their analysis, to be used when staff as a whole rated the work climate as demoralized and when they endorsed more stigmatizing beliefs about clients with mental illness.

Although the TLS Scale was an important early effort, the scale had interpretation difficulties because it weighted different types of behaviours equally, including hypothetical actions such as 'considering hospitalization' alongside concrete actions such as petitioning for involuntary commitment. In addition, it contained practices that are not necessarily coercive, such as representative payeeship, which may or may not result in the use of contingent withholding or leverage. Angell (2005) adapted the scale's items to exclude hypothetical behaviours and to focus more narrowly on practices reported to be used to increase medication adherence; they administered the scale to two samples, one consisting of ACT providers and the other a broader sample of mental health staff in a community mental health centre. As was the case in the original Neale and Rosenheck study (1999), the frequency of lower-pressure strategies such as providing reasons in order to persuade clients to adhere to medication, were more common than higher-pressure strategies such as withholding money or cigarettes to leverage adherence. Using techniques from item response theory, the scale items were used to form a continuum that could be used to define the intensity of pressure used to promote adherence with a given client. Using the resulting measure, Angell found that the intensity of pressure tended to be higher if the provider perceived the client as less adherent to medication and less cooperative.

Examining the presence of coercive behaviours at a more organizational level of analysis, Moser and Bond (2009) administered a measure to 23 ACT teams in Indiana, USA, assessing practices reported at a team rather than individual provider level. Agency control practices referred to the maintenance of supervisory responsibility over clients, such as serving as a payee or leasing housing to them. Restrictive practices represent using that supervisory responsibility to set limits on client behaviour. Agency control practices, which create the possibility for but do not necessarily result in coercion, were more common than limit setting. Within types of agency control, representative payeeship and intensive medication monitoring were more commonly used than leasing housing to clients and the use of IOC orders. Contrary to the authors' expectations, fidelity to the ACT model bore no relationship to the frequency of agency control practices.

Qualitative studies of leverage in ACT

Provider perspectives on the use of leverage and limit setting in ACT has likewise been examined in the context of qualitative studies, which allow pressure and coercion to be examined within the context of interpersonal interactions and organizational context. Angell et al. (2006) studied how two US ACT teams promoted adherence in their everyday practice, using both interviews with the providers and observations of their interactions with clients. She found that a significant level of adherence management occurs in programme design, including routine delivery of medication. Providers also sought to use methods of logical and relational persuasion, such as giving reasons and expressing that they cared about the patient as frequently as possible. However, the clinicians' perceived responsibility for ensuring client safety and well-being induced them to resort to more directive tactics (e.g. arranging money disbursement to occur simultaneously with medication delivery; directing the client to take medication under watchful supervision) at certain times, such as when they perceived that a client was beginning to decompensate. The propensity to exert greater pressure on clients was heightened in certain contexts, such as living in a small community in which the client was known to many, and also in situations where clients were receiving treatment under a court mandate.

Salyers et al. (2011), in an ethnographic study of two ACT teams in Indiana, sought to identify the elements of a 'recovery orientation' in ACT, with findings that illustrate the ways in which paternalistic practices run counter to the recovery philosophy. For example, programmes lacking a recovery philosophy tended to speak about clients in parental ways, make decisions for them rather than with them, and insisted on intensive monitoring of medication until clients 'earned' their way off of it. Providers characterized as low in recovery orientation also revealed that they sought to use IOC frequently and to communicate the terms of the orders in vague terms so that clients were not fully aware of their rights and obligations.

Two studies using focus groups of ACT providers examined questions of how these professionals manage adherence issues in practice. Appelbaum and LeMelle (2008) studied 23 staff from four ACT teams in New York City. In contrast to other studies, the providers involved took issue with the suggestion that they behaved strategically to improve patient compliance; instead, they saw themselves as facilitators who helped patients work on self-determined goals. They did, however, acknowledge that they would use subtle methods to encourage clients to take medications, and one provider mentioned that the team would schedule money disbursement following appointments to provide a subtle inducement to attend. Rugkåsa et al. (2014) conducted focus groups with staff from six community teams in the UK with regard to their methods of influencing reluctant patients. Like the providers in the Angell et al. (2006) study, the community team staff sought to use negotiation instead of force (e.g. sectioning via the Mental Health Act) in order to preserve their relationships with their patients and build their trust. To do otherwise, they reported, would sabotage their own efforts to negotiate with their clients in the future and undermine the clients' level of motivation to care for their own well-being by taking medications consistently.

In a recently conducted ethnographic study, Brodwin (2012) examined efforts of ACT staff to influence adherence, but sought to locate these processes within the internal logic of ACT, and indeed psychiatry as an institution, rather than isolating them as individual provider behaviours. In doing so, he proposes the concept of 'assemblage' to theorize that providers accept the need for limit-setting behaviours because treatment practices such as medication management and informed consent make up a package of taken-for-granted understandings and practices that are embedded in the logic of intensive community treatment. Practitioners' tacit acceptance of the underlying logic of the programme obviates the need for them to weigh up the ethical ramifications of everyday decisions.

Conclusion and implications

The proliferation of studies on coercion in psychiatry over the past 20 years suggests the presence of hidden forms of influence and control in the practice of mental health treatment. The review in this chapter reveals that providers perform an important role in the enactment of practices used to pressure patients with mental illness to adhere to treatment. Although some of these practices are driven by laws and policies, others grow out of the professional discretion of individuals and teams. It is important to take into consideration the dilemmas of these professionals, who are often considered the fixed point of responsibility for ensuring that patients do not cause harm to themselves or to others, and also for promoting patient wellbeing to the greatest extent possible. To this end, the range of mechanisms discussed here are deployed as tools in a difficult and unpredictable job.

With some exceptions, formal opportunities to acquire knowledge and skills in the ethical and judicious use of leverage are often very limited or absent. The studies reviewed here show that providers commonly report that they need more information about the capacities and limits of different forms of leverage. In the literature on CTOs, for example, the problem of enforcement and the breadth of the powers provided by the law are nearly ubiquitous questions that call for greater attention to codify legal procedure and to train providers about which interventions are possible under what circumstances. So too, the apparent conflict between the discourses of recovery and of leverage begs for reconciliation, as providers face institutional pressures both to protect clients from harm and to grant them autonomy over treatment decisions. Thus, the field is ripe for innovation in training, decision aids, and treatment guidelines that serve to encourage providers to reflect upon the ethics, benefits, and harms of using leverage to promote adherence in clients with serious mental illness.

References

Angell B (2005). Measuring strategies used by mental health providers to encourage medication adherence. *Journal of Behavioral Health Services and Research*, 33:53–72.

Angell B, Mahoney CA, Martinez NI (2006). Promoting treatment adherence in assertive community treatment. *Social Service Review*, 80:485–526.

Angell B, Martinez NI, Mahoney C, et al. (2007). Payeeship, financial leverage, and the client-provider relationship. *Psychiatric Services*, 58:365–372.

Angell B, Matthews E, Barrenger S, et al. (2014). Engagement processes in model programs for community re-entry from prison for people with serious mental illness. *International Journal of Law and Psychiatry*, 37:490–500.

Appelbaum PS, Le Melle S (2008). Techniques used by assertive community treatment (ACT) teams to encourage adherence: patient and staff perceptions. *Community Mental Health Journal*, 44:459–464.

Bond GR, Drake RE, Mueser KT, et al. (2001). Assertive community treatment for people with severe mental illness: critical ingredients and impact on patients. *Disease Management and Health Outcomes*, 9:141–159.

Brodwin P (2012). *Everyday ethics: voices from the front line of community psychiatry*. Berkeley, CA: University of California Press.

Brodwin P (2014). The ethics of ambivalence and the practice of constraint in US psychiatry. *Culture, Medicine, and Psychiatry*, 38:527–549.

Burns T, Yeeles K, Molodynski A, et al. (2011). Pressures to adhere to treatment ('leverage') in English mental healthcare. *British Journal of Psychiatry*, 199:145–150.

Canvin K, Rugkåsa J, Sinclair J, et al. (2014). Patient, psychiatrist and family carer experiences of community treatment orders: qualitative study. *Social Psychiatry and Psychiatric Epidemiology*, 49:1873–1882.

Christy A, Petrila J, McCranie M, et al. (2009). Involuntary outpatient commitment in Florida: case information and provider experience and opinions. *International Journal of Forensic Mental Health*, 8:122–130.

Churchill R, Owen G, Singh S, et al. (2007). *International experiences of using community treatment orders*. London: Department of Health.

Coyle D, Macpherson R, Foy C, et al. (2013). Compulsion in the community: mental health professionals' views and experiences of CTOs. *The Psychiatrist*, 37:315–321.

Currier G (1997). A survey of New Zealand psychiatrists' clinical experience with the Mental Health (Compulsory Assessment and Treatment) Act of 1992. *New Zealand Medical Journal*, 110:6–9.

Davidson G, Campbell J (2007). An examination of the use of coercion by assertive outreach and community mental health teams in Northern Ireland. *British Journal of Social Work*, **37**:537–555.

Dawson J, Romans S (2001). Uses of community treatment orders in New Zealand: early findings. *Australian and New Zealand Journal of Psychiatry*, **35**:190–195.

Diamond RJ (1996). Coercion and tenacious treatment in the community. In: *Coercion and aggressive community treatment: a new frontier in mental health law* (ed. DL Dennis, J Monahan), pp. 51–72. New York: Plenum.

Dixon L, Turner J, Krauss N, et al. (1999). Case managers' and clients' perspectives on a representative payee program. *Psychiatric Services*, **50**:781–786.

Elbogen EB, Swanson JW, Swartz MS, et al. (2003). Characteristics of third-party money management for persons with psychiatric disabilities. *Psychiatric Services*, **54**:1136–1141.

Eno Louden J, Skeem JL, Camp J, et al. (2012). Supervision practices in specialty mental health probation: what happens in officer–probationer meetings? *Law and Human Behavior*, **36**:109–119.

Epperson MW, Canada K, Thompson J, et al. (2014). Walking the line: specialized and standard probation officer perspectives on supervising probationers with serious mental illnesses. *International Journal of Law and Psychiatry*, **37**:473–483.

Fisher DB, Ahern L (2000). Personal assistance in community existence (PACE): an alternative to PACT. *Ethical Human Sciences and Services*, **2**:87–92.

Floersch J (2002). *Meds, money, and manners: the case management of severe mental illness*. New York: Columbia University Press.

Gibbs A, Dawson J, Mullen R (2006). Community treatment orders for people with serious mental illness: a New Zealand study. *British Journal of Social Work*, **36**:1085–1100.

Gomory T (1999). Programs of assertive community treatment (PACT): a critical review. *Ethical Human Sciences and Services*, **1**:147–163.

Henwood BF, Stanhope V, Padgett DK (2011). The role of housing: a comparison of front-line provider views in housing first and traditional programs. *Administration and Policy in Mental Health and Mental Health Services Research*, **38**:77–85.

Iyer S, Banks N, Roy MA, et al. (2013). A qualitative study of experiences with and perceptions regarding long-acting injectable antipsychotics: part I-patient perspectives. *Canadian Journal of Psychiatry-Revue Canadienne de Psychiatrie*, **58**(5 Suppl 1):14S–22S.

Manning C, Molodynski A, Rugkåsa J, et al. (2011). Community treatment orders in England and Wales: national survey of clinicians' views and use. *The Psychiatrist*, **35**:328–333.

Manuel J, Appelbaum P, Le Melle S, et al. (2014). Use of intervention strategies by assertive community treatment teams to promote patients' engagement. *Psychiatric Services*, **64**:579–585.

Maughan D, Molodynski A, Rugkåsa J, et al. (2014). A systematic review of the effect of community treatment orders on service use. *Social Psychiatry and Psychiatric Epidemiology*, **49**:651–663.

Monahan J, Bonnie RJ, Appelbaum PS, et al. (2001). Mandated community treatment: beyond outpatient commitment. *Psychiatric Services*, **52**:1198–1205.

Monahan J, Redlich AD, Swanson J, et al. (2005). Use of leverage to improve adherence to psychiatric treatment in the community. *Psychiatric Services*, **56**:37–44.

Morrissey JP, Desmarais SL, Domino ME (2014). Outpatient commitment and its alternatives: questions yet to be answered. *Psychiatric Services*, **65**:812–815.

Moser L, Bond G (2009). Scope of agency control: assertive community treatment teams' supervision of consumers. *Psychiatric Services*, **60**:922–928.

Moser LL, Bond GR (2011). Practitioner attributes as predictors of restrictive practices in assertive community treatment. *Journal of the American Psychiatric Nurses Association*, **17**:80–89.

Mullen R, Dawson J, Gibbs A (2006). Dilemmas for clinicians in use of community treatment orders. *International Journal of Law and Psychiatry*, **29**:535–550.

Neale MS, Rosenheck RA (2000). Therapeutic limit setting in an assertive community treatment program. *Psychiatric Services*, **51**:499–505.

O'Reilly RL, Keegan DL, Elias JW (2000). A survey of the use of community treatment orders by psychiatrists in Saskatchewan. *Canadian Journal of Psychiatry–Revue Canadienne de Psychiatrie*, **45**:79–81.

Pinfold V, Rowe A, Hatfield B, et al. (2002). Lines of resistance: exploring professionals' views of compulsory community supervision. *Journal of Mental Health*, **11**:177–190.

RA Malatest and Associates Ltd (2012). *A legislated review of community treatment orders.* Toronto, ON: Ontario Ministry of Health and Long Term Care.

Rawala M, Gupta S (2014). Use of community treatment orders in an inner-London assertive outreach service. *Psychiatric Bulletin*, **38**:13–18.

Romans S, Dawson J, Mullen R, et al. (2004). How mental health clinicians view community treatment orders: a national New Zealand survey. *Australian and New Zealand Journal of Psychiatry*, **38**:836–841.

Rooney RH (ed.) (2013). *Strategies for work with involuntary clients.* New York: Columbia University Press.

Rosenheck RA, Neale MS (2004). Therapeutic limit setting and six-month outcomes in a Veterans Affairs assertive community treatment program. *Psychiatric Services*, **55**:139–144.

Rugkåsa J, Canvin K, Sinclair J, et al. (2014). Trust, deals and authority. Community mental health professionals' experiences of influencing reluctant patients. *Community Mental Health Journal*, **50**:886–895.

Salyers MP, Stull LG, Rollins AL, et al. (2011). The work of recovery on two assertive community treatment teams. *Administration and Policy in Mental Health and Mental Health Services Research*, **38**:169–180.

Scheid-Cook TL (1993). Controllers and controlled: an analysis of participant constructions of outpatient commitment. *Sociology of Health and Illness*, **15**:179–198.

Serowik KL, Bellamy CD, Rowe M, et al. (2013). Subjective experiences of clients in a voluntary money management program. *American Journal of Psychiatric Rehabilitation*, **16**:136–153.

Skeem JL, Emke-Francis P, Louden JE (2006). Probation, mental health, and mandated treatment: a national survey. *Criminal Justice and Behavior*, **33**:158–184.

Solomon P, Draine J (1995). Issues in serving the forensic client. *Social Work*, **40**:25–33.

Swanson JW, Swartz MS (2014). Why the evidence for outpatient commitment is good enough. *Psychiatric Services*, **65**:808–811.

Swartz MS, Swanson JW (2013). Economic grand rounds: can states implement involuntary outpatient commitment within existing state budgets? *Psychiatric Services*, **64**:7–9.

Swartz MS, Swanson JW, Wagner HR, et al. (1999). Can involuntary outpatient commitment reduce hospital recidivism? Findings from a randomized trial with severely mentally ill individuals. *American Journal of Psychiatry*, **156**:1968–1975.

Swartz MS, Swanson JW, Hannon MJ (2003). Does fear of coercion keep people away from mental health treatment? Evidence from a survey of persons with schizophrenia and mental health professionals. *Behavioral Sciences and the Law*, 21:459–472.

Swartz MS, Wilder CM, Swanson JW, et al. (2010). Assessing outcomes for consumers in New York's assisted outpatient treatment program. *Psychiatric Services*, 61:976–981.

Szmukler G, Appelbaum PS (2008). Treatment pressures, leverage, coercion, and compulsion in mental health care. *Journal of Mental Health*, 17:233–244.

Wilson A, Draine J (2006). Collaborations between criminal justice and mental health systems for prisoner reentry. *Psychiatric Services*, 57:875–878.

Wolff N, Epperson M, Shi J, et al. (2014). Mental health specialized probation caseloads: Are they effective? *International Journal of Law and Psychiatry*, 37:464–472.

Part 4

The context

Chapter 12

Psychiatric coercion: some sociological perspectives

David Pilgrim

Introduction

In developed societies today some people who are deemed by others to be psychologically abnormal are detained without trial and may receive imposed interventions, which are life-inhibiting and at times even life-threatening. This is a contentious socio-ethical scenario *par excellence*. Not only are few social groups detained without trial in democratic societies (terrorists and psychiatric patients being the main groups that break the legal mould in this regard), but not *all* people deemed to be mentally disordered are detained and treated coercively. Thus a double distinction is in play within a social process: normal and abnormal conduct is distinguished and some, but not all, abnormal conduct is met with coercion from those who are sane by common consent. That peculiar scenario should invite some sociological insights. In this chapter I summarize and offer some of these but, for reasons of space, only so much can be said.

Sociology and psychiatric coercion

Sociology is a broad discipline containing a range of historically bequeathed currents of thought. A longer description of its implications for the study of mental health and illness is offered in Rogers and Pilgrim (2014), but here I draw upon that summary selectively in order to explore the relevance of sociology to the particular topic of psychiatric coercion. Here I single out three main types of sociological exploration of relevance to this book.

Social causationism

Some sociologists have little to say about coercion as such but instead focus on the social forces of aetiology, within Durkheimian or Marxian orientations (Pilgrim 2014). Those forces are multiple and vary from context to context: diagnosed mental disorder is socially patterned. It is inflected strongly by membership of social groups, with social class being the best predictor of mental health status, followed by age, with the very young and very old being more vulnerable to mental disorder or its attribution. Gender is important in the limited arena of coercion, where this is slanted heavily towards male targets; so too with race, with some, but not all, non-White groups suffering disproportionately enforced detention.

Moreover, within this social causationist tradition, 'intersectionality' has become *de rigueur* when analysing complex open human systems (Walby 2007). Not only is mental health status shaped or explained by the intersection of different social processes linked to class, age, race, and gender, but also *within-group differences* are important, especially the micro-social implications of intra-familial neglect and abuse. This has been increasingly confirmed in recent years by both retrospective and prospective investigations of the link between childhood adversity or trauma and consequent vulnerability to mental disorder (e.g. Ogata et al. 1990; Read et al. 2003; Varese et al. 2012).

This 'traumogenic model' is important, but it has nothing itself to say about coercion, except by implication. If traumatized children are at greater risk of subsequent mental disorder, then a sub-group of them will be at greater risk of coercive detention and treatment. The prospects of re-traumatization in this scenario are self-evident. This is one reason why critiques of coercion by service users and some dissenting professionals are sensitive to the repeated scenario of the powerful coercing the powerless.

Labelling theory

Labelling theory was developed by the 'symbolic interactionism' wing of the Chicago School of Sociology, which aimed to understand society by studying the ways in which humans exchange meanings in their interactions. The other, 'ecological', wing of this school provided the first large-scale studies of social causationism (social epidemiology) and still finds its expression in the sociological literature (e.g. Almog et al. 2004). Labelling theory instead focuses not primarily on aetiology but on how the reaction of others maintains 'secondary deviance'.

'Primary deviance' emerges from a range of biological, psychological, and social causes and is often trivial, transient, and ignored by others for a while. Thus labelling theorists have been interested in the particular contingencies under which labelling does or does not happen. For example, Yarrow et al. (1955) found that the wives of men eventually labelled as schizophrenic ignored and rationalized their husbands' symptoms for varying periods of time before seeking help. In a seminal study of labelling in the professional arena, Rosenhan (1973) showed that 'pseudo-patients' were admitted to psychiatric facilities for simply reporting hearing the words 'empty', 'hollow', and 'thud'. In all other respects, they behaved rationally but the staff recorded all of their behaviour as if it were indicative of mental illness.

Labelling theorists at times focus on the lay arena, with professionals 'rubber-stamping' decisions already made by the family or strangers in fear or exasperation (Coulter 1973). Others, such as Scheff (1966), emphasize the power of psychiatry to label. Goffman (1961) argued that both lay and professional powers formed an alliance of those who were sane by common consent. This created a 'betrayal funnel', as the patient was subjected to a 'degradation ritual'. This process of labelling alters the person's identity and social status—once a person is seen to have lost their reason, then their credibility is permanently undermined (Garfinkel 1956).

Some sociologists criticized labelling theory for understating the underlying power of the (biological, psychological, and social) causes of primary deviance (in this case this refers to mental disorder) and noted that labelling can have the positive consequence of giving patients access to help to reduce their deviance (Gove 1970, 1975). This matter of actual or putative *warranted* medical paternalism is thus an important consideration with regard to psychiatric coercion within the sociological discourse (Pols 2001).

Another criticism of labelling theory is that we would expect an alignment between everyday stereotypes of mental illness and professional action. Jones and Cochrane (1981) found that stereotypes conform very poorly to the prevalence of psychiatric labelling. Depression is the commonest diagnosis but is rarely emphasized by lay people, who stereotype mental illness. The dominant typical lay stereotype is of a wild, deranged patient, manic and violent and beyond all reason about anything. Also, note that Rosenhan's pseudo-patients mentioned above did not go on to actually adopt the role of psychiatric patients after their discharge from hospital.

Because of doubts among sociologists about the power of labelling explanations, labelling theory fell out of favour for a while. However, subsequent empirical evidence emboldened a new generation to return with a modified theory. Link and Phelan (1999) summarized a number of studies which clearly demonstrate the negative effects of labelling. Some studies indicate that disvalued social statuses, such as prostitution, epilepsy, and substance, abuse form a hierarchy of stigma (e.g. Skinner et al. 1995).

Moreover, some experimental studies showed that knowledge of a person's psychiatric history predicts social rejection, and that these tendencies start in childhood (e.g. Harris et al. 1990). The general public manifest that fear of violence, and the need to keep a social distance diminishes with increasing contact with people with a psychiatric diagnosis (Alexander and Link 2003). Also, some de-stigmatization campaigns, which focus on mental illness 'being an illness like any other', may have paradoxical impacts, highlighting why lay labelling remains very important (Pescosolido 2013). Note that even at the very time that labelling theory was losing its popularity, there was evidence that a psychiatric history reduced a person's access to housing and employment (e.g. Farina and Felner 1973).

In the light of this sort of research, Link and Phelan (1999) suggested a 'modified labelling theory' supported by two main findings in a series of studies. First, provided that best practice is offered in mental health services, people with mental health problems can derive positive benefits. This supports Gove's claim about the positive opportunity created by labelling. Second, whether or not specialist mental health services have positive or negative effects (a function of their range of quality), stigma and social rejection tend to persist in the community.

This second type of finding does not entail the direct prejudicial and rejecting action of others (the 'classical' position of labelling theory). Instead, Link and Phelan suggest that stigma and rejection emerge from a shared cultural expectation. For all parties mental disorder can lead to mutual suspicion. This shared view then leads to both parties lacking confidence during their personal encounters (what Goffman called 'face work'). This creates a self-fulfilling prophecy of mutual avoidance. The patient keeps his or her distance and the non-patient expects this and so is complicit in the social distancing. This then is the path to an ongoing process of social rejection, with patients often routinely and mainly relating to psychiatric staff (who expect and tolerate mentally disordered conduct, contra Scheff's focus above) and other patients in their lives.

This emphasis on the internal and interpersonal work done by patients about expectations is also supported by other findings about rule breaking and self-labelling.

Thoits (1985) demonstrates how we learn from a young age to self-monitor emotional deviance. We begin to learn when it is appropriate to be happy, sad, or fearful and when we must conform to the expectations of others in particular situations. By late childhood we are typically in a position to identify in ourselves when our emotional conduct might be considered inappropriate by others; we know what constitute 'feeling rules' and their transgressions. However, if we fail to learn the meta-rule of ongoing social accountability relevant to our particular cultural context, then others will react negatively. Those deemed to be 'psychotic' (who live in a world of their own) or 'personality disordered' (who live incorrigibly and egocentrically) may well then feel the force of those reactions. Psychiatric coercion is one possible outcome in our current times.

But psychiatry has only been in existence since the middle of the nineteenth century and practice is only extensively in the developed world. Consequently some historical and cultural relativism about the social control of mental disorder is required for a fuller context, starting with our current assumptions.

Social history

Self-evident ways of regulating daily life are part of our socialization and constitute the Aristotelian notion of *doxa* in any particular culture. We learn to behave in this way, not that, in this particular setting and take this for granted unreflectively with our present norms and mores. But we transgress those expectations at our peril, and we only tend to notice things when they go wrong in social scenarios. And when they do go wrong, if we are the transgressor we are expected to explain ourselves (Scott and Lyman 1968; Antaki 1981).

When and if we fail to account for our rule transgressions or role failures then others may consider that we are immoral, criminal, or insane (or even some ambivalent combination of the three). Only psychoanalysis and ethnomethodology problematize normality. Most of us most of the time are oblivious to, and unreflective about, the routine flow of our particular culture. But that is also why when we enter a different culture we notice the oddity (to us) of some of its norms and why we risk getting things wrong (to natives).

But within our own culture most of us have a very fine-tuned understanding about what conduct should appear in which social context in everyday life. The option of psychiatric coercion then emerges in some societies faced with rule transgressions and role failures of certain sorts. And some sociologists have even argued that the 'social dystonia' created by madness *legitimately warrants* psychiatric patients being sequestrated forcibly from the general population, for the protection of *the latter* (Kecmanovic 2013; cf. Pilgrim 2013).

Because human societies are open systems and vary across time and space, self-evident assumptions and their consequent self-evident mandates (in this case to coercively interfere with the lives of risky people who are also deemed to be psychologically deviant) are contestable, both in fact and in principle. For example, some stereotypes of madness, such as a proneness to violence and aimless wandering, were present in Ancient Greece (Rosen 1968). However, Socrates also noted that madness, like sanity, was given by the gods, and so its virtues not just its vices must be appraised. He argued that madness was not merely random pathology and social threat but that it also inspired lovers, poets, and prophesiers (Screech 1985).

But, historically, the most important rupture of relevance here was the Enlightenment. This was the watershed in which reason and science were to emerge, as the new defining features of civilized humanity, displacing religion and superstition (Doerner 1969). Thereafter unreason, whether it was at the aggregate level (religion) or individual level (lunacy), came under particular suspicion. However, as the reforms of the early nineteenth century were to reveal, the residue of religious means of managing madness remained strong. This was evident at the Retreat in York run by Quakers who were 'lay administrators'. There madness was seen as a moral challenge not as a disease of the brain (the post-Kraepelinian orthodoxy to emerge later). Patients were treated in a kindly manner with a mixture of forbearance and expectations of helpful but corrective daily routines in order to coax lunatics back into the moral fold (Scull 2011).

In Britain by the end of the nineteenth century coercive detention was comprehensive. All patients were 'certified' when entering asylums, a legal routine that was not challenged or disrupted until the 1930 Mental Treatment Act, when the term 'community care' first emerged and 'voluntary boarders' were introduced as a social administrative category. At the turn of the twentieth century the cultural image of the deranged lunatic, noted earlier, dominated the public imagination and the fear of 'unfair detention' was a motif of legislative and other policy debates (Bean 1980, 1986). Bean notes that psychiatry may well be a medical discipline but its core social function is one of rule enforcement; so too with other public servants such as police officers and social workers, both of which accordingly are now key actors in psychiatric coercion.

Even today it may be difficult for psychiatric professionals to accept that they are agents of social control, but indeed they are, whether that role is played out coercively or voluntarily. Whether the benign aspirations or rhetoric of medical paternalism ('treating patients under the Mental Health Act') are achieved or not (see later), the primary mandate for professional coercion is based upon the need for 'something to be done' in some sort of difficult situation in which social flow has been disrupted (non-criminally). As Bean notes, all psychiatric crises are social crises. However, coercion can be used more routinely outside conditions of social crisis, for example in the long-term warehousing of mentally disordered offenders in high-security hospitals.

The matter of psychiatric social control was highlighted by the crisis in psychiatry created when some practitioners were dutifully deployed to control political dissidents in the old Soviet Union, with a favoured diagnosis of 'sluggish schizophrenia' (Bloch and Reddaway 1977). This raised an important logical point: was this an abuse of psychiatry? And, if so, did this mean that routine psychiatry outside the Soviet Union (which was also coercive and also enacted by state-employed practitioners) was *not* abusive in form and content?

At the centre of this contention was the dissenting psychiatric position (which by the 1970s had become a sociological point of reference) that an adult citizen, who was not a criminal, should be free to speak and act as he or she pleased (Szasz 1963; Laing 1967). 'Mental health law', especially under what are known as 'civil sections' in Britain, is actually about the negation of this core principle. Szasz therefore designated modern state psychiatry as a form of witch-finding, which habitually crushed citizenship and personhood. Thus, since the mid twentieth century, psychiatry has witnessed a plurality of debates about its role in society and diverse positions about its theory and practice (Fussinger 2011).

The main sociological point here is at that people who are deemed by those who are sane by common consent to be not only mentally disordered but also risky to self or others, warrant coercive control according to some parties to this debate but not others, both inside and outside of psychiatry. It is not surprising, then, that the matter of coercion has continued to be a rallying call for angry and disaffected service users who, as professional 'anti-psychiatry' lost its energy as a cultural force, coalesced into a new social movement in the 1980s (Rogers and Pilgrim 1991; Crossley 2008; Rose 2009). To this day, the role of psychiatry in society remains precarious, both for its internal defenders and detractors (e.g. Craddock et al. 2012; cf. Bracken and Thomas 2006). The question of coercion is one of several reasons for this professional angst; hence the emergence of this book. It is not the only reason but it is one of them (Pilgrim and Rogers 2009).

Discussion

I have drawn upon three traditions of sociological work. The first is from social causationism driven mainly by the ecological wing of the Chicago School of Sociology around the time of the World War II. Its relevance is not directly obvious, but its dogged environmentalism, represented in more recent times by the popularity of the traumogenic model to explain the existence of mental disorder, is consequentially relevant. If, actuarially, those who develop mental health problems have already suffered disproportionately at the hands of *both* social forces *and* oppressive intra-familial relationships, then the use of coercion in their lives will have a compounding and resonating experiential character.

The second, and more obvious and relevant contribution, came from labelling theory. Its first incarnation, from the other wing of the Chicago School by Erving Goffman and his followers, set out the case that the role of others has to be addressed; we cannot simply focus on the actual or assumed indwelling skin-encapsulated psychopathology of identified patients. Those patients exist in social relations, which include the enacted powers of third parties, especially psychiatric professionals, significant others, and occasionally strangers (see later).

I noted that following its fall from fashion in the wake of empirical criticisms about its explanatory value, labelling theory was resurrected more persuasively in modified form. If mental disorder emerges from a social negotiation, then within that the option of coercion is one amongst many on a continuum. We can start with the patient being self-identified and then propelled into help-seeking by their distress. Further along others may suggest the latter course. When someone is identified in the lay arena as having a problem but does not admit to it, then other options emerge. Significant others may apply pressure and may even threaten to break off support unless some help is sought. They may indeed approach services themselves, as it were to 'report' the incipient but reluctant patient.

And finally they (or strangers and the police) may look to psychiatry to 'do something' about what has become a social crisis. Within that final scenario professionals can deploy a range of threats and levers which fall just short of formally recording the 'involuntary' or 'formal' status of the patient under 'mental health law' (Szmukler and Appelbaum 2008). By the time though that psychiatry becomes involved, a range of social transactions have occurred which have been transmitted to 'statutory services'.

This point about transmission as a complex social process in open systems is important. While coercion is seemingly in the sole hands of statutory professionals, any micro-social analysis entails more than their ethical dilemmas and the courses of action they choose. So too with other analyses, such as studying the knowledge and biases of the police under Section 136, when it is members of *the public* who alert them to a problem and so their anxieties (not those of the police) must be part of any sociological formulation.

Similarly when families ask professionals to get involved, coercively or otherwise, they are not really reacting to the presence of mental illness in their relative but to their *conduct*. It is the way that incipient patients behave, not their symptoms of mental disorder per se, that prompt the concerns and actions of others. After all, most mentally disordered patients are not subjected to coercion, and those who are, even episodically, are rarely subjected to it at great length (if we exclude mentally disordered offenders, and even they typically leave services eventually).

If social causationists, via the traumogenic model, alert us to the social context of coercion in one way and labelling theorists in another, then social history puts the topic into a much larger framework of time and place. As far as the historical context is concerned, coercion has an ambiguous medical history. Philippe Pinel, a medical man, allegedly struck the chains from the lunatics of the Hospice de Bicêtre. However, he always conceded that what was to pre-figure 'moral treatment' (what we now know as the therapeutic community movement) was instigated by the lay governor of the madhouse, Pinel's de facto mentor Jean-Baptiste Pussin (Schuster et al. 2011). And subsequently the non-medical management of lunacy at the York Retreat was also at the hands of 'lay administrators', not doctors.

By the end of the nineteenth century, with psychiatry named and newly established, the medical superintendents of asylums simply took it as part of their normal role to hold and treat 'certified' patients against their will. At that point, the emphasis within the medical discourse shifted from the patient's right to liberty to the doctor's right to treat. By then coercion and its necessity became modern psychiatric *doxa*; a position shared by most of the public, provided they were assured of safeguards against 'unfair detention', given its imagined or real enough risks to human welfare.

And the issue of the impact of psychiatric detention on human welfare then returned in the middle of the twentieth century. First, the Nazi medical killing centres murdered psychiatric patients, using eugenic grounds as an overture to the 'Final Solution', an option also seriously entertained by the American psychiatric profession in the 1940s (Joseph 2005; Pilgrim 2008). Second, in the wake of this Kraepelinian eugenic discourse, after the war dissident colleagues like Szasz accused his profession of a form of witch-finding. Third, during the 1970s Russian psychiatrists embarrassed their international colleagues, creating a link for some critics between coercion and clinical iatrogenesis. Secretly shot documentary footage showed dissidents trembling, drooling, and shuffling zombie-like, when being detained and treated for their 'sluggish schizophrenia'.

By the 1970s, this uncomfortable scenario for psychiatry invited this question: why was it OK for patients in the West to suffer Parkinsonism and tardive dyskinesia under the 'proper' deployment of 'mental health law', but it was a human rights' outrage when exactly the same iatrogenic symptoms were being experienced by political dissidents detained 'improperly'? Was this evident psychiatric iatrogenesis suddenly acceptable in the West but not in the Soviet regime it criticized and, if so, on what clinical or political grounds (Brown and Funk 1986)? If psychiatric treatment was so acceptable and effective, then why was coercion needed at all, and why, since Victorian times, had the general public feared 'unfair detention'? Given that psychotropic medication lacked the treatment specificity of, say, insulin for diabetes, and given that it was often ineffective, its use under conditions of coercion was proving to be understandably problematic.

It is in the light of these problems about coercive psychiatry being exposed by debates in the 1970s that I now place 'mental health law' in quotation marks: it is a euphemism. It is not about mental health gain but specifiable conditions of social control. This became an official position (not merely a mundane observation of pernickety sociologists) when the British government was warding off attempts by critics of legal reforms to link law to service quality. A Department of Health statement complained that critics of the reforms were arguing:

> ... that the legislation should be about improving services. The Bill is not about service provision. It is about the legal process for bringing people under compulsion.

> Department of Health (2005, p. 4, para. 10)

Thus 'mental health law' is not about treating people optimally but about the detail of lawful compulsion. Without that detail, agents of the state would be guilty of false imprisonment and assault. 'Mental health law' protects psychiatric staff from that eventuality. And this is acceptable, by and large, to those who are sane by common consent, its episodic beneficiaries. The demand for social control comes from below; it is not a paternalistic medical whim. If a profession, other than medicine, were to be responsible for the coercive control of rule transgressions, then the demand from the public would still be there (Cohen and Scull 1985).

The first summary point made by Phelan and Link above was a concession to the criticism from Gove that coercion may bring benefits not just costs. Provided that optimal mental health care ensues for the patient, they could eventually experience a good outcome in their life. However, this potential benefit has to be cautioned by other facts. If coercive detention brings with it (typically but not necessarily) coercive *treatment*, then iatrogenesis invoked without consent is risked. And given that psychiatric drugs have a blunderbuss impact on the central nervous system, and consequently the functioning of major organs and both smooth and striated muscles, then a range of unwanted effects are possible for all recipients. This is the case whether or not they ask for the treatment and whether or not they experience a reduction in their symptoms (Breggin 1993; Moncrieff 2007).

Moreover, in the British context we do not have strong grounds for promising optimal care. The final report of the Mental Health Act Commission noted that over a 20-year period, from the mid 1980s, involuntary detention more than doubled for civil sections of the Mental Health Act. It also noted that the average standard of care in acute psychiatry was so poor that the then President of the Royal College of Psychiatrists (Professor Dinesh Bhugra) would not have been happy for his family to be admitted to it (Pilgrim 2012).

What the debates from social history have pointed out is that current norms of coercive practice are just that: they are (1) current and (2) norms. They are historically contingent and not trans-historically inevitable. They are taken-for-granted forms of practice that, like all forms of human action, are open to contestation and possible revision or even abandonment hereafter. To put this normative point into a real and immediate comparative context, let me mention a thought experiment that I use as a deliberate provocation with the psychology, sociology, and social work students I teach (Pilgrim and Tomasini 2012).

Supposing the governments of current developed societies passed a law which imposed a curfew on all people under the age of 30 years from dusk on Friday to dawn on Monday. In one dramatic move, this would have a number of immediate impacts on public health, crime, injury, deaths, and health service utilization. The imagined curfew would reduce: sexual and non-sexual assaults, road traffic accidents, suicides, homicides, intimate violence, A&E costs to the health service, police deployments, sexually transmitted diseases, and unwanted pregnancies. This is a fairly impressive list of benefits. So why does it seem such a bizarre proposal? My students, biased of course by their age profile, generally think that it is a preposterous suggestion (though intriguingly a few agree with it). I then put it to the majority of scoffers that if it is preposterous, then why does 'mental health law' exist, when the great majority of psychiatric patients are not a risk to others and self-harm and suicide are not an illegal acts?

This thought experiment forces us all to reflect very seriously on the political or moral mandate that we take for granted about the current norm of psychiatric coercion in society. If it is risk to self that is the issue, then why not 'section' people who smoke or eat fatty foods or have unprotected sexual intercourse? Or how about racing-car drivers, boxers, and rock climbers: should we detain them for their own protection, because their actions are lacking in insight and blatantly risky?

These points return us to Szasz (1963), to the irritation of his colleagues exasperated by his arguments. He makes the simple point that in modern societies it is not dangerousness that is the issue *but the manner in which one is dangerous*. The drunk with a cut lip and bloody nose from his previous night's brawl is released under caution from his police cell, with a hangover but his liberty intact. Indeed if his liberty is curtailed any further, he must be charged and his innocence potentially advanced by a legal advocate.

No such advantage is offered to the sectioned psychiatric patient. The only state employees involved are judging the correctness of detention. There is no ensured 'other side' paid to argue against that consensus formation, in order to protect the liberty of the patient and to pre-empt the risk of coerced iatrogenesis.

Conclusion

This chapter has offered a selective overview of the sociological literature relevant to the topic of psychiatric coercion. In particular, the implications of the traumogenic model, derived from social causationist assumptions, modified labelling theory, and social history were outlined. Coercion always occurs in particular social contexts and the latter contain social processes, which are both peculiar to a time and place and reflect the history of that cultural setting. Those studying psychiatric coercion, from any discipline, can use these points to reflect on both their topic of interest and their own acculturated expectations about it.

References

Alexander LA, Link BG (2003). The impact of contact on stigmatizing attitudes toward people with mental illness. *Journal of Mental Health*, **12**:271–290.

Almog M, Curtis S, Copeland A, et al. (2004). Geographical variation in acute psychiatric admissions within New York City 1990–2000: growing inequalities in service use? *Social Science and Medicine*, **59**:361–376.

Antaki C (ed.) (1981). *The psychology of ordinary explanations of social behaviour*. London: Academic Press.

Bean P (1980). *Compulsory admissions to mental hospital*. Chichester: Wiley.

Bean P (1986). *Mental disorder and legal control*. Cambridge: Cambridge University Press.

Bloch S, Reddaway P (1977). *Russia's political hospitals*. London: Gollancz.

Bracken P, Thomas P (2006). *Postpsychiatry: mental health in a postmodern world*. Oxford: Oxford University Press.

Breggin P (1993). *Toxic psychiatry*. London: HarperCollins.

Brown P, Funk SC (1986). Tardive dyskinesia: barriers to the professional recognition of iatrogenic disease. *Journal of Health and Social Behaviour*, **27**:116–132.

Cohen S, Scull A (eds) (1985). *Social control and the state*. Oxford: Basil Blackwell.

Coulter J (1973). *Approaches to insanity*. New York: Wiley.

Craddock N, Antebi D, Attenburrow MJ, et al. (2008). Wake-up call for British psychiatry. *British Journal of Psychiatry*, **193**:6–9.

Crossley N (2008). *Contesting psychiatry: social movements in mental health*. Abingdon: Routledge.

Department of Health (2005). *Government response to the report of the Joint Committee on the Draft Mental Health Bill 2004*. London: Stationery Office.

Doerner K (1969). *Madness and the bourgeoisie*. Oxford: Oxford University Press.

Farina A, Felner RD (1973). Employment interview reactions to former mental patients. *Journal of Abnormal Psychology*, **82**:268–272.

Fussinger C (2011). 'Therapeutic community', psychiatry's reformers and anti-psychiatrists: reconsidering changes in the field of psychiatry after World War II. *History of Psychiatry*, **22**:146–163.

Garfinkel H (1956). Conditions of successful degradation ceremonies. *American Journal of Sociology*, **61**:420–424.

Gove W (1970). Societal reaction as an explanation of mental illness: an evaluation. *American Sociological Review*, **35**:873–884.

Gove W (1975). The labeling theory of mental illness: a reply to Scheff. *American Sociological Review*, 40:242–248.

Harris MJR, Millich EM, Johnson DW (1990). Effects of expectancies on children's social interactions. *Journal of Experimental Social Psychology*, 26:1–12.

Jones L, Cochrane R (1981). Stereotypes of mental illness: a test of the labelling hypothesis. *International Journal of Social Psychiatry*, 27:99–107.

Joseph J (2005). The 1942 'euthanasia' debate in the *American Journal of Psychiatry*. *History of Psychiatry*, 16:171–179.

Kecmanovic D (2013). Psychotic patients and other social deviants. *Australian and New Zealand Journal of Psychiatry*, 47:805–810.

Laing RD (1967). *The politics of experience and the bird of paradise*. Harmondsworth: Penguin.

Link BG, Phelan JC (1999). The labeling theory of mental disorder (II): the consequences of labeling. In: *A handbook for the study of mental health* (ed. AV Horwitz, TL Scheid), pp. 73–86. Cambridge: Cambridge University Press.

Moncrieff J (2007). *The myth of the chemical cure: a critique of psychiatric drugs*. Basingstoke: Palgrave.

Ogata SN, Silk KR, Goodrich S, et al. (1990).Childhood sexual and physical abuse in adult patients with borderline personality disorder. *American Journal of Psychiatry*, 147:1008–1012.

Pescosolido BA (2013). The public stigma of mental illness: what do we think; what do we know; what can we prove? *Journal of Health and Social Behavior*, 54: 1–21.

Pilgrim D (2008). The eugenic legacy in psychiatry and psychology. *International Journal of Social Psychiatry*, 54:272–284.

Pilgrim D (2012). Final lessons from the Mental Health Act Commission for England and Wales: the limits of legalism-plus-safeguards. *Journal of Social Policy*, 41:61–81.

Pilgrim D (2013). Social dystonia and psychosis: an alternative perspective. *Australian and New Zealand Journal of Psychiatry*, 47:811–814.

Pilgrim D (2014). *Understanding mental health: a critical realist exploration*. London: Routledge.

Pilgrim D, Rogers A (2009). Survival and its discontents: the case of British psychiatry. *Sociology of Health and Illness*, 31:947–961.

Pilgrim D, Tomasini F (2012). On being unreasonable in modern society: are mental health problems special? *Disability and Society*, 27:631–646.

Pols J (2001). Enforcing patients' rights or improving care: the interference of two modes of doing good in mental health care. *Sociology of Health and Illness*, 25:325–347.

Read J, Agar K, Argyle N, et al. (2003). Sexual and physical abuse during childhood and adulthood as predictors of hallucinations, delusions and thought disorder. *Psychology and Psychotherapy: Theory, Research and Practice*, 76:1–22.

Rogers A, Pilgrim D (1991). 'Pulling down churches'—accounting for the British mental health users' movement. *Sociology of Health and Illness*, 13:129–148.

Rogers A, Pilgrim D (2014). *A sociology of mental health and illness*, 5th edn. Maidenhead: Open University Press.

Rose D (2009). Survivor produced knowledge. In: *This is survivor research* (ed. A Sweeney, P Beresford, A Faulkner, et al.), pp. 15–30. Ross-on-Wye: PPCS Books.

Rosen G (1968). *Madness in society*. New York: Harper.

Rosenhan DL (1973). On being sane in insane places. *Science*, 179:250–258.

Scheff T (1966). *Being mentally ill: a sociological theory.* Chicago: Aldine.

Scott MB, Lyman SM (1968). Accounts. *American Journal of Sociology,* **33**:12–18.

Schuster J-P, Hoertel N, Limosin F (2011). The man behind Philippe Pinel: Jean-Baptiste Pussin (1746–1811)—psychiatry in pictures. *British Journal of Psychiatry,* **198**:241.

Screech MA (1985). Good madness in Christendom. In: *The anatomy of madness* (ed. WF Bynum, R Porter, M Shepherd), pp. 25–39. London: Tavistock.

Scull A (2011). Institutionalization and deinstitutionalization. In: *The Sage handbook of mental health and illness* (ed. D Pilgrim, A Rogers, B Pescosolido), pp. 430–452. London: Sage.

Skinner LJ, Berry KK, Griffiths SE, et al. (1995). Generalizability and specificity of the stigma associated with the mental illness label: a reconsideration twenty five years later. *Journal of Community Psychology,* **23**:3–17.

Szasz TS (1963). *Law, liberty, and psychiatry: an inquiry into the social uses of mental health practices.* New York: Syracuse University Press.

Szmukler G, Appelbaum P (2008). Treatment pressures, leverage, coercion and compulsion in mental health care. *Journal of Mental Health,* **17**:233–244.

Thoits P (1985). Self-labeling processes in mental illness: the role of emotional deviance. *American Journal of Sociology,* **91**: 221–249.

Varese F, Smeets F, Drukker M, et al. (2012). Childhood adversities increase the risk of psychosis: a meta-analysis of patient-control, prospective- and cross-sectional cohort studies. *Schizophrenia Bulletin,* **38**:661–671.

Walby S (2007). Complexity theory, systems theory and multiple intersecting social inequalities. *Philosophy of the Social Sciences,* **37**:449–470.

Yarrow MJ, Schwartz C, Murphy H, et al. (1955). The psychological meaning of mental illness. *Journal of Social Issues,* **11**:12–24.

Chapter 13

Human rights in community psychiatry

Genevra Richardson

Concern for human rights has crept up the global mental health policy agenda in recent years. This chapter considers why this might be, and what value human rights might add in relation to the use of coercion in community mental health.

Law and 'coercion' in an international context

There is no single generally applicable definition of coercion in law. Typically, in the interests of self-determination, the law will not allow A to force B to act against B's will in the absence of some overriding objective. In that sense the law will prohibit coercion. But not all external pressure or influence can be regarded as sufficiently *coercive* as to be illegal in domestic law, or even to render the consequent decision or action invalid. The same is true of international human rights. Much will depend on context.

In relation to the provision of treatment and care for mental disabilities, many domestic legal systems expressly authorize the use of coercion in the form of involuntary treatment and detention. (The term mental disability is being used here to include both intellectual or learning disabilities and more psychiatric diagnoses. It has been chosen because it is the term now employed in the international human rights literature and is preferred by service users internationally.) Patients subject to such involuntary powers can be said to experience formal coercion. However, the vast majority of people receiving care for a mental disability are not subject to formal legal powers but might none the less feel coerced, in the sense that their choices are influenced either by the knowledge that the legal powers exist, by the hierarchical nature of psychiatric institutions, or by any of the other obvious sources of power imbalance (Bean 1986). This form of perceived coercion is often termed 'informal coercion' and has received a lot of attention in the literature (Monahan et al. 1995; Poulsen 1999, 2002; Høyer et al. 2002). Again there is no generally accepted definition, but most studies have emphasized the patient's belief that she is not free to refuse (Monahan et al. 1995, p. 252). In addition to informal coercion, so understood, there is the increasingly common practice of leverage, the 'attempt to influence patients' treatment adherence by, for example, making patients' access to subsidised housing conditional upon adherence to treatment or by making treatment adherence a condition of patients' avoidance of financial control' (Canvin et al. 2013, p. 100; see also Szmukler 2009; Dunn et al. 2012).

Finally there is the question of decision-making capacity and the extent to which coercion can be said to exist if the person is unaware of the external pressure being brought to bear upon them. Thus, in order to assess the role of international human rights in relation to coercion it is necessary to consider at least these three forms, i.e. formal and informal coercion and leverage, and to consider the relevance or otherwise of decision-making capacity.

The enormous burden of mental disabilities worldwide is now widely acknowledged. In 2013, an article in the *New England Journal of Medicine* reported that the aggregate burden of [years lived with disability] resulting from mental and behavioural disorders continues to be higher than that resulting from any other disease category (Becker and Kleinman 2013). More than 75% of people with a serious mental illness in less-developed countries do not receive treatment for it. This burden of disease is then commonly set in the context of the level of expenditure on mental health care in various regions of the world. According to the *Mental health atlas* published by the World Health Organization (WHO) in 2011, median expenditures on mental health per capita are US$1.63 with a large variation among income groups, ranging from US$0.20 in low-income countries to US$44.84 in high-income countries (World Health Organization 2011). Similar discrepancies are seen in relation to human resources. The median number of psychiatrists per 100,000 of population is 0.05 in low-income countries and 8.59 in high-income countries, and across all mental health professionals the median in low-income countries is 1.3 while in high-income countries it is 50.8.

Mental disorder and abuse of human rights

Not all commentators agree with the data on disease burden as typically presented, and the emphasis placed on both the expenditure figures and the human resource ratios can be seen as an inappropriate imposition of criteria applicable to a Western medical model of care (Summerfield 2011; Read 2012; Lewis 2014; White and Sashidharan 2014). Nonetheless, few can deny that the reality faced by people with mental disabilities in many low- and middle-income counties is extremely poor. Many gross human rights abuses have been reported by bodies including the WHO and the UN Special Rapporteur on Torture both within psychiatric institutions and in the community itself (World Health Organization 2012; United Nations 2013). An article in *The Lancet* in 2011 listed the following as the most common human rights violations suffered by people with mental disabilities (Drew et al. 2011):

+ exclusion, marginalization, and discrimination in the community
+ denial or restriction of employment rights and opportunities
+ physical abuse/violence
+ inability to access effective mental health services
+ sexual abuse/violence
+ arbitrary detention
+ denial of opportunities for marriage/right to found a family
+ lack of means to enable independent living in the community

* denial of access to general health/medical services
* financial exploitation

In response to this grim picture there have been a number of international initiatives. Since its call to action in 2001 the WHO has published a resource book (World Health Organization 2005), a qualityrights tool kit (World Health Organization 2012), and a mental health action plan (World Health Organization 2013). In 2005 the UK Department for International Development initiated its Mental Health and Poverty Project (Department for International Development 2010) and in 2007 the Movement for Global Mental Health was launched in a series of articles in *The Lancet* (Patel 2008), followed up by a further special issue in 2011 (Patel 2011).

Many of these initiatives have placed considerable emphasis on law and human rights. The WHO's action plan, for example, requires states to have mental health laws and policies that comply with the UN Convention on the Rights of Persons with Disabilities (CRPD) (World Health Organization 2013). It sets a global target for 50% of countries to have mental health laws in line with international and regional human rights instruments by 2020. The Global Movement for Mental Health, in its 2007 incarnation, did not place particular emphasis on human rights, but the editorial to the 2011 special issue of *The Lancet* indicated a distinct change in tone: 'First and foremost, the issue of the human rights of people with mental health problems should be placed at the foreground of global health' (Patel 2011).

Reference to human rights may have become commonplace, but what does the WHO expect human rights to achieve? What do those who support the Global Movement understand by human rights as possessed by people with mental disabilities? In a telling critique of the use made of human rights rhetoric Oliver Lewis expressed the fear that for 'some leaders of world psychiatry, human rights boil down to imposing treatment whether the patient likes it or not. Theirs is an idiosyncratic and intolerant view that is challenged by firmly established notions of human rights'. He does not place the Global Movement in that category but he cautions that those 'who speak on behalf of the Global Movement for Mental Health would be well advised to distance themselves from those who seek to use rhetoric of human rights to legitimise forced treatment' (Lewis 2014, p. 257). This may be vivid language, but it reflects a real fear that if 'human rights' are not carefully specified they can be used to serve widely disparate causes.

The nature of traditional human rights

In many jurisdictions the law has had a long and significant role in relation to the provision of mental health care. The position in England and Wales is typical of the structure adopted in many jurisdictions. It:

(1) imposes obligations on authorities to provide care;

(2) provides both a power to treat involuntarily in hospital and a structure for community treatment orders (the Mental Health Act 1983);

(3) establishes an inspectorate (the Care Quality Commission);

(4) provides a structure for decision making on behalf of people who lack mental capacity (the Mental Capacity Act 2005).

To some degree the presence of legal regulation can be regarded as good in and of itself. It provides mechanisms for accountability and nurtures the rule of law. But the domestic legal framework in any specific jurisdiction may or may not be compliant with the demands of international human rights, and the WHO expressly emphasizes the need to comply with those international demands.

A great deal has been written on the nature of international human rights, their origins, content, and status. This is not the place to review that literature, but it is at least worth recalling the traditional split between first-generation, or negative, rights on the one hand and second-generation, or positive, rights on the other (Berlin 1969). So-called negative rights are designed primarily to protect the individual from interference, mainly from the state. They include the right to personal liberty, bodily integrity and security, religious freedom, etc. Positive rights, on the other hand, include the right to material goods, education, shelter, food, etc. Increasingly, the distinction between the two has been seen to be imperfect. Security of the person, for example, demands expenditure on such material goods as police, courts, and prisons. But in the context of mental disability the distinction can at least serve to illustrate some recurrent tensions. Here the distinction can be expressed as being between the right to health, the positive right, and the more traditional protective rights to be free from inhuman and degrading treatment and from unlawful detention. In its essence, the right to health might be designed to address the desperate absence of care while the protective rights provide safeguards against direct abuse. Again the distinction is highly permeable, as attested by the levels of malnutrition in some psychiatric facilities.

The right to health

This right, which found its first indirect articulation in the UN Declaration of 1948, takes its current, more direct, form in Article 12(1) of the International Covenant on Economic, Social and Cultural Rights 1976: 'the States Parties to the present Covenant recognise the right of everyone to the enjoyment of the highest attainable standard of physical and mental health'. It has been highly controversial from the start, particularly insofar as it includes entitlements, and has attracted an extensive literature (Wolff 2012; Gostin 2014). It is not a right to be healthy. It is a right to facilities, goods, services, and conditions that are conducive to the realization of the highest attainable standard of physical and mental health. It is also in the main subject to progressive realization rather than immediate compliance (United Nations 2000). For the present purposes it should be sufficient to agree with those who argue that, whatever its shortcomings, we should take the right to health seriously as one way of tackling the global burden of disease (Wolff 2012).

Protective rights or freedoms

These are the rights familiar from the UN Covenant on Civil and Political Rights and the European Convention on Human Rights (ECHR). The African Charter on Human and Peoples' Rights 1981, known as the Banjul Convention, is more expansive and contains both protective rights and the right to enjoy the best attainable state of physical and mental health (Article 16). Protective rights constitute rights to be free from abuse by the state and state actors and include the right to liberty and security, to the peaceful enjoyment of family life, and to freedom of expression and religion. The model of mental health legislation familiar in many jurisdictions is typically devised to comply with such rights and freedoms. In England and Wales, for example, the Mental Health Act 1983 (MHA) authorizes interference with fundamental rights in relation to involuntary hospital detention and treatment but is broadly compliant with the ECHR which permits detention on grounds of unsoundness of mind and has been interpreted as allowing involuntary treatment in certain circumstances. The Mental Capacity Act 2005 (MCA), which provides for substitute decision making on behalf of adults who lack mental capacity, is also generally compliant with the ECHR, even when its powers are used to deprive a person of his or her liberty. The implications of a recent decision on the interpretation of the ECHR by the UK Supreme Court (2014) which has particular relevance to community provision are considered later.

The current structure of international human rights thus contains both positive rights or entitlements, and protective rights to be free from abuse. But people with mental disabilities still experience unacceptable conditions in the community as well as in institutions. Do we have any reason to believe that this will change or that international human rights can be a useful part of the engine of change, given the reservations expressed earlier concerning the use of human rights rhetoric (Lewis 2014)? In relation to coercion specifically, I have argued elsewhere that the ECHR 'fails to capture much of the coercion experienced by patients in practice' (Richardson 2008). The important question now is whether the CRPD can do any better. After setting out the principles underlying the CRPD, the rest of this chapter will consider its potential impact in relation to the provision of care within the community.

A new legal landscape: the UN Convention on the Rights of Persons with Disabilities

The CRPD is a significant development in international human rights and considerable emphasis has been placed upon it (World Health Organization 2012, 2013). It was adopted by the UN in 2006 and came into force in 2008. As of April 2014, 158 states had signed the CRPD and 143 had ratified it. As its name implies the CRPD relates to all disabilities. It expressly includes mental disabilities and adopts a social, rather than a medical, model of disability:

> Persons with disabilities include those who have long-term physical, mental, intellectual or sensory impairments which in interaction with various barriers may hinder their full and effective participation in society on an equal basis with others.

CRPD, Article 1

In traditional terminology it contains both positive and protective rights and may therefore have the potential to deal with both inadequate provision and direct abuse. At its heart is the principle of non-discrimination on grounds of disability:

> The purpose of the present Convention is to promote, protect and ensure the full and equal enjoyment of all human rights and fundamental freedoms by all persons with disabilities, and to promote respect for their inherent dignity.

CRPD, Article 1

and:

> Equality and non-discrimination
>
> 1. States Parties recognise that all persons are equal before and under the law and are entitled without any discrimination to the equal protection and equal benefit of the law.
>
> 2. States Parties shall prohibit all discrimination on the basis of disability and guarantee to persons with disabilities equal and effective legal protection against discrimination on all grounds.
>
> CRPD, Article 5

On the face of it these provisions do not appear particularly controversial, but much will turn on the interpretation of discrimination and whether and in what circumstances differential treatment is permissible. According to Article 2:

> Discrimination on the basis of disability' means any distinction, exclusion or restriction on the basis of disability which has the purpose or effect of impairing or nullifying the recognition, enjoyment or exercise, on an equal basis with others, of all human rights and fundamental freedoms in the political, economic, social, cultural, civil or any other field.

This would appear to indicate a strong approach to discrimination prohibiting any distinction made on the grounds of disability which interferes with a human right, however benign in intent (United Nations 2014). Under such an interpretation any legal provisions which interfere with rights on the grounds of disability would be unacceptable. In furtherance of this approach, the CRPD introduces the notion of universal legal capacity and requires that persons with disabilities 'enjoy legal capacity on an equal basis with others in all aspects of life' (CRPD, Article 12(2)), specifies that 'the existence of a disability shall in no case justify a deprivation of liberty' (CRPD, Article 14(1)(b)), and states that 'every person with disabilities has a right to respect for his or her physical and mental integrity on an equal basis with others' (CRPD, Article 17).

Unlike the ECHR, the UN CRPD does not have a specific court to provide interpretation nor to enforce its provisions. Like other UN conventions it has instead a special committee to monitor its implementation, the Committee on the Rights of Persons with Disabilities. This Committee conducts country reviews, investigates individual complaints, and issues General Comments on aspects of the CRPD. It is therefore the most authoritative non-national body when it comes to interpreting the Convention. The Committee has produced a number of concluding comments following individual country reports and a General Comment on Article 12 (United Nations 2014). The concluding comments have consistently adopted a strict interpretation, assuming that legislation which denies legal capacity to those who lack mental capacity and provides instead for substitute decision making on their behalf (the model adopted by the MCA) and legislation which provides powers of involuntary hospitalization and treatment in the case of those with mental disabilities is non-compliant with the requirements of the CRPD (United Nations 2011a,b). Accordingly these concluding comments have urged states parties to repeal legislation which provides for substitute decision making on behalf of persons with mental disabilities and legislation which provides powers to treat involuntarily or to detain on grounds of mental disability. Its General Comment on Article 12 is equally clear that legislation which denies legal capacity to adults on the grounds of a lack of mental capacity will be in breach of the CRPD (United Nations 2014).

The implications of such a strict interpretation, particularly in relation to Article 12 and the right to legal capacity, have been the subject of much debate internationally, and in England and Wales a review is currently under way to consider the question of the compliance of the MCA (House of Lords 2014; Martin et al. 2014). The controversy surrounding these provisions of the CRPD and the difficulties they are thought to present for states parties has tended to divert attention from its more positive features. In the context of community provision this is particularly unfortunate.

The CRPD evolved through a process which was unusual in the level of participation achieved by service users, and as a consequence directly reflects many of their priorities (Dhanda 2006). Most significantly for the present discussion it establishes a clear right to independent living. It is worth setting this out in full:

> States Parties to the present Convention recognise the equal right of all persons with disabilities to live in the community, with choices equal to others, and shall take effective and appropriate measures to facilitate full enjoyment by persons with disabilities of this right and their full inclusion and participation in the community, including by ensuring that:
>
> (*a*) Persons with disabilities have the opportunity to choose their place of residence and where and with whom they live on an equal basis with others and are not obliged to live in a particular living arrangement
>
> (*b*) Persons with disabilities have access to a range of in-home, residential and other community support services, including personal assistance necessary to support living and inclusion in the community, and to prevent isolation or segregation from the community;
>
> (*c*) Community services and facilities for the general population are available on an equal basis to persons with disabilities and are responsive to their needs.
>
> Article 19 [of the CRPD]: Living independently and being included in the community

According to Thomas Hammerberg, then Council of Europe Commissioner for Human Rights, 'Recognising the right to live in the community is about enabling people to live their lives to their fullest within society and access the public sphere, including "small places, close to home." It is a foundational platform for all other rights: a precondition for anyone to enjoy all their human rights is that they are within and among the community' (Hammerberg 2012). It is closely linked to other essential human rights such as the right to liberty and the quiet enjoyment of family life, but Article 19 of the CRPD captures the right to live independently in the community as a distinct right. Hammerberg traces the evolution of this right via a number of UN and European legal norms and political commitments. As articulated in Article 19, the right has three key elements: choice, individualized supports that promote inclusion and prevent isolation, and making services for the general public accessible to people with disabilities (Hammerberg 2012, p. 5).

Article 19 is therefore closely linked to the right under Article 12 to legal capacity, or to make your own decisions, and the right to the supports necessary to enable you to do so. It contains both positive obligations and negative protective rights of direct relevance to the use of coercion in the community, particularly when it is read alongside other articles within the CRPD:

(1) In the first place, in a fully CRPD-compliant structure some would argue that all formal coercive powers available on grounds of disability would be prohibited whether in hospital or in the community (United Nations 2011a,b, 2014). On such a view it must follow that any form of informal coercion that relied on the threat of formal powers would also fall.

(2) More positively, Article 19 imposes an obligation on states to provide the supports necessary to facilitate independent living in the community. This right, coupled with the protective rights to be free from detention, is obviously violated when people with disabilities are accommodated in large isolated institutions, as has been and still is the case in a number of Council of Europe jurisdictions (Hammerberg 2012; Mental Disability Advocacy Centre 2014; see also *Stanev v Bulgaria* [2012] ECHR 46). But isolation does not depend on the size of the institution, as Hammerberg (2012) explains, Article 19 can equally be violated when accommodation is provided in much smaller units in the community. This issue is discussed further later.

(3) In addition the Article 19 right can be violated when there is no provision made to support a person with disabilities within the community and as a consequence that person is isolated and possibly detained within her family setting.

(4) Article 19 may also be violated in situations where a person has no real choice as to where she lives or with whom, where her access to the services provided to others within the community is restricted, or where her support is provided as a package and is dependent on her acceptance of the whole. This latter aspect is particularly relevant to the use of leveraged pressure, as defined by Canvin et al. (2013).

(5) Article 19 gives the person the right to choose where and with whom to live, and Article 12 guarantees respect for the person's will and preferences. Supports are to be provided to enable the person to express her will but there is obvious scope here for conflicts of interest, informal coercion, and leverage. While the CRPD recognizes this and the consequent need to provide for 'appropriate and effective safeguards' (Article 12(4)), there is a danger that the coercion experienced by people with disabilities will simply change in nature rather than disappear. As Hammerberg (2012) insists, effective monitoring will be essential, but effective monitoring is notoriously hard to achieve even in an institutional setting within a high-income country (Hammerberg 2012; Mental Disability Advocacy Centre 2006; House of Lords Select Committee 2014).

Informal coercion and the limits of 'support'

While the emphasis on community living is directly in tune with current models of service provision in high-, medium-, and low-income countries, the underlying principles of non-discrimination on grounds of mental disability, universal legal capacity, and patient choice may meet with more resistance from mental health professionals. According to the principles of the CRPD, people with disabilities certainly have rights to support and to services but they also have the right to choose, and their choices must be respected. Care cannot be provided through the use of formal coercion, through informal coercion by way of an implicit threat to use formal powers, or through the use of leveraged pressure. This is a long way from the understanding of human rights which Lewis (2014) attributes to 'some leaders of world psychiatry', but more significantly it would demand a fundamental revision of the traditional legal framework. The implications flowing from this raise issues far beyond the scope of this chapter, but whatever the conclusion on formal coercive powers in general, many questions of direct relevance to community mental health remain: is it ever possible to remove all aspects of informal coercion, even in a world free from formal coercion? Would such a reality truly serve the interests of all those with mental disabilities? How do we guard against conflicts of interest? How do we understand coercion in relation to those whose decision-making abilities are impaired?

The practical relevance of these questions to the provision of community mental health care is clearly illustrated by the situation described in a study conducted in southern India (Srinivasan and Thara 2002). It concerned the covert administration of medication but raises issues of much wider application. The majority of people with schizophrenia in India live with their families, and those families supervise their medication. A study of patients attending an urban outpatient clinic noted that when patients were acutely ill and were refusing medication many families would administer that medication to them without their knowledge. The report of the study considers the complex and often conflicting clinical and ethical implications of such a practice. Looked at through the lens of the CRPD the situation becomes even more complex. The CRPD emphasizes the person's right to choose, and insists that their will and preference be respected. The covert administration of medication in the face of the individual's objection would appear to be in direct breach of these requirements, whatever its clinical justification. However, it might be argued that the refusal of medication is not a reflection of the person's true will and preference. The CRPD establishes a right to the supports necessary to enable the person to express her choice and someone with schizophrenia would thus be entitled to support to help her make her decision about medication. With this support she may adjust her view on medication. But equally she may not, and if she remains adamant in her refusal any covert administration would be prohibited whatever the consequences for her health. The CRPD certainly imposes the obligation on states to provide support, but ultimately the decision belongs to the person.

Deprivation of liberty and the ECHR

While the Indian study reveals the questions raised by the non-consensual administration of medication, a recent UK Supreme Court decision (UK Supreme Court 2014) illustrates the human rights implications of community supervision more generally. The case involved three people with different forms of learning disability, but its potential significance extends far beyond those specific disabilities. It would apply to anyone whose mental disability, whether intellectual or 'psychiatric', had adversely affected their decision-making abilities and who required intense levels of care. Two of the appellants were housed in small units within the community while one lived with foster parents. All three required high levels of support, the provision of which led to significant restrictions on their movement and choice. P, in particular, required 24-hour care to meet his personal needs. He wore a 'body suit' of all-in-one underwear to prevent him pulling at his incontinence pads and putting pieces in his mouth (UK Supreme Court 2014, p. 17). All three attended educational or social facilities during the day but none was allowed out without supervision. While none of the three was objecting to their housing nor to most aspects of their care, they cannot to be said to have chosen it, and their daily lives were subject to significant restrictions. Whether or not these restrictions amount to coercion, formal or informal, they certainly raise questions of compliance with the CRPD, as discussed below. But for the UK Supreme Court the central question was compliance with the ECHR, as it would be for any court in a jurisdiction bound by that convention.

The ECHR prohibits 'deprivation of liberty' except in certain specific situations. 'Deprivation of liberty' is permitted in the case of 'unsoundness of mind' if certain conditions are met and it is properly authorized by law (Article 5(4), *Winterwerp v The Netherlands* (1979) 2 EHRR 387). In England and Wales, in order to comply with these human rights requirements a statutory framework has been introduced to provide safeguards and review for those who lack mental capacity but need, in their own best interests, to be deprived of their liberty—the Deprivation of Liberty Safeguards (DoLS). The central question before the Supreme Court was whether the three appellants had been deprived of their liberty, in which case the DoLS would have to be applied. Lady Hale gave the lead judgement. Human rights she explained are universal, people with disabilities have the same human rights as everyone else. The criteria for what constitutes a deprivation of liberty must be the same for everyone. From previous case law she derived an 'acid test': was the individual under continuous supervision and control and not free to leave? If so they would be deprived of their liberty. All seven judges agreed that P's situation met this test, but three considered that the test was not met in the case of the other two appellants, MEG and MIG. Thus the finding of a deprivation in their cases was by majority only.

Beyond trying to clarify the definition of a deprivation of liberty under the ECHR, the case is significant in a number of ways:

(1) In the first place it has raised concerns that the combination of a wide definition and its application to small community settings, including foster care, will greatly extend the potential scope of Article 5 and thus its procedural requirements. While this may be of particular concern to those caring for people with dementia or learning disabilities, as greater emphasis worldwide is placed on community provision in mental health care more generally the distinction between forms of coercion which merely restrict liberty and those that amount to a deprivation will become increasingly important in jurisdictions bound by the ECHR.

(2) In reaching her judgment Lady Hale emphasized the protective role of Article 5 of the ECHR. She was confident that those caring for the three appellants had 'done the best they could to make their lives as happy and fulfilled, as well as safe, as they possibly could be'. But this would not prevent there being a deprivation of liberty, 'the purpose of Article 5 is to ensure that people are not deprived of their liberty without proper safeguards, safeguards which will secure that the legal justifications for the constraints which they are under are made out' (UK Supreme Court

2014, p. 56). To declare the provision of care a deprivation of liberty should not be seen as stigmatizing or as an indication of a failure on the part of mental health services. It should simply be the trigger for the application of the safeguards necessary to protect the interests of very vulnerable people.

(3) In further reflection of the protective role of the Article 5 safeguards it is evident that a restriction can amount to a deprivation whether or not the person is aware of it or objects to it. Coercion does not have to be perceived as such in order to engage the law.

(4) The case illustrates very directly the difference in approach between the ECHR and the CRPD. Lady Hale quoted the CRPD in support of her assertion that people with disabilities have the same human rights as everyone else (UK Supreme Court 2014, p. 45). The definition of deprivation of liberty could not differ on grounds of disability as the Court of Appeal had suggested (see *Cheshire West and Chester Council v P* [2011] EWCA Civ 1257). However, by virtue of Article 5(1)(e), a deprivation of liberty can be justified under the ECHR on grounds of 'unsoundness of mind'. So the definition may be universal but the prohibition can be lifted on grounds of mental disability. This appears to conflict directly with the principles of the CRPD, particularly Articles 12 and 14.

(5) In addition, whether or not the restrictions placed on the choices available to the appellants amounted to a deprivation of liberty, they certainly raise questions with regard to Article 19 of the CRPD and the right to live independently in the community. In MEG's case, for example, the staff exercised control 'over every aspect of her life. She would not be allowed out without supervision, or to see people whom they did not wish her to see, or to do things which they did not wish her to do' (UK Supreme Court 2014, p. 52). The same was true for MIG (UK Supreme Court 2014, p. 53) and P was 'completely under the control of members of staff at Z house'. He could not 'go anywhere or do anything without their support and assistance' (UK Supreme Court 2014, p. 51). Such circumstances, however understandable and benign in intent, are hard to reconcile with the state's obligation under Article 19 to 'recognise the equal right of all persons with disabilities to live in the community, with choices equal to others'.

This case illustrates contradictions in the approach of international human rights to the use of coercion in the provision of mental health care in the community. All three appellants needed extensive support, and as far as is evident from the reports there was no criticism of the level of that support from any of the judges. But it is also evident that the support as provided involved elements of coercion. Under the provisions familiar from the ECHR such coercion, or interference with fundamental rights, can be justified in relation to the right to peaceful enjoyment of family life (Article 8) and the right to liberty and security (Article 5) if it is proportionate and in the interests of health (Article 8) or in the case of unsoundness of mind (Article 5). By contrast, the CRPD, strictly interpreted, prohibits any difference in treatment on grounds of disability, however benign in intent, which interferes with fundamental rights (Article 2) (United Nations 2014), although other interpretations are possible (Martin et al. 2014). It further establishes a clear positive right to the support and services necessary to enable independent living in the community (Article 19).

Conclusions

The position exemplified by the ECHR, which allows proportionate interference with rights in the interests of health, may present some challenges to community-based mental health care even in high-income countries. The presence of abuse and the need to provide for the adequate monitoring of services have now been recognized in the UK and elsewhere within the European Union, even if solutions remain elusive (Mental Disability Advocacy Centre 2006; House of Lords Select Committee 2014). But the challenge presented by the approach of the CRPD is far more fundamental. In the first place, the expressed will and preference of the person with disabilities must be respected. On the face of it this would appear to prohibit all formal coercive powers and the informal coercion that is derived from them. Whether this absolute prohibition ultimately prevails remains to be seen but, in any event, the use of informal coercion and leveraged pressure might also conflict with the obligation placed on states to provide the safeguards necessary to guard against undue influence and conflicts of interest. In addition to these negative prohibitions, Article 19 imposes the positive obligation on states to take 'effective and appropriate measures to facilitate full enjoyment' of the right to independent living in the community. In combination, these negative prohibitions and positive obligations, whatever the details of their ultimate interpretation, constitute a radical shift in emphasis the full implications of which have yet to be grasped. They present a fundamental challenge to mental health professionals, many of whom may fear that they will restrict their ability to act in their patients' interests. But there can be no doubt that the CRPD contains an articulation of human rights that places the wishes and preferences of the person with a mental disability centre stage. As such it must be taken seriously, and every effort should be made to build on its positive aspects and to construct community mental health care in reflection of its underlying principles.

References

Bean P (1986). *Mental disorder and legal control*. Cambridge: Cambridge University Press.

Becker A, Kleinman A (2013). Mental health and the global agenda. *New England Journal of Medicine*, **369**:66–73.

Berlin I (1969). Two concepts of liberty. In: *Four essays on liberty*, pp. 118–172. Oxford: Oxford University Press.

Canvin K, Rugkåsa J, Sinclair C, et al. (2013). Leverage and other informal pressures in community psychiatry in England. *International Journal of Law and Psychiatry*, **36**:100–106.

Department for International Development (2010). *The Mental Health and Poverty Project: mental health policy development and implementation in four African countries*. Available at: http://r4d.dfid.gov.uk/pdf/outputs/mentalhealth_rpc/mhapp_final_report_forr4d.pdf

Dhanda A (2006). Legal capacity in the Disability Rights Convention: stranglehold of the past or lodestar for the future? *Syracuse Journal of International Law and Commerce* 34:429.

Drew N, Funk M, Tang S (2011). Human rights violations of people with mental and psychosocial disabilities: an unresolved global crisis. *The Lancet*, **378**:1664–1675.

Dunn M, Maughan D, Hope T, et al. (2012). Threat and offers in community mental health. *Journal of Medical Ethics*, **38**:204–209.

Gostin L (2014). *Global health law*. Cambridge, MA: Harvard University Press.

Hammerberg T (2012). *The right of people with disabilities to live independently and be included in the community*. Issue Paper published by the Council of Europe Commissioner for Human Rights. Strasbourg: Council of Europe.

House of Lords Select Committee [on the Mental Capacity Act 2005] (2014). *Mental Capacity Act 2005: post-legislative scrutiny*. Report of Session 2013–14. London: The Stationery Office.

Høyer G, Kjellin L, Engberg M, et al. (2002). Paternalism and autonomy: a presentation of a Nordic study on the use of coercion in the mental health care system. *International Journal of Law and Psychiatry*, **25**:93–108.

Lewis O (2014). The role of global psychiatry in advancing human rights. In: *Torture in health care settings: reflections on the Special Rapporteur on Torture's 2013 thematic report*, pp. 247–262. Washington, DC: American University Washington College of Law, Centre for Human Rights and Humanitarian Law. Available at: http://antitorture.org/wp-content/uploads/2014/03/PDF_Torture_in_Healthcare_Publication.pdf

Martin W, Michalowski S, Jutten T, et al. (2014). *Achieving CRPD compliance: a report to the UK Ministry of Justice*. University of Essex, Essex Autonomy Project. Available at: http://autonomy.essex.ac.uk/uncrpd-report

Mental Disability Advocacy Centre (2006). *Inspect! Inspectorates of mental health and social care institutions in the European Union*. Budapest: Mental Disability Advocacy Centre.

Mental Disability Advocacy Centre (2014). *Mental Disability Advocacy Centre biennial report, 2011–12*. Budapest: Mental Disability Advocacy Centre. Available at: http://www.mdac.info/sites/mdac.info/files/biennialreport_2011-12_web.pdf

Monahan J, Hoge S, Lidz C, et al. (1995). Coercion and commitment: understanding involuntary hospital admission. *International Journal of Law and Psychiatry*, **18**:249–263.

Patel V (2008). *The Lancet*'s series on mental health: 1 year on. *The Lancet*, **372**:1354–1357.

Patel V (2011). A renewed agenda for global mental health. *The Lancet* **378**:1441–1442.

Poulsen H (1999). Perceived coercion among committed, detained and voluntary patients. *International Journal of Law and Psychiatry*, **22**:167–175.

Poulsen H (2002). The prevalence of extralegal deprivation of liberty in a psychiatric hospital population. *International Journal of Law and Psychiatry*, **25**:29–36.

Read U (2012). 'I want the one that will heal me completely so it won't come back again': the limits of antipsychotic medication in rural Ghana. *Transcultural Psychiatry*, **49**:438–460.

Richardson G (2008). Coercion and human rights: a European perspective. *Journal of Mental Health*, **17**:245–254.

Srinivasan T, Thara R (2002). At issue: management of medication noncompliance in schizophrenia by families in India. *Schizophrenia Bulletin*, **28**:531–535.

Summerfield D (2011). Afterword: against 'global mental health'. *Transcultural Psychiatry*, **49**:519–530.

Szmukler G (2009). Financial incentives for patients in the treatment of psychosis. *Journal of Medical Ethics*, **35**:224–228.

UK Supreme Court (2014). *P v Cheshire West and Chester Council and P and Q v Surrey County Council* [2014] UKSC 19.

United Nations (2000). *CESCR General Comment no. 14. The right to the highest attainable standard of health*. Office of the High Commissioner for Human Rights.

United Nations (2011a). *Concluding observations of the Committee on the Rights of Persons with Disabilities: Tunisia*. UN document CRPD/C/TUN/CO/1.

United Nations (2011b). *Concluding observations of the Committee on the Rights of Persons with Disabilities: Spain*. UN document CRPD/C/ESP/CO/1.

United Nations (2013). *Report of the Special Rapporteur on torture and other cruel, inhuman or degrading treatment or punishment, Juan E.Méndez*. A/HRC/22/53.

United Nations (2014). *Committee on the Rights of Persons with Disabilities, General Comment No. 1*. Available at: http://daccess-dds-ny.un.org/doc/UNDOC/GEN/G14/031/20/PDF/G1403120.pdf?OpenElement

White R, **Sashidharan S** (2014). Towards a more nuanced global mental health. *British Journal of Psychiatry*, **204**:415–417.

Wolff J (2012). *The human right to health*. New York: WW Norton.

World Health Organization (2005). *WHO resource book on mental health, human rights and legislation*. Geneva: World Health Organization.

World Health Organization (2011). *Mental health atlas 2011*. Geneva: World Health Organization.

World Health Organization (2012). *WHO qualityrights tool kit: assessing and improving quality and human rights in mental health and social care facilities*. Geneva: World Health Organization.

World Health Organization (2013). *Mental health action plan 2013–2020*. Geneva: World Health Organization.

Chapter 14

The ethics of coercion in community mental health care

Tania Gergel and George Szmukler

Introduction

How we reconcile an individual's right to liberty with coercive interventions is a fundamental question in medical ethics and psychiatry, especially given psychiatry's chequered history. Current measures within developed countries are generally quite tightly regulated and there is a relatively strong evidence base to support the use of modern-day psychiatric interventions. Nevertheless, many ethical questions remain, particularly in relation to coercion within community mental healthcare, a growing and relatively underexplored phenomenon (as described in earlier chapters).

The last 70 years have seen major reforms of mental health laws and practices throughout the developed world, motivated by a mixture of risk-based, libertarian, and economic factors. In general, mental health law is now preventative and status-based, allowing forcible detention and treatment where there is perceived risk to individuals themselves or others resulting from a diagnosed mental disorder (Dawson and Szmukler 2006). While the need for legal provision to enforce treatment is widely accepted, its form remains controversial. Strong arguments can be made that status- and risk-based laws are intrinsically discriminatory against those with mental disorder, and that a fairer measure would be based on decision-making capacity, regardless of diagnosis (Dawson and Szmukler 2006; Bach and Kerzner 2010). At present, even in jurisdictions with capacity-based laws applying to non-consensual medical treatment, coercive measures are usually introduced through separate legislation specific to mental disorder, with restrictions that do not apply to the broader population.

Until recently debate centred on the use of enforced treatment and detention within a controlled inpatient environment. Now, however, as psychiatry moves increasingly towards community care, the question is far broader, in terms of both setting and the conditions judged as warranting coercive measures. While community care may have been envisioned as a step towards greater liberty within psychiatry, use of coercion in many countries is currently increasing (Salize and Dressing 2004; Keown et al. 2008; Health and Social Care Information Centre 2013; Robiliard 2013; Zielasek and Gaebel 2015).

Formal coercion within the community typically takes the form of a community treatment order (CTO) mandating enforced recall to hospital for those who are non-compliant with treatment. Many jurisdictions permit the application of an order, even for those patients who retain decision-making capacity, and CTOs may function to impose continuing treatment on an individual who, once stabilized, is regarded as sufficiently 'safe' to live within the community (Dawson 2006; Lawton-Smith et al. 2008). In addition, other forms of leverage also occur, such as withdrawal or withholding of particular benefits in order to promote adherence, and the 'coercion context' of mental health care (see Chapter 8) can increase their coercive pressure. Essentially the ongoing justification for CTOs stems from anticipated risk, should an individual, usually with a history of defaulting on prescribed treatment, default again.

Thus community coercion appears to cover a new 'grey area', with an individual being deemed well enough to live within the community but not to make his or her own decisions about matters such as treatment. CTOs could therefore be seen to take the pre-emptive and speculative dimension of anticipated risk one step further (Szmukler 2014). The 'risk' criterion embedded in mental health laws makes mental disorder the only situation in most societies in which involuntary detention (or the threat of involuntary detention) can be invoked, not because a dangerous act constituting a criminal offence has taken place but because it is believed that there is a high probability of a dangerous act occurring. If we extend this to an individual subject to an ongoing CTO, but now sufficiently stable to live outside of a controlled inpatient environment, we are not simply allowing coercion based on risk of some kind of harm in the near future; we are, effectively, extending this to a judgement that, should a stable individual decide to discontinue treatment, the risk from discontinuation is sufficiently high to over-ride their right to make treatment decisions. Given the moral imperative to limit coercion and respect the right to self-determination wherever possible, we need to think very carefully about whether such an extension is justifiable.

In this chapter, we will lay out a framework of ethical assumptions underlying coercion in community psychiatric care and explore the inherent difficulties. We will not focus on individual jurisdictions, but on a range of examples and some general principles applicable to countries with reasonably well-developed legal systems. We will consider the justifications for such measures, the mechanisms through which they are imposed, their potential consequences, and the significance of their effectiveness. We shall not be considering provisions in forensic practice concerning patients who have committed a serious offence.

Overall, we would like to suggest that coercion within a community, as opposed to the inpatient environment, does not raise radically new questions, but can be seen to heighten the complexity of the ethical concerns surrounding coercive treatment, and thereby highlight some major ethical difficulties within existing mental health legislation and practices. To conclude, we will offer some ideas for reforms that could incorporate coercion, where necessary, into a framework more adequately suited to the human rights of patients.

Conventional justifications for involuntary treatment

The need for some provision for compulsory treatment of mental disorders is generally accepted. It is usually justified on the basis that severe episodes of illness may cause an individual to be unable to understand the need for interventions to help treat a condition that may result in serious harm to themselves or others if untreated. The threat to individual freedom of choice is viewed as outweighed by the risk to oneself or others. A legal framework gives structural validity to such measures and also entails safeguards intended to prevent abuse. In practice, however, appraisal of risk is often disproportionate and inaccurate.

It is also important to acknowledge that formal coercion, even when deemed necessary, still involves an experienced loss of liberty which may be deeply traumatic and can never be a 'perfect' solution. Any provision for coercion must be accompanied by a moral obligation to ensure that it is only carried out in circumstances where it is deemed necessary and with the minimum degree of perceived violation.

Coercion within the community—liberalist justifications

Liberalist motivations played a large role in the move towards community care, with hopes for improved quality of life and human rights. With asylums being viewed as a form of social segregation allowing greater opportunity for unregulated coercion, many hoped that community care could increase integration and social contact and allow greater control and restriction of coercion while encouraging patients to take a more willing and active role in their own care.

If accepted unreservedly such justifications may well appear to suggest that care within the community, when safe, is automatically better an individual than inpatient treatment. One might draw a further conclusion that a community setting, even when the treatment involves coercion, is preferable to hospitalization. It is also often argued that community coercion can lead to an improved and more stable quality of life amongst vulnerable 'revolving-door patients' if it can induce adherence to treatment and thus decrease admissions.

However, there are various problems with these arguments. First, while the asylum system may have been flawed in many respects, the security and support of an inpatient environment can be a valuable resource during severe episodes, and care in the community should not be seen as a near replacement. Nonetheless, inpatient provision is rapidly diminishing. Inpatient care is extremely costly and, as resources are stretched, increased community care, which allows for shorter admissions, can be seen as one dramatic way to reduce the cost of mental health care by facilitating vast reductions in beds by cutting the duration and number of admissions. In the UK, for example, bed numbers fell by 31% between 2003 and 2013, with extremely deleterious consequences (NHS England 2014). Similar reductions have occurred in other countries, such as the USA (Treatment Advocacy Centre 2014). Those in crisis may be denied inpatient treatment or, with no bed available locally, may be admitted to a hospital far away from home. Patients may not be admitted until symptoms have escalated to crisis point and detention might be necessary. All too often, discharge occurs before it is therapeutically ideal.

Far from decreasing coercion, the reduction in psychiatric beds has been accompanied by increased formal coercion. During the same period UK mental health detentions have increased (Keown et al. 2008; Health and Social Care Information Centre 2013). A recent UK parliamentary report, for example, identified 'an inverse relation between the number of beds currently available and the number of people being detained' and recommended urgent investigation into the reported phenomenon of clinicians using formal detention to secure a bed (Health Committee 2013).

Coercion within the community—risk-based justifications

The difficulties intensify when we examine the further consequences of this treatment shift. If society relocates mental health care into the community, concerns are raised for public security. High-profile, but extremely isolated, cases of homicides by patients are sensationalized by the media and spark disproportionate public alarm and recrimination against clinicians. Thus, despite hopes that coercive measures in psychiatry should reflect the patient's best interests, all too often it appears that inaccurate and unsubstantiated estimation of risk becomes the over-riding motivation. The procedures for assessing the risk of serious harm to the individual give extremely poor results (Hart et al. 2007; Large et al. 2011a; Wand and Large 2013; Singh et al. 2014). For rare events such as suicide, homicide, or even serious violence to others, even with the very best risk assessment procedures and propitious research conditions, the 'false positives' (i.e. those predicted to be 'high risk' but not committing such an act) hugely outnumber the 'true positives'. For example, in the year following discharge from hospital, only 2% of patients predicted to be at 'high risk' of suicide actually committed suicide (Large et al. 2011b). In the UK around 1% per year of serious violence in the community is committed by patients treated by community mental health teams, and a similar tiny percentage of those rated as 'high risk', using the best available risk assessment instruments, act violently. Predicting a homicide involves a false positive rate in the thousands for each correct prediction. These are the examples of the statistical 'base rate' problem: events that are rare are extremely difficult to predict accurately, even with the best available methods (Szmukler 2003; Large et al. 2011a).

Risk aversion and risk management have become increasing features of decision and policy making within the developed world, and are increasingly influential within psychiatry and public debate on mental illness (Turner 2014), with risk assessment now being a standard part of mental health service provision. For psychiatric patients deemed to be well enough to live long-term within the community, perceived risk provides a major impetus for invoking coercive measures and outweighs consideration of statistical probabilities, best interests, or civil liberties. The increased use of such measures could also be seen to increase stigma by giving structural reinforcement to prejudicial and stereotype-based beliefs about mental illness and dangerousness (Undrill 2007).

Risk-based measures justify coercion by considering the individual, if untreated, to be such a serious risk to themselves or others that treatment, even if involuntary, is in the best interests of themselves and society. In addition to the problems of inaccuracy, such measures also constitute unfair discrimination against those with mental illness. As Kisely et al. (2005) suggest: 'It is, nevertheless, difficult to conceive of another group in society that would be subject to measures that curtail the freedom of 85 people to avoid one admission to hospital or of 238 to avoid one arrest'. Psychiatric patients are the only group within society who can be constrained on a basis of a perceived *risk* of harmful actions, rather than by committing a violent and illegal act (Dawson and Szmukler 2006). Furthermore, given that community coercion is not constrained by a 'ceiling effect' limiting the numbers of involuntary patients to available hospital beds, it may be opening the floodgates for subjecting increasing numbers to such measures.

Mechanisms for community coercion

The extension of the 'coercive context' and its ethical ramifications

Once a legal system has unique and status-based provision for the formal coercion of those with mental illness, the shared knowledge of such provision amongst both patients and those involved in their care creates a context within which the patient can be pressured in various ways—for example to make treatment decisions—even when formal measures are not actually invoked:

> The very possibility that coercive measures can be used will be part of the situational context in cases in which staff and patients differ in their opinions about what is the best course of treatment to undertake. Hence, there is a subtle interrelationship between coercion and compliance in all realms of psychiatric care.
>
> Sjöström (2006)

This is all the more pertinent within a community setting, where the possibilities for coercive practices can be extended beyond those available within a controlled inpatient environment in a number of related respects: (1) the people who can be involved in implementation; (2) the type of coercive interventions which can be used; (3) the lower level of severity of the condition; and (4) the length of time for which the patient is exposed.

Within mental health law coercive interventions are usually clinically driven. Decisions are based on judgements by mental health professionals, variously approved by a judge or tribunal at the outset, or after a time interval, or following an appeal by the patient (or carers or supporters). In principle, decisions are based upon the expert opinion of more than one mental health professional, involve clinical objectivity, and are formulated within a very distinct legal framework designed to protect the rights of the patient. Once coercion moves into the community, those contributing to the coercive process may well expand beyond the clinical team. With CTOs, for example, depending on jurisdiction, restrictions governing factors such as place of residence or behaviours may be imposed, and carers or other members of the public may be drawn into the monitoring process (Dawson 2006). Non-clinicians (e.g. social services and housing association staff and families) can also use the 'coercion context' to exert pressure upon patients. The involvement of non-professionals raises questions not only about objectivity and the understanding of mental disorders, but also about the patient's relationships with his or her community. Involving members of an individual's social network with the implementation of coercive measures, whether formal or informal, and however indirectly, has the potential to create a power imbalance which may compromise those relationships. However useful the involvement of the wider community in psychiatric care, it raises clear ethical questions surrounding issues such as trust, equality, and abuse, even if unintentional.

Broadening the 'coercion context' within the community also extends the processes through which coercion is implemented. Formal CTOs have been introduced to impose treatment adherence on those outside an inpatient setting, while leverage through factors such as housing or finance are also increasing. Moreover, such processes can be seen to extend the applicability of coercive measures beyond periods of illness, when safety is severely compromised, to periods when the individual is sufficiently stable to live outside the hospital environment.

A hierarchy of coercive measures

Although ethical debate is dominated by issues surrounding formally sanctioned compulsion or CTOs, the range of ways in which coercive measures can be implemented is far broader and the implementation of coercive pressures involves a range of different mechanisms. 'Treatment pressures' can be seen as a spectrum, involving progressively stronger levels of coercion (Szmukler and Appelbaum 2008). This spectrum can be presented in the following way, going from less to more coercive measures:

(1) persuasion

(2) interpersonal leverage

(3) inducements

(4) threats (including deception)

(5) compulsory treatment (community or inpatient)

For each of these categories it is important to consider the types of processes used and how interventions are classified and evaluated in relation to each other.

Compulsion (formal coercion)

At the most severe end comes compulsion. Not only does this involve the strongest levels of coercion, it also requires formal sanction and is, for both these reasons, the subject of the most sustained discussion. CTOs are the most common form of compulsion ('backed up force supported by legal statute'; Szmukler and Appelbaum 2008) exerted within a community setting. Typically, they mandate that a patient who fails to comply with treatment can be forcibly returned to hospital, sometimes directly to an inpatient environment. In general, statutes vary concerning whether medication can then be automatically administered by force.

As with so many changes in psychiatric practices, CTOs have both liberal and more restrictive motivations. One can differentiate between 'least restrictive types' and the 'preventative' types. In the former the criteria for the CTO are more or less identical to those for inpatient treatment orders and the CTO is imposed when the person's mental state has already deteriorated, as a less restrictive alternative to forced hospitalization. 'Preventative' CTOs, broaden the applicability of the order and are used within psychiatric management with the aim of preventing deterioration. While 'least restrictive types' present no substantial additional ethical challenge to existing statutes, they are less easy to use. In effect, they are little different from existing practices of, for example, 'trial leave' or 'supervised discharge' from hospital (Churchill et al. 2007).

'Preventative' types offer a new range of possible applications, but greater ethical challenges, since they move away from imminent risk or danger to pre-emptive measures to prevent the possibility of such dangers and broaden the stages of illness to which compulsion can apply. The types of CTOs vary between jurisdictions (Dawson 2006). In the USA, statutes are moving increasingly from 'least restrictive' to 'preventative', while in a number of other jurisdictions orders are mixed, boundaries unclear, and the type instituted may depend upon clinical discretion in individual cases.

From an ethical point of view the main concern is with 'preventative' types, although 'mixed' types can also present challenges, since a lack of clarity may well lead a patient to perceive greater levels of compulsion or consequences for failure to follow the conditions of the order than are in fact in place. Even with 'preventative' CTOs, contravention usually has only limited consequences, and further assessment, often accompanied by transfer to an inpatient order, is generally required before compulsory treatment can be given. The major effect of 'preventative' CTOs appears to be to facilitate the swift return of non-compliant patients to a hospital environment, often with police involvement. When orders are 'mixed' and boundaries unclear, leading patients to believe that their choices are more limited than they in fact are, compulsion may effectively happen through deception rather than statute. This is a major point to consider, as CTOs may enable a situation where a lack of clarity enables a greater perception of restriction and lack of choice than are actually instantiated within the law. Not only is the range of those who can be subject to compulsion through an order being broadened, but patients may be experiencing elevated coercion through deception about the actual power of the law. One clinician reports a patient's confusion: 'I don't think it's made any difference to her. I think actually she still thinks that she has to take medication. I'm not sure that she realised the difference between the Section 3, Section 17 leave and the CTO and not being under any restrictions at all' (Stroud et al. 2013). Thus the ethical issues here do not simply concern what is dictated by the law, but the worrying consequences of legal obfuscation.

The use of CTOs might also have a number of other potentially problematic consequences, and considerable opposition and concern has been raised by clinicians (Lawton-Smith et al. 2008; Manning 2013). Firstly, they might affect the quality of treatment. Treatment options may well be limited to those which are enforceable under such schemes, with intramuscular 'depot' injections often the only treatment option that can be confidently monitored, even if it is not necessarily the most desirable (Patel et al. 2011). Over-reliance on the use of CTOs may well mean that care shifts from attention to the quality of available community services and an exploration of alternative options for engagement to enforcement (or threats) (Sinaiko and McGuire 2006). The pressure to enforce orders may also result in resources being diverted to groups subject to such orders and away from others.

Living in the community while subject to such an order might contribute to feelings of social isolation in a number of ways, such as: increased feelings of stigmatization (RA Malatest and Associates 2012); altering dynamics in relationships with non-clinicians, such as carers or hostel workers who play a part in assessing adherence; and increasing fear of further coercion which may discourage an individual from seeking help. CTOs have been unpopular with many patients for increasing coercion and decreasing legitimate debate about the problems associated with certain medications. One patient, for example, described the change in their relationships with family and carer that occurred after the imposition of a CTO as 'instead of them being concerned out of care and compassion for the problem I was having, there was reason for them to be responsible and have authority over me', and also reported feeling criminalized and stigmatized and with restricted choices (Manning 2013).

Moreover, the issuing of a CTO is not a rare occurrence, as was initially envisaged. Factors such as the absence of a 'ceiling effect', already mentioned, have led to increasing numbers of patients being subject to formal compulsion. The 2012 statistics for Ontario, Canada, for example, show that the 'prevalence of CTOs (issues or renewals) has risen from an estimate of less than five per 100,000 to 36 per 100,000 in 2010/11' (RA Malatest and Associates 2012), while the use of CTOs is high and increasing in Australia (Health and Social Care Information Centre 2012). Similar marked increases can be seen in the UK and elsewhere, where the number of CTOs issued has far exceeded initial estimates (Taylor 2010).

There is also good reason to question the true effectiveness of such interventions. A 2011 Cochrane review states that 'compulsory community treatment results in no significant difference in service use, social functioning or quality of life compared with standard care' (Kisely et al. 2011). Similarly Rugkåsa and Dawson (2013) argue that the current evidence from randomized controlled trials suggests that CTOs do not reduce readmission rates over 12 months, even though a decrease in readmission among 'revolving-door patients' is a primary justification given for their use.

Given that coercive interventions compromise the principles of liberty and the right to self-determination in a number of important dimensions, effectiveness could be a factor which might be argued to outweigh some disadvantages and render such interventions more morally justifiable. If it is the case that such interventions are not effective and yet their use is increasing then there are serious ethical ramifications. As Rugkåsa and Dawson (2013) put it: 'when CTOs restrict patients' autonomy, however, and there is a duty to provide the least restrictive form of treatment, the RCTs must give pause for thought'. Likewise, McCutcheon (2013) writes: 'we have to ask ourselves what are the ethics of treating a patient with an intervention that they will often not desire when we have no evidence of its benefit?' (Taylor 2010; McCutcheon 2013).

Informal leverage mechanisms

By leverage we refer to a pressure to accept a course of action—this 'is distinct from persuasion and compulsion'. It is a concept that is increasingly identified with the informal pressures commonly used to influence patients, and involves three key components: 'use of a specific identifiable lever', such as finances, housing, or access to children; attachment of explicit conditions to the acceptance or declining of the proposal; and a proposal made by those 'perceived [by the patient] to have the power to act upon the conditions they impose' (Dunn et al. 2014). Although quantitative data on the use of leverage are harder to gather than for formal measures, patient surveys suggest that leverage is a commonplace experience within community mental health (Monahan et al. 2005; Canvin et al. 2013; Dunn et al. 2014). Despite its prevalence, however, there are virtually no formal or accepted guidelines, which makes it far harder to deal with ethical concerns and establish consistent practice.

Threats

Threats are commonly viewed as imposing conditions which would leave an individual worse off than their 'pre-proposal baseline' if they fail to comply with the proposal. According to Wertheimer's influential account, this baseline involves a consideration of the broad moral context within which the proposal is made, and whether an individual will be significantly disadvantaged in this respect (Wertheimer 1989). In contrast to compulsion, the use of threats may depend more heavily on an individual's awareness of the possibility that non-compliance may result in compulsion. A typical example might be the patient who is informed that their refusal of voluntarily admission to hospital will result in forced admission.

In ethical discussions, threats are usually placed at the very worst end of the spectrum, and it is generally accepted, on an institutional level, that formally sanctioned compulsion is more ethically acceptable than threats. The UK Mental Health Act (MHA) Code of Practice 2007 (4.12), for example, states: 'the threat of detention must not be used to induce a patient to consent to admission to hospital or to treatment (and is likely to invalidate any apparent consent)'. In practice, however, this is far from the reality of what occurs, a fact which might seem alarming (Health Committee 2013). The threat of involuntary admission, whether explicit or implicit (i.e. believed by the patient), is probably commonly used within psychiatry to convince patients to accept treatment or hospitalization. Even in those instances where a clinician may believe that their words technically constituted 'persuasion' or 'unwelcome prediction' rather than 'threat', the 'coercion context' means that the recipient may understand this as a threat that voluntary status will be removed if they fail to comply. This gap between ethical guidelines and clinical practice poses something of an ethical conundrum, as the prevalence of threats might seem to suggest that theory does not reflect our ethical intuitions about their use. Analysis of what threats involve can show that it might be worth reconsidering the conventional evaluation.

We can divide instances that are usually categorized as threats into three broad categories. First there are threats that involve deception—the patient is threatened with consequences which, unknown to them, cannot in fact be implemented. As we have suggested in the case of CTOs, this type of threat might be better categorized as a type of 'compulsion via deception' with the subjective experience of compulsion, even where compulsion is not formally sanctioned. Second, there are threats which stipulate conditions involving the deprivation of something to which an individual is unconditionally entitled by law or duty of care. Both types of threat are clearly ethically unacceptable (Bonnie and Monahan 2005; Dunn et al. 2012). The third, and probably most common, use of threats is to produce compliance without implementing formal compulsion when the threatened outcome would be both possible and legal. The term 'threat' carries negative associations of intimidation and exploitation, while compulsion is perhaps seen to involve greater transparency. Yet, are we being influenced by this to push aside what could conceivably be judged a preferable course of action, in terms of both subjective experience and consequences? For example, would it necessarily be worse for a manic patient to accept treatment purely because refusal would result in forced hospitalization, rather than being subject to formal admission and treatment?

Threats are often judged as inferior to inducements on the basis that the threatened party will be worse off if the threat is carried out. However, the same argument might also suggest that a threat can be preferable to compulsion. If the patient resumes medication, recovers, and avoids deterioration and formal hospital admission, this would surely seem preferable to the alternative in terms of outcome. Although the subjective experience of being threatened may be disturbing, it is unlikely that this would be worse for the individual than the subjective experience of forced admission and treatment. A threat, even if complied with, may offer the patient more remaining freedoms than would a compulsory admission.

Another major concern about threats is the lack of established guidelines. However, as long as it is maintained on a structural level that threats must be avoided, a lack of scrutiny or regulation will remain, even if usage is widespread. In particular, if it is truly judged to be preferable for the individual to remain within the community and retain voluntary status, it seems that this distinction should be re-examined and that we need a framework that can properly accept discussions and guidelines surrounding the use of threats.

Inducements

The use of inducements, incentives, or offers varies by region and is currently far more widely used, for example, in the USA than the UK, although the increased shift towards community care does seem to be leading to an increase in the actual or proposed usage of inducements. Within community mental health care, examples of inducements might be offers that could leave the person better off in terms of housing or other benefits in return for adherence to medication or other aspects of their prescribed treatment. In principle, an inducement is an offer of something without which the individual to whom the offer is made will be no worse off than they were prior to the offer; in this respect an inducement is often seen as less problematic than a threat (Wertheimer 1989; Dunn et al. 2012). Their increased use in the USA is perhaps linked to patients being diverted from the criminal justice or social care systems (Sinaiko and McGuire 2006), through, for example, 'mental health courts'. Here a sentence after conviction for an offence is suspended if an offer of psychiatric treatment is accepted (this is an offer, not a threat, since its rejection would leave the person as convicted and sentenced, and thus no worse off, than if the offer had never been made). There have been calls for greater attention to be given to examining the ethical dimensions of such interventions (Monahan et al. 2005; Appelbaum and Redlich 2006).

We will briefly consider the particular ethical challenges presented by inducements and how these compare with those presented by threats and coercion. There are a number of ethical concerns with inducements themselves, while the gap between inducements and interventions perceived to be more coercive may also not be as clear-cut as one might assume.

First, there is the issue of fairness in allocating resources. Why should those patients who are reliably compliant with treatment be denied privileges, and why should the resources of services or finances be diverted disproportionately to less compliant patients? Those who are not offered incentives may be discouraged from accepting treatment, while a reliance on incentives could foster a culture of dependence by encouraging patients to take a more passive role in their care. If clinicians stand to gain from patients' compliance, there is also a risk of exploitation, insofar as benefits to the clinician, rather than patients' best interests, could become a significant motivation for offering inducements (Dunn et al. 2012).

Inducements involve 'relations of power', although the assumption of an 'economic' rather than a 'power-structure' paradigm means that the associated ethical issues are often overlooked (Grant and Sugarman 2004). This is particularly relevant within mental health care, where the 'authority-relationship' of clinician and service user is already framed within a coercive context that will very likely affect the individual's degree of voluntariness in decision making. Furthermore, in jurisdictions where, for example, the law is ambiguous on the rights of a representative payee to withhold or dispense benefits or where the patients are themselves unsure (Elbogen et al. 2005), the boundaries between offer and threat become blurred (Bonnie and Monahan 2005).

A key element of inducements is also that they offer an 'extrinsic benefit' rather than being 'the natural or automatic consequence of an action or a deserved reward or compensation' (Grant and Sugarman 2004), and we can see this aspect as being problematic in terms of best interests and 'incommensurability of values'. The primary and intrinsic aims of medical interventions are to improve health and human flourishing. Clinicians are expected to offer independent health-related guidance. Offers of secondary material gains from medication, such as money or housing, may come to corrupt or degrade the value of the primary aim, as well as affecting the patient's sense of agency by disrespecting what they consider to be in the best interests of their own health. To use material incentives to convince a patient with capacity who has decided not to comply not only undermines their own decision making concerning their best health interests (Szmukler 2009) but also endorses a commodification of medical treatment instead of its value lying in its promotion of wellbeing. We would argue, *contra* Dunn et al. (2012), that this is the case, regardless of the eventual possibility of relapse.

In addition, there is the risk of discrimination against poorer patients, insofar as any resulting decrease in voluntariness will be greatest for those to whom the material benefit on offer would make the greatest degree of difference. Material inducements might even be seen to be exploiting the typically low socio-economic status of those with long-term mental health conditions to influence their decision making. There is also the risk that such transactions alter the nature of the relationship between caregiver and recipient, whether personal or professional (Elbogen et al. 2005). A UK survey of clinicians' attitudes to offering financial incentives for adherence revealed widespread reservations surrounding the use of such measures, in terms of all of these concerns (Claassen 2007).

Finally, if we reconsider the common assumption that inducements are less coercive than threats, problems may emerge in the ethical division usually posited between them. It is undeniable that benefits, as well as penalties, have the potential to influence how individuals make decisions, especially within a 'coercive context'. Yet, inducements might still seem distinct from, and less morally troubling than, threats and penalties, since the latter appear to leave those who do not accept them in a worse position than they were prior to the proposal being made. The relative ability of threats and inducements to influence decision making would be supported by well-attested theories of 'loss aversion', where threats of deprivation exert more influence than offers of benefits, even where material outcomes are the same (Kahneman et al. 1991).

Nevertheless, just as we have suggested that threats may be morally acceptable if the threatened consequences are legal and acceptance of the proposal could be advantageous, we might also wish to question the idea that inducements, whether declined or accepted, do not leave those to whom they are offered unharmed. First, there are the multiple concerns already detailed, such as the possible disempowerment, dependency, inequality, and perceived coercion due to context, which may result simply from offering inducements, whatever the choice. These concerns are raised in other discussions of the use of incentives, for example in the context of political or medical research (Collier and Collier 1979; Grant and Sugarman 2004; Emanuel et al. 2005).

It is also important to consider the fact that many inducements considered within a psychiatric context are a long-term and iterative intervention, and this in itself complicates the issues involved. For example, in a recent trial of inducements, patients were paid inducements of £15 on either a weekly, fortnightly, or monthly basis when they received anti-psychotic medication (Priebe et al. 2013). Given the low economic status of the majority of those on long-term antipsychotics for the maintenance of a psychotic disorder, this amount may well represent a substantial increase to their monthly income in the long term. Indeed, the most significant result was a perceived improvement in quality of life amongst those who received the intervention, and, given that there was no appreciable difference in health outcomes between the control and intervention group, it seems possible that this change might be attributed to the increased income.

If the individual accepts for a period of time and then wishes to reconsider, they are now making this decision within a framework where receiving payment for medication has become the norm. Any decision to discontinue will be now be perceived as involving a loss of income or benefits, which may well have made a substantive difference to their quality of life. The argument that without the offer having been given they would have received no payment regardless of choice is less compelling once the payment is iterative and remuneration has, for them, become the accepted norm in return for taking medication.

Moreover, this leads to further questions about long-term adherence. Inducements are offered to those who may be reluctant to comply in order to encourage adherence. If compliance is now secured, unless the individual experiences a radical shift in their views about the health benefits of medication, their motivation for adherence very likely stems to a great degree from the financial benefits. If the inducements are then subsequently discontinued, they may well lose their motivation to continue with treatment. The consideration of whether to use inducement schemes must therefore take into account not simply the effects while the scheme is in place but the potential problems it might cause for participants after discontinuation.

Within a psychiatric context, there are some very clear problems, therefore, in the idea that offers leave those who decline them, or even those who accept, them unharmed in some significant ways. Moreover, the potential disadvantages of inducements are far less transparent than those that accompany a threat; this, in itself, might be seen to render them ethically problematic.

For all the above reasons it appears that, from an ethical standpoint, it becomes hard to justify the use of inducements within psychiatry. Though exposure to financial incentives may be commonplace in many spheres of life in our market-orientated society, the particular context of mental health care requires special recognition. Mental health patients commonly experience a lack of respect from many sources for their preferences and values, and are marginalized as participants in society. There is a clear risk that inducements will serve as a structural reinforcement of this marginalization and disempowerment.

Interpersonal leverage and persuasion

Similar problems occur even at the lowest end of the coercive spectrum if we consider the use of interpersonal leverage and persuasion. With persuasion, an appeal is made to reason to convince an individual that a particular course of action would be in their best interests. Interpersonal leverage might be seen as an emotion-based addition to persuasion, in which an individual uses a well-established and positive relationship with someone to influence their decision, for example by showing signs of distancing or disappointment if the recommended course of action is rejected.

Both are means of influencing decision making. As we have argued, within the 'coercive context' of much mental health-care practice any such influence runs the risk of being perceived by the patient as coercive. Moreover, there may be a 'grey area' where even these modes of persuasion could seem to imply, from the patient's perspective, an element of underlying threat. For example, a clinician in an outpatient clinic might argue that, based on several similar past instances, the likely consequence for the patient of withdrawing from medication would be involuntary admission. One might call this an 'unwelcome prediction', a prediction based on evidence and not intended as a threat. However, there may in practice be a fine line between the reasoned arguments suggesting likely consequences and what might be perceived as a threat, especially when the individual expressing these arguments would be likely to be part of the team that makes the decision to invoke involuntary treatment.

A range of difficulties

There are clear ethical difficulties across the range of coercive and 'leverage-based' interventions employed in mental health care. An examination of these difficulties shows that, within the coercive context of mental health, there is greater overlap between the different categories of intervention than there might first appear, so that their relative classification and evaluation needs careful consideration.

Nevertheless, despite the prevalence of the varying types of leverage within current mental health-care systems, there has been little attention to guidelines or sustained ethical discussion of those interventions that do not involve formal compulsion. If we are seriously to consider the relative ethics of all mechanisms of leverage, we need a structural approach to mental health care which can make space to accommodate guidance for the whole range of treatment pressures employed in practice.

An alternative approach to involuntary treatment

Severe mental disorder can lead to clinical situations where a patient appears to lack true autonomy, so that coercive interventions may well reflect their best interests even if they incur short-term loss of liberty. Despite the numerous ethical difficulties, it seems that we need provision for coercive interventions and that individual types or instances must be examined in terms of what might maximize their ethical coherence. This is all the more pressing within a community context, where the complexity and scope for such interventions has broadened considerably.

Many current difficulties appear to stem from the underlying risk- and status-based structure of mental health legislation. Not only does its dependence on status render it fundamentally discriminatory, but the emphasis on risk leads to overuse of coercive measures based on prejudicial, over-protective, and highly inaccurate justifications (Dawson and Szmukler 2006; Szmukler and Rose 2013). It also leaves gaps surrounding the use of informal coercive interventions, often used as an alternative to formal measures, to obtain compliance. Further problems arise from a lack of clarity and consistency, which increases the likelihood of greater degrees of coercion being experienced by a patient because of confusion about their rights.

A recent development in international law, the 2006 United Nations Convention on the Rights of Persons with Disabilities (CRPD) is highly relevant here. With its move from substitute to supported decision making (see Chapter 13), it is pushing us towards an urgent reconsideration of existing laws regarding coercion. The CRPD rejects substitute decision making, and there is currently extensive debate surrounding the difficulties of applying this principle to a mental health context (Kelly 2014). However, it also stipulates our obligations to respect the 'current will and preferences' of an individual and to support them in reaching a valid expression of these.

A better approach to mental health legislation might therefore be to use a 'decision-making capacity and best interests' approach, where best interests are determined by trying to attain the closest possible understanding of the *authentic will and preferences* of the individual (Dawson and Szmukler 2006; Szmukler et al. 2013). Assessment would take into account a patient's current mental state and abilities but would also involve a fuller picture of their beliefs and values, drawn from their past history—for example, the consistency of the person's decision-influencing beliefs with their broader life choices, the support such beliefs have, whether they are amenable to revision or argument, their stability over time, their evolution, the extent of their self-endorsement, past commitments they have engendered, and their cultural meaningfulness and rationality, to name but a few possible considerations—together with any advance statements they themselves might have written, to assess whether their current preferences are consistent within this broader framework. To a certain extent such ideas are represented within the framework of legislation such as the Mental Capacity Act (MCA) 2005, which stipulates that determination of best interests must take into account, where 'reasonably ascertainable', 'past and present wishes and feelings', likely beliefs, values, or other considerations if the individual had capacity (MCA 2005, 1.4.6). However, the individual's will and preferences are still only used post-assessment to determine their best interests, rather than being integrated into the capacity assessment, while capacity-based legislation is, in practice, almost always trumped by mental health legislation.

An approach based on an assessment of 'will and preferences' would reflect the language and values of the CRPD more closely than current frameworks. By making 'will and preferences' central to determining capacity, the 'best interests' criterion, used to determine what action should be taken, will be reframed far more in terms of the subjective beliefs and values of the patient. This would force us to interpret the person's own beliefs and values and perhaps help in the move towards a model which can incorporate greater degrees of supported decision making. Ultimately, decisions about whether to bring in substitute decision making might still depend on the likely harm from non-compliance, the 'adverse effects' anticipated, for example, by Bach and Kerzner (2010). However, this understanding of harmful consequences would be determined by the deeply held values of individuals themselves, as opposed to general and unsubstantiated estimates of risk.

This approach is highly suitable to making decisions about 'coercive' interventions in a community mental health-care setting. One would aim for the least coercive option, while the more coercive the intervention the stronger the justification must be. This framework offers a structure for clinical discussion and fosters greater clarity and transparency in decision making.

In theory, the aim of coercive interventions would no longer be the avoidance of putative risk, which is both inaccurate and discriminatory, but the maximization of will and preference-based best interests and, through this, the maximization of self-determination. Some ways to achieve this in practice might be to encourage increased use of advance statements and their incorporation within a legal and clinical framework. Although the aim of advance decision making is often seen as decreased coercion or hospitalization, it could also be used by the patient to determine a means of including coercive measures in their care in a manner acceptable to them, by specifying preferences for treatment or management of their affairs during periods when they might be lacking in capacity. They might even incorporate coercion into their own supported decision-making process. For example, could a person include a request for a set period under a CTO, either to shorten the period of hospitalization or because they know from past experience that they will discontinue treatment even when apparently 'well enough' to be discharged? Similarly, a patient who anticipates future episodes of mania, for example, might use a self-binding advance directive (a Ulysses contract) to ensure that they receive treatment, even if they are unwilling at that time, at the advent of precursor symptoms which they themselves have identified and accepted in agreement with their clinical team. In this way, they could use their experience of past episodes and treatments to dictate a strategy involving coercion, as a form of damage limitation, whether this be compulsion or using the contract as leverage.

These considerations present a major challenge to mental health services. The potential for an expansion of coercive interventions in response to community fears and diminishing resources is substantial. Mental health professionals rightly accept an obligation to act to protect their patients and those around them from serious harm. However, if abuses are to be avoided, they must not allow unrealistic views either of risk or the effectiveness of coercive interventions amongst the wider community or professionals to obstruct any modifications to current law and practice that can enhance their ethical acceptability.

References

Appelbaum PS, Redlich A (2006). Use of leverage over patients' money to promote adherence to psychiatric treatment. *Journal of Nervous and Mental Diseases*, **194**:294–302.

Bach M, Kerzner L (2010). *A new paradigm for protecting autonomy and the right to legal capacity*. Available at: http://www.lco-cdo.org/disabilities/bach-kerzner.pdf

Bonnie RJ, Monahan J (2005). From coercion to contract: reframing the debate on mandated community treatment for people with mental disorders. *Law and Human Behavior*, **29**:485–503.

Canvin K, Rugkåsa J, Sinclair J, et al. (2013). Leverage and other informal pressures in community psychiatry in England. *International Journal of Law and Psychiatry*, **36**:100–106.

Churchill R, Owen GS, Singh S (2007). *International experiences of using community treatment orders*. London: Department of Health.

Claassen D (2007). Financial incentives for antipsychotic depot medication: ethical issues. *Journal of Medical Ethics*, **33**:189–193.

Collier R, Collier D (1979). Inducements versus constraints: disaggregating 'corporatism'. *American Political Science Review*, **73**:967–986.

Dawson J (2006). Fault-lines in community treatment order legislation. *International Journal of Law and Psychiatry*, **29**:482–494.

Dawson J, Szmukler G (2006). Fusion of mental health and incapacity legislation. *British Journal of Psychiatry*, **188**:504–549.

Dunn M, Maughan D, Hope T, et al. (2012). Threats and offers in community mental healthcare. *Journal of Medical Ethics*, **38**:204–209.

Dunn M, Sinclair JM, Canvin KJ, et al. (2014). The use of leverage in community mental health: ethical guidance for practitioners. *International Journal of Social Psychiatry*, **60**:759–765.

Elbogen EB, Soriano C, Van Dorn R (2005). Consumer views of representative payee use of disability funds to leverage treatment adherence. *Psychiatric Services*, **56**:45–49.

Emanuel EJ, Currie XE, Herman A (2005). Project Phidisa. Undue inducement in clinical research in developing countries: is it a worry? *The Lancet*, **366**:336–340.

Grant RW, Sugarman J (2004). Ethics in human subjects research: do incentives matter? *Journal of Medicine and Philosophy*, **29**:717–738.

Hart SD, Michie C, Cooke DJ (2007). Precision of actuarial risk assessment instruments. Evaluating the 'margins of error' of group v. individual predictions of violence. *British Journal of Psychiatry*, **190**:s60–s65.

Health Committee (2013). *Health Committee—first report. Post legislative scrutiny of the Mental Health Act 2007*. Available at: http://www.publications.parliament.uk/pa/cm201314/cmselect/cmhealth/584/58402.htm

Health and Social Care Information Centre (2012). *Number of mental health detentions and community treatment order rises*. Available at: http://www.hscic.gov.uk/article/2282/Number-of-Mental-Health-detentions-and-Community-Treatment-Order-rises

Health and Social Care Information Centre (2013). *Inpatients formally detained in hospitals under the Mental Health Act 1983 and patients subject to supervised community treatment, England—2012-2013, annual figures.* Available from: http://www.hscic.gov.uk/catalogue/PUB12503

Kahneman D, Knetsch JL, Thaler RH (1991). Anomalies: the endowment effect, loss aversion, and status quo bias. *Journal of Economic Perspectives*, 5:193–206.

Kelly BD (2014). An end to psychiatric detention? Implications of the United Nations Convention on the Rights of Persons with Disabilities. *British Journal of Psychiatry*, 204:174–175.

Keown P, Mercer G, Scott J (2008). Retrospective analysis of hospital episode statistics, involuntary admissions under the Mental Health Act 1983, and number of psychiatric beds in England 1996–2006. *British Medical Journal*, 337:a1837.

Kisely S, Campbell LA, Preston N (2005). Compulsory community and involuntary outpatient treatment for people with severe mental disorders. *Cochrane Database of Systematic Reviews*, (3):CD004408.

Kisely SR, Campbell LA, Preston NJ (2011). Compulsory community and involuntary outpatient treatment for people with severe mental disorders. *Cochrane Database of Systematic Reviews*, (2):CD004408.

Large MMBS, Ryan CJM, Singh SPM, et al. (2011a). The predictive value of risk categorization in schizophrenia. *Harvard Review of Psychiatry*, 19:25–33.

Large M, Sharma S, Cannon E, et al. (2011b). Risk factors for suicide within a year of discharge from psychiatric hospital: a systematic meta-analysis. *Australian and New Zealand Journal of Psychiatry*, 45:619–628.

Lawton-Smith S, Dawson J, Burns T (2008). Community treatment orders are not a good thing. *British Journal of Psychiatry*, 193:96–100.

McCutcheon R (2013). Community treatment orders for patients with psychosis. *The Lancet*, 382:501.

Manning S (2013). Psychiatric asbos were an error. *The Independent*, 14 April. Available at: http://www.independent.co.uk/life-style/health-and-families/health-news/psychiatric-asbos-were-an-error-says-key-advisor-8572138.html

Monahan J, Redlich AD, Swanson J, et al. (2005). Use of leverage to improve adherence to psychiatric treatment in the community. *Psychiatric Services*, 56:37–44.

NHS England (2014). *Bed availability and occupancy data—overnight.* Available at: http://www.england.nhs.uk/statistics/statistical-work-areas/bed-availability-and-occupancy/bed-data-overnight/

Patel MX, Matonhodze J, Baig MK, et al. (2011). Increased use of antipsychotic long-acting injections with community treatment orders. *Therapeutic Advances in Psychopharmacology*, 1:37–45.

Priebe S, Yeeles K, Bremner S, et al. (2013). Effectiveness of financial incentives to improve adherence to maintenance treatment with antipsychotics: cluster randomised controlled trial. *British Medical Journal*, 347:f5847.

RA Malatest and Associates (2012). *The legislated review of community treatment orders (final report).* Toronto, ON: Ministry of Health and Long-Term Care. Available at: http://www.health.gov.on.ca/en/common/ministry/publications/reports/mental_health/cto_review_report.pdf

Robiliard D (2013). *CRPA: Sur l'internment psychiatrique abusif et illégal.* Available at: http://psychiatrie.crpa.asso.fr/341

Rugkåsa J, Dawson J (2013). Community treatment orders: current evidence and the implications. *British Journal of Psychiatry*, **203**:406–468.

Salize HJ, Dressing H (2004). Epidemiology of involuntary placement of mentally ill people across the European Union. *British Journal of Psychiatry*, **184**:163–168.

Sinaiko AD, McGuire TG (2006). Patient inducement, provider priorities, and resource allocation in public mental health systems. *Journal of Health Politics, Policy and Law*, **31**:1075–1106.

Singh JP, Fazel S, Gueorguieva R, et al. (2014). Rates of violence in patients classified as high risk by structured risk assessment instruments. *British Journal of Psychiatry*, **204**:180–187.

Sjöström S (2006). Invocation of coercion context in compliance communication—power dynamics in psychiatric care. *International Journal of Law and Psychiatry*, **29**:36–47.

Stroud J, Doughty K, Banks L (2013). *An exploration of service user and practitioner experiences of community treatment orders*. Available at: http://sscr.nihr.ac.uk/PDF/5_12_13_Insights/Stroud%20CTOs%20(14.20).pdf

Szmukler G (2003). Risk assessment: 'numbers' and 'values'. *Psychiatric Bulletin*, **27**:205–207.

Szmukler G (2009). Financial incentives for patients in the treatment of psychosis. *Journal of Medical Ethics*, **35**:224–248.

Szmukler G (2014). Fifty years of mental health legislation: paternalism, bound and unbound. In: *Psychiatry: past, present, and prospect* (ed. S Bloch, S Green, J Holmes), pp. 133–153. Oxford: Oxford University Press.

Szmukler G, Appelbaum PS (2008). Treatment pressures, leverage, coercion, and compulsion in mental health care. *Journal of Mental Health*, **17**:233–244.

Szmukler G, Rose N (2013). Risk assessment in mental health care: values and costs. *Behavioral Sciences and the Law*, **31**:125–140.

Szmukler G, Daw R, Callard F (2013). Mental health law and the UN Convention on the rights of persons with disabilities. *International Journal of Law and Psychiatry*, **37**:245–252.

Taylor M (2010). Community treatment orders and their use in the UK. Commentary on compulsion in the community and supervised community treatment. *Advances in Psychiatric Treatment*, **16**:260–262.

Treatment Advocacy Centre (2014). *No room at the inn: trends and consequences of closing public psychiatric hospitals*. Available at: http://tacreports.org/bed-study

Turner T (2014). Improving mental health services in England. *British Medical Journal*, **348**:g1907.

Undrill G (2007). The risks of risk assessment. *Advances in Psychiatric Treatment*, **13**:291–297.

Wand T, Large M (2013). Little evidence for the usefulness of violence risk assessment. *British Journal of Psychiatry*, **202**:468.

Wertheimer A (1989). *Coercion*. Princeton, NJ: Princeton University Press.

Zielasek J, Gaebel W (2015). Mental health law in Germany. *BJPsych International*, **12**:14–16.

Part 5

International perspectives

Chapter 15

Coercion in community mental health treatment in the Americas

Richard O'Reilly and John Gray

Introduction

The Americas consist of the combined continental land mass of North America and South America and their associated islands. The total population of the Americas is over 950 million (Wikipedia, Americas). The two northernmost countries, Canada and the USA, are developed industrialized countries with lengthy democratic traditions. The countries to the south of the USA have undergone variable degrees of industrialization and most are democracies, though some of relatively short duration. There are a total of 35 countries in the Americas in addition to several protectorates of Western countries.

In Canada and the USA health care is a joint responsibility of federal and provincial or state governments. However, mental health legislation is enacted at the provincial and state level, resulting in 13 Canadian mental health acts and 51 mental health acts in the USA. Canada, the USA, and a number of Caribbean countries were originally British colonies and have maintained many elements of British legal tradition. In contrast, most South American countries had periods of Spanish colonization. Brazil, which was originally a Portuguese colony, is a notable exception.

Health-care spending varies considerably in the Americas. The USA spends 17.9% of its gross domestic product (GDP) on health care (http://www.who.int/countries/usa/en/), which is the highest percentage of any country in the world. In contrast, Venezuela spends 4.7% of its GDP on health care, which is the lowest of all countries in the Americas (http://www.who.int/countries/ven/en/). As the USA has a higher GDP than other countries, the absolute difference in spending per capita is even larger.

Mental health services are better developed and more comprehensive in Canada and the USA than in South American countries. The early development of mental health services in Canada and the USA was primarily in large psychiatric hospitals. Many individuals with the most severe mental illness lived their lives in these hospitals. Deinstitutionalization had dramatic consequences for individuals with serious mental illness in Canada and the USA (Torrey 1997). Most other countries in the Americas did not hospitalize the mentally ill at the same rates as occurred in Canada and the USA, and some of the changes associated with deinstitutionalization have not been as dramatic in those countries.

The objective of this chapter is to provide an overview of how coercion is used to ensure adherence to treatment for people with mental illness living in community settings. We review both formal laws and informal methods used to pressure individuals to accept treatment outside hospital settings. Where relevant, we refer briefly to procedures to involuntarily hospitalize individuals with mental illness.

First, we examine the situation in the two northernmost countries, Canada and the USA. These are both federal states, in which most jurisdictions have formal legislation that requires people to take treatment in the community when specific criteria are met. The subsequent analysis of compulsory treatment in the community in Latin America and the Caribbean poses major problems. We are unaware of any jurisdictions in the Americas, apart from some Canadian provinces and US states, that have statutes specifically authorizing involuntary treatment of individuals who are not inpatients. However, we are not able to confirm this on a country by country basis. As has been noted elsewhere, most of the literature on coercion comes from developed countries such as Canada and the USA (Molodynski et al. 2014). We also note that the World Health Organization (WHO) has acknowledged similar difficulties in gaining a clear perspective on arrangements for compulsory care in the community in Europe (Strachan 2009).

Our approach is to describe some of the major differences in the delivery of mental health services in Canada and the USA compared with Latin American and Caribbean countries. We discuss how service differences affect the management of patients who would probably be viewed as candidates for community treatment orders (CTOs) in Canada and the USA. We then provide a description of services, legislation, and practices in three jurisdictions: Brazil and Argentina, which are two of the largest Latin American countries, and Jamaica, a Caribbean country. In our descriptions of practice in Latin American countries, we have relied on personal communication with psychiatrists and other mental health clinicians working in these countries, supplemented where possible with additional citable sources.

Canada

Canada is the northernmost country in the Americas and comprises 10 provinces and three territories. The population is approximately 35 million (Statistics Canada 2014). Across Canada's jurisdictions, it is estimated that 7.2% of total government health expenditure is spent on mental health (Institute of Health Economics 2010). Canada has 31 mental hospital beds per 100,000 population (World Health Organization, Canada). Canada's Mental Health Commission has endorsed the long-standing Canadian trend of shifting services and resources from mental hospitals to community mental health facilities. Deinstitutionalization was extensive through the 1980s and 1990s (Sealy and Whitehead 2004), and continues, albeit at a slower pace, in most Canadian jurisdictions. Similar to the situation in the USA (Lamb and Bachrach 2001), there has been criticism in Canada that closure of large mental hospitals has not been accompanied by the establishment of promised services in the community (O'Reilly 2001).

Canada has 13 mental health acts because each of the provinces and territories is responsible for its own health laws and services. In Canadian jurisdictions, inpatient and various forms of outpatient involuntary treatment fall under these mental health acts (O'Reilly and Gray 2014). As with all Canadian laws, mental health acts must conform to the overarching Canadian Charter of Rights and Freedoms, which is part of the country's constitution. In most Canadian jurisdictions, apart from the province of Quebec, legislation is based on common law; whereas in Quebec it is based on a civil code, as is the case in France.

All Canadian provinces except New Brunswick and Prince Edward Island have legislated CTOs or similar mechanisms for compulsory community treatment, such as conditional leave. Canada's three northern territories do not have such legislation either. Apart from Quebec, where a judge must authorize a CTO, the Canadian system for authorizing CTOs resembles that used in Scotland and in England and Wales. Depending on the jurisdiction, one or more physicians must complete the required forms and a CTO can be initiated either when the patient is in hospital or living in the community. In practice, the great majority are initiated while a person is awaiting discharge from involuntary inpatient admission.

With the exception of the province of Alberta, all Canadian provinces require that a person must have had a stipulated amount of inpatient psychiatric care before being placed on a CTO (Gray et al. 2012). For example, Newfoundland and Labrador requires that the person has been involuntarily hospitalized on three or more occasions in the previous 2 years.[1] Thus, from a policy perspective, Canadian CTO statutes attempt to solve the revolving-door phenomenon rather than adhering to the principle of providing care in the least restrictive setting.

Alberta has incorporated flexibility in its CTO provision. The basic CTO requires that the person has had two or more involuntary admissions or has had one admission of 30 or more days in hospital in the previous 3 years. However, in Alberta, a person can be placed on a CTO without previous hospital admissions if the person has already exhibited a recurrent pattern of behaviour that indicates that he or she is likely to cause harm or to deteriorate if not on a CTO (Gray et al. 2012).

Saskatchewan recently reduced its requirements for past hospitalization from three involuntary admissions or a total of 60 days of involuntary hospitalization in the past 2 years, to one voluntary or involuntary admission of any length.[2] Thus in Saskatchewan, an individual who is hospitalized for the first time and whose inpatient detention can be shortened by a CTO can be placed on a CTO during that admission.

Formal treatment planning is a required part of the CTO in most jurisdictions and all jurisdictions require that the services necessary to support the CTO are available to the patient.

The introduction of CTOs has been controversial in some Canadian jurisdictions, especially in Ontario. In 2013, an application that CTOs contravened the Canadian Charter of Rights and Freedoms was dismissed by the Ontario Superior Court.[3]

A number of Canadian jurisdictions have incorporated into their CTO legislation a requirement for a formal review of the legislation. In Ontario, Canada's largest

---

[1] *Mental Health Care and Treatment Act*, S.N.L. 2006, c. M-9.1, s. 40.

[2] *Mental Health Services Act*, S.S. 1984-85-86, c. M-13.1, s. 24.3(1)(a)(ii).

[3] Karlene Thompson and Empowerment Council, Systemic Advocates in Addiction and Mental Health v. Attorney General of Ontario. Docket: 05-cv-293285. 2013. See: http://digital.ontarioreports.ca/ontarioreports/20140214?pg=123# (accessed 11 August 2014).

province, the two completed reviews concluded that CTOs provide benefits to patients and their families and recommended their continued use (Dreezer & Dreezer Inc. 2005, RA Malatest and Associates 2012). The second of these reports noted that CTOs are used at a rate of approximately 36 per 100,000 population (RA Malatest and Associates 2012). This indicates that Ontario has medium to high utilization of CTOs compared with other international jurisdictions (Lawton-Smith 2005). The legislated review in Nova Scotia commented positively on the effect of CTOs, and recommended their continued use (LaForest and Lahey 2013). The legislated review from the province of Newfoundland and Labrador indicated a very low use of CTOs, with three individuals on a CTO in 2012 in a jurisdiction with a population of just over 500,000 (Newfoundland and Labrador Centre for Health Information 2012).

The limited research on CTOs in Canada has reported that their use is associated with reduced hospitalization (Frank et al. 2005; O'Brien and Farrell 2005; Hunt et al. 2007; Nakhost et al. 2012).

Informal coercion of individuals with mental illness to comply with psychiatric treatment occurs in Canada, as it presumably does in all countries. Informal coercion is more difficult to quantify than coercion resulting from legal statutes. Several Canadian provinces have adopted the Program of Assertive Community Treatment (Stein and Test 1980). Clinicians from assertive community treatment (ACT) teams visit individuals with severe and persistent mental illness in community settings. One of their key roles is to encourage adherence to treatment. Scholars have noted that a significant degree of informal coercion accompanies ACT (Moser and Bond 2009).

Many jurisdictions in Canada attempt to divert individuals with mental illness from the legal system into the mental health system. Individuals may have charges stayed or avoid a period of incarceration in jail if they can commit to an appropriate course of treatment (Thompson et al. 2007).

In Canada many individuals with severe and persistent mental illness live with their families. We are aware of many cases in which the family insists on adherence to treatment in return for the continued provision of food, lodging, and other care.

The United States

The USA comprises 50 states and a federal district, Washington, DC. With a population of 316 million, the USA is the third most populous country in the world and the most populous in the Americas (World Population Review 2014a).

The USA has a developed health-care system. However, despite spending almost 18% of its GDP on health care, which is the highest proportion of GDP spent on health care of all the countries in the world, many people in the USA are uninsured and unable to afford basic health-care services (AMSA 2007). As of 2005, mental health spending represented 6.1% of the total health budget (Mark et al. 2011). The USA has 19 mental hospital beds and 14 psychiatric beds in general hospitals per 100,000 population (World Health Organization, USA). Large psychiatric hospitals have mostly been closed, resulting in a marked reduction in the proportion of psychiatric care that is provided in inpatient settings (Torrey 1997). There has been a vigorous debate in the USA about deinstitutionalization, with a consensus view that poor implementation has resulted in homelessness, imprisonment, or the death of many people with severe mental illness (Torrey 1997; Lamb and Bachrach 2001).

In the USA a physician must petition a court to have a patient placed on a CTO. These court orders are usually referred to as outpatient committal, but occasionally as assisted outpatient treatment. Legal requirements that patients who are not involved with the criminal justice system must follow a plan of treatment in the community were first used in the USA. It seems possible that the first patient was committed to outpatient treatment from the wards of St Elizabeth's Hospital in Washington, DC in 1972 (Torrey 2011).

Forty-five states have now enacted outpatient committal legislation, but in 12 states it is rarely if ever used (Stettin et al. 2014). The duration of an individual outpatient commitment order varies between 2 and 12 months, and they are typically renewable if the need persists (Stettin et al. 2014).

Some US jurisdictions such as Washington, DC require that a patient who is placed on a CTO must meet the jurisdiction's inpatient criteria—the diversionary or least restrictive model, whereas others such as New York use a preventive model of CTO, in which the criteria for placement on outpatient committal are less stringent than for placement on inpatient committal.

There has been much academic debate in the USA about the need for and the ethical underpinnings of CTOs (Morrissey et al. 2014; Swanson and Swartz 2014). The USA has also been the site of many studies of CTOs, including the first two randomized controlled trials (Swartz et al. 1999; Steadman et al. 2001), which arrived at different conclusions about the efficacy of CTOs.

The USA has also spawned many informal types of coercion to assist with treatment adherence. We have already described ACT teams, which were first developed in the state of Wisconsin (Stein and Test 1980). Other approaches include: representative payeeship, leverage through subsidized housing, and court diversion programmes.

The US Social Security Administration allows a representative payee to be appointed for an individual with severe mental illness who has difficulty managing their money. This representative is often a family member or mental health worker. After paying for accommodation and food the representative may make access to remaining funds from disability cheques dependent on the recipient adhering to treatment regimens (Monahan et al. 2001). In a study of five US cities, between 7% and 19% of patients receiving outpatient mental health services reported that at some time access to money had been dependent on treatment adherence (Monahan et al. 2005).

Similar leverage may be applied by group homes or other subsidized housing programmes (Monahan et al. 2001). These services are often managed by community mental health agencies. Applicants are sometimes required to give an undertaking to continue psychiatric treatment as part of their lease, whereby failure to do so may result in eviction (Monahan et al. 2005). In Monahan's study of five US cities, between 23% and 40% of patients receiving mental health services said that their housing had been linked to a requirement to accept treatment.

In the USA many individuals with serious mental disorders find themselves in trouble with the law. Courts will frequently impose a lenient disposition of a mentally ill person's case if that person agrees to adhere to treatment. In the five-city study 15–30% of adult patients receiving outpatient services reported experiencing this type of judicial leverage (Monahan et al. 2005).

As is the case in Canada, the USA has many courts that deal specifically with people with mental illness who have been charged with a criminal offence. These courts routinely encourage treatment adherence by linking it to the staying of criminal charges for minor offences. Such mental health courts operate in different ways and intervene at different points in the judicial process (Thompson et al. 2007). Overall, they appear to be effective and to be preferred by people with mental illness who are facing charges (Poythress et al. 2012).

Latin America

The term 'Latin America' is often used to describe the American continent south of the USA. While there is considerable variation in the politics and culture of the countries forming Latin America there are commonalities that distinguish these countries from Canada and the USA. Two distinctions are relevant to the management of individuals with severe mental illness who do not adhere to treatment regimes. First, mental health services in Latin American countries are not as well developed or comprehensive as they are in Canada and the USA. Second, families play a more important role in providing support for ill relatives in Latin America than in North America, where a higher value is placed on individualism.

As is the case in many low- and middle-income countries in other areas of the world, most psychiatric beds in Latin American countries are in large mental hospitals rather than in general hospital psychiatric units (McKenzie et al. 2004). Despite efforts to reduce the centralization of mental health services in many countries, funding for psychiatric hospitals still constitutes a large component of the total mental health budget. However, the number of psychiatric beds per capita in Latin American countries has always been lower than the levels in higher-income countries (Belfort and González 2005; Berenzon et al. 2009).

In many low- and middle-income Latin American and Caribbean countries, up to 75% of individuals who need psychiatric care do not receive it (Kohn et al. 2005). Formal counselling services and standard classes of medications for major mental illnesses are not available to many citizens. For example, many psychotropic drugs listed by the WHO as essential medications are unavailable to the average citizen outside large urban centres in Peru. The lack of such basic services in Peru led one scholar to observe that 'the unavailability and inaccessibility of mental healthcare is the most important rights issue' (Rondon 2009). When gaining access to needed and wanted services is difficult, less attention is paid to providing needed, but unwanted, services.

Latin American countries generally lack formal laws that require individuals to adhere to treatment and follow-up services in community settings. As noted, they also lack inpatient services to treat individuals who have severe mental illness, which impairs their capacity to voluntarily accept treatment in the community. In consequence, informal coercion in community settings is likely to be much higher in these countries than it is in Canada and the USA.

The culture of many Latin American countries differs from that of Canada and the USA. There is a greater emphasis on the family, and correspondingly a decreased emphasis on the individual. Families are required to provide a greater portion of the care and treatment for their relatives, and in turn families usually expect their ill members to adhere to treatment regimes. When an ill relative lacks understanding and appreciation of the need for treatment, family pressure may be exerted to ensure adherence. If the authority of the spokesperson for the family is insufficient, specific leverage may be used, such as linking the ongoing provision of shelter to treatment adherence. The threat of withdrawal of the provision of shelter in these countries is likely to be more significant than in Canada or the USA, where the state will provide funds for indigent individuals who are not living with their families.

Brazil

With a population of just over 200 million, Brazil is the fifth most populous country in the world and second in the Americas (World Population Review 2014b). Unlike other South American countries, the dominant language is Portuguese, not Spanish. Brazil is a federation of a federal district, 26 states and 5564 municipalities (Wikipedia, Brazil). The Federal Constitution allows three levels of legislation to apply: federal, state, and local law. However, since the higher levels have primacy, there is conformity of laws (Taborda 2013).

All Brazilians have a right to receive health care free of charge (World Health Organization 2007). Mental health spending represents 2.4% of the total health budget (World Health Organization, Brazil). Brazil has 18 mental hospital beds per 100,000 population and 1.3 psychiatric beds in general hospitals per 100,000 population (World Health Organization, Brazil). Large psychiatric hospitals are being phased out in Brazil, and psychiatric care is increasingly being provided in general hospitals and in the community. However, services are unequally distributed across different regions of the country. Although access to basic psychotropic drugs is guaranteed to Brazilian citizens, access is limited in some remote rural areas (World Health Organization 2007). One commentator laments that closure of hospital beds without the establishment of sufficient community services has resulted in a situation in which people with mental illnesses '... remain at home in an impoverished state, wander the streets, are locked in prisons or present at general emergency rooms' (Taborda 2013).

The Brazilian mental health act does not define mental illness, but speaks of 'people with mental disorders'. In practice this means disorders included in the ICD-10 system. There are processes and criteria in Law 10.216 for three types of hospitalization, all of which require authorization by a doctor that the person needs inpatient treatment. The three types of hospitalization are: voluntary hospitalization if the person is competent, involuntary hospitalization if the person requires a proxy consent, and compulsory hospitalization if the person is refusing hospitalization.

Involuntary hospitalization requires a judicial order. The criteria for involuntary hospitalization are not specified in the current law: rather they are outlined in the 1934 legislation and include risk of aggression to self or others, 'moral exposure' (social/ moral risk in financial, sexual, or behavioural areas), and lack of capacity for self-care.

Except for voluntary admissions, the decision to discharge is at the discretion of the physician. There are no defined renewal or review periods. The law does not address involuntary treatment as such, but the implication is that the patient has no right to refuse treatment. For more intrusive treatments, such as electroconvulsive therapy, the law requires consent from the patient's representative unless there is an imminent risk to the patient.

Brazil does not have any legislation to support involuntary treatment of patients in the community apart from provisions for offenders with a mental disorder or other forensic patients (Taborda 2103). However, under the Brazilian Civil Code, a person can be declared incompetent and placed under guardianship if the person has a mental disorder which results in impaired judgement (Taborda 2013). In theory, this law might be used like a CTO in other countries. However, it requires the effort and expense of obtaining a judicial order and is not significantly used in that way.

Informal coercion by families, professionals, and social agencies is used in Brazil, as it is in other countries, to encourage people to receive treatment in the community.

Argentina

Argentina has a population of 40 million (World Health Organization, Argentina). Argentina has 26 mental hospital beds per 100,000 population and two psychiatric beds in general hospitals per 100,000 population (World Health Organization, Argentina). The official mental health policy, revised in 2010, calls for a shift of services and resources from mental hospitals to community mental health facilities (World Health Organization, Argentina).

In Argentina, mental health laws can be enacted by different levels of government including the National Congress, some provinces, and the autonomous city of Buenos Aires. In 2010, the Argentinean Congress approved a new mental health law (Law 26657) that 'establishes principles for human rights and the protection of patients, and aims to develop approaches to mental health that are compatible with the most advanced views and legislation from high income countries' (Moldavsky et al. 2011; Moldavsky and Cohen 2013).

Law 26657 stresses human rights including a presumption of capacity, the right to be informed, a requirement for informed consent to treatment, and promotion of treatment in the least restrictive environment. The law mandates 'positive' rights to services in the community and requires that 10% of health expenditure must be for mental health services. The provision of services in general hospital psychiatric units is encouraged and the building of new asylums is forbidden. Hospital admissions can be voluntary or compulsory. All admissions, whether voluntary or compulsory, must be reported to a review and regulatory body if they are over 60 days and compulsory admissions must be reported within 10 hours. The criteria for involuntary admission are that 'outpatient approaches are not possible' and that a 'clear and present danger to the person or third parties exists'.

CTOs are not included in this law and there does not appear to be a leave provision, which in some jurisdiction is used like a CTO. We do not know if there are mechanisms for coercing community treatment such as guardianship.

The Caribbean

Many of the small island states in the Caribbean do not have mental hospitals (World Health Organization 2011b). Some jurisdictions have psychiatric beds in the general hospital system. The availability of inpatient care in either general or psychiatric hospitals is limited in many Caribbean countries. Despite the shortage of inpatient services, most jurisdictions with mental hospitals are committed to reducing their size (World Health Organization 2011b). Mental health services are underfunded, and most jurisdictions are committed to reallocating scarce resources to the currently poorly developed community services.

All Caribbean countries and territories have a mental health act. However, several jurisdictions have not amended their mental health acts since the 1950s before the adoption of relevant international conventions and standards (World Health Organization 2011b; Abel et al. 2012). There are no Caribbean countries with CTO legislation.

Jamaica

Jamaica has a population of almost 3 million (World Health Organization, Jamaica). Mental health expenditure by the government health department/ministry comprises 6% of the total health budget, with approximately 80% of spending going to hospital-based services (World Health Organization, Jamaica). Jamaica has 14 mental hospital beds per 100,000 population and three psychiatric beds in general hospitals per 100,000 population (World Health Organization, Jamaica). The services are in transition and the ministry of health has been scaling back on Bellevue, the country's biggest psychiatric hospital. There are psychiatric units in many general hospitals and patients with psychiatric illnesses are often treated in the medical wards of general hospitals (Abel et al. 2011). The country has also developed community-based services that rely on specialist nurses who have been designated as mental health officers (McKenzie 2008; Abel et al. 2011). As is the case in many South and Central American countries, there is limited availability of psychotropic medications that are considered standard in Canada and the USA (McKenzie 2008).

The mental health services make an effort to limit the duration of inpatient care, and patients with psychosis are usually discharged when their acute agitation has settled. Mental health officers provide follow-up treatment in the community. Families play a critical role in ensuring that that the patient attends follow-up appointments and complies with medication treatment (McKenzie 2008).

One result of limiting the duration of inpatient stay is that patients who have significant psychotic symptoms are treated in the community and are expected to adhere to the prescribed treatment regimen. The amendments to the mental health act in 1974 made provisions for a mental health officer to enter the home of a person with a mental illness and take the person to a clinic or hospital for evaluation and treatment by medical practitioners. This authorization fell under the common law system which governs the treatment of physically ill persons who are incapacitated (McKenzie 2008). Mental health services often keep a list of patients who are prone to default on their appointments and treatment and who, as a result, are likely to deteriorate to the point of dangerousness. Mental health officers visit these patients if they fail to show up for appointments.

In cases where a person is not known to the local mental health services, written consent from relatives is necessary to allow a mental health officer to enter the person's home for assessment.

Discussion

While epidemiological studies show some variation in the prevalence of schizophrenia and affective psychosis between different world regions, these disorders are ubiquitous (Bresnahan et al. 2003; McGrath et al. 2008). Consequentially, all countries in the Americas face the quandary of what to do when individuals with severe mental illness who require treatment and assistance to live safely in community settings do not follow-up with treatment services.

Canadian and US jurisdictions have passed legislation in an attempt to limit the harm that occurs when individuals with severe mental illness do not adhere to treatment while living in the community. Similar legislation does not appear to be available in other countries in the Americas. In addition to legislated schemes, non-legislated leverage to encourage treatment adherence is used in Canada and the USA. Based on our discussions with clinicians and families, it seems that the informal mechanisms are more widely applied in Latin America and the Caribbean than they are in Canada and the USA. Most of these countries have cultures in which the family plays a more prominent role than in North America, and insistence by the family is the key factor ensuring that individuals adhere to a treatment regimen.

An advantage of formal legal mechanisms is that there is regulatory oversight, including the right to appeal. Research has shown that individuals on CTOs view them as coercive (Swartz et al. 2002). However, qualitative studies indicate that many people who are, or have been, on CTOs say that they have been beneficial and justified (Gibbs et al. 2005). We are unaware of any studies comparing perceived coercion under formal legislative schemes with informal coercion. However, research linking higher levels of perceived coercion to a lack of procedural justice (Galon and Wineman 2011) suggests that informal measures, lacking regulatory oversight, are more likely to be perceived negatively.

A variety of legislative schemes requiring adherence to psychiatric treatment and follow-up in community settings exist in North America and there are wide disparities in the rates with which these schemes are employed. From our perspective, it appears that schemes that are more complex and burdensome on clinicians tend to be used less frequently.

Most of the Canadian schemes have incorporated prior hospitalization requirements. As we have noted, the province of Newfoundland and Labrador requires that for a person to be eligible for placement on a CTO they must have had three involuntary admissions in the previous 2 years. Canada has seen extensive deinstitutionalization, with it being increasingly difficult to access the shrinking number of inpatient beds. Three involuntary admissions within a 2-year period is a significant barrier limiting the number of people who would be eligible to be placed on a CTO. Thus, the prior hospitalization requirement is probably a factor accounting for the very low utilization of CTOs in the province of Newfoundland and Labrador. In contrast, in 2015 Saskatchewan abandoned a hospitalization requirement similar to that of Newfoundland and Labrador because it was restricting access to CTOs for patients who could benefit from their use.

If the purpose of CTOs is to stop revolving-door admissions, a high prior utilization requirement is logical. However, many clinicians view CTOs as a tool to prevent deterioration and to promote recovery (O'Reilly et al. 2012). If this is the purpose of the CTO, prior hospitalization requirements are unnecessary, as is the situation in most US states.

Canada favours a diversionary model of CTOs in which the patient must meet the inpatient committal criteria to be eligible for placement on a CTO. In contrast, many US states use a preventative model. Some scholars have argued that a preventative model is harder to justify from a legal and ethical perspective (Winick 2003). Psychiatrists are presumably wary of allowing a patient to live in the community when they have identified him or her as being at risk to themselves or to others. Therefore, a diversionary model is likely to work best in jurisdictions that have an inpatient committal criterion based on a risk of mental or physical deterioration in addition to criteria based on the risk of dangerousness.

Apart from Quebec, all Canadian provinces use a physician to initiate a CTO. Quebec and all US states use a judge. It has been suggested that the authority of a judge provides a 'black robe effect' that makes adherence to the treatment order more likely. There is no empirical evidence to support this view. Initiation by a physician emphasizes the clinical nature of the decision and is less intrusive. Avoidance of a court appearance may be less upsetting for the patient, while still maintaining regulatory oversight and the right of appeal.

References

Abel W, Sewell C, Thompson E, et al. (2011). Mental health services in Jamaica: from institution to community. *Ethnicity and Inequalities in Health and Social Care*, 4:103–111.

Abel WD, Kestel D, Eldemire-Shearer D, et al. (2012). Mental health policy and service system development in the English-speaking Caribbean. *West Indian Medical Journal*, 61:475–482.

AMSA (2007). *The case for universal health care* [written 2005/6 updated 2007/8]. http://www.amsa.org/wp-content/uploads/2015/03/CaseForUHC.pdf (last accessed 11 November 2015).

Belfort E, González J (2005). Psychiatry in Venezuela. *International Psychiatry*, 2(9):11–13.

Berenzon S, Senties H, Medina-Mora E (2009). Mental health services in Mexico. *International Psychiatry*, 6(4):93–95.

Bresnahan M, Menezes P, Varma V, et al. (2003). Geographical variation in incidence, course and outcome of schizophrenia: a comparison of developing and developed countries. In: *The epidemiology of schizophrenia* (ed. RM Murray, PB Jones, E Susser, et al.), pp. 34–49. Oxford: Oxford University Press.

Dreezer & Dreezer Inc. (2005). *Report on the legislated review of community treatment orders, required under section 33.9 of the* Mental Health Act. Toronto, ON: Ministry of Health and Long-Term Care. Available at: http://www.health.gov.on.ca/en/common/ministry/publications/reports/dreezer/dreezer.aspx (accessed 11 August 2014).

Frank D, Perry JC, Kean D, et al. (2005). Effects of compulsory treatment orders on time to hospital readmission. *Psychiatric Services*, 56:867–869.

Galon P, Wineman NM (2011). Quasi-experimental comparison of coercive interventions on client outcomes in individuals with severe and persistent mental illness. *Archives of Psychiatric Nursing*, 25:404–418.

Gibbs A, Dawson J, Ansley C, et al. (2005). How patients in New Zealand view community treatment orders. *Journal of Mental Health*, 14:357–368.

Gray JE, Shone MA, O'Reilly RL (2012). Alberta's community treatment orders: Canadian and international comparisons. *Health Law Review*, 20(2):13–21.

Hunt AM, da Silva A, Lurie S, et al. (2007). Community treatment orders in Toronto: the emerging data. *Canadian Journal of Psychiatry*, 52:647–656.

Institute of Health Economics (2010). *The cost of mental health and substance abuse services in Canada*. A report to the Mental Health Commission in Canada. Available at: http://www.ihe.ca/advanced-search/the-cost-of-mental-health-and-substance-abuse-services-in-canada (accessed 23 July 2014).

Kohn R, Levav I, de Almeida JM, et al. (2005). Mental disorders in Latin America and the Caribbean: a public health priority. *Revista Panamericana de Salud Pública*, 18:229–240.

La Forest GV, Lahey W (2013). *Report of the independent panel to review the Involuntary Psychiatric Treatment Act and community treatment orders*. Halifax, Nova Scotia: Nova Scotia Department of Health and Wellness. Available at: http://novascotia.ca/dhw/mental-health/reports/IPTA-Review-2013.pdf (accessed 11 August 2014).

Lamb HR, Bachrach LL (2001). Some perspectives on deinstitutionalization. *Psychiatric Services*, 52:1039–1045.

Lawton-Smith S (2005). *A question of numbers. The potential impact of community-based treatment orders in England and Wales*. London: Kings Fund. Available at: http://www.kingsfund.org.uk/sites/files/kf/field/field_publication_file/question-numbers-potential-impact-community-based-treatment-orders-england-wales-simon-lawton-smith-kings-fund-20-september-2005.pdf (accessed 11 August 2014).

McGrath J, Saha S, Chant D, et al. (2008). Schizophrenia: a concise overview of incidence, prevalence, and mortality. *Epidemiologic Reviews*, 30:67–76.

McKenzie K (2008). Jamaica: community mental health services. In: *Innovative mental health programs in Latin America and the Caribbean* (ed. JM Caldas de Almeida, A Cohen), pp. 79–92. Washington, DC: Pan American Health Organization. Available at: http://www.gulbenkianmhplatform.com/conteudos/00/83/00/01/Innovative-programms_6775.pdf (accessed 11 August 2014).

McKenzie K, Patel V, Araya R (2004). Learning from low income countries: mental health. *British Medical Journal*, 329:1138–1140.

Mark TL, Levit KR, Vandivort-Warren R, et al. (2011). Changes in US spending on mental health and substance abuse treatment, 1986–2005, and implications for policy. *Health Affairs (Millwood)*, 30:284–292.

Moldavsky D, Cohen H (2013). The new mental health law in Argentina. *International Psychiatry*, 10(1):11–13.

Moldavsky D, Savage C, Stein E, et al. (2011). Mental health in Argentina. *International Psychiatry*, 8(3):64–66.

Molodynski A, Turnpenny L, Rugkåsa J, et al. (2014). Coercion and compulsion in mental healthcare—an international perspective. *Asian Journal of Psychiatry*, 8:2–6.

Monahan J, Bonnie RJ, Appelbaum PS, et al. (2001). Mandated community treatment: beyond outpatient commitment. *Psychiatric Services*, **52**:1198–1205.

Monahan J, Redlich AD, Swanson J, et al. (2005). Use of leverage to improve adherence to psychiatric treatment in the community. *Psychiatric Services*, **56**:37–44.

Morrissey JP, Desmarais SL, Domino ME (2014). Outpatient commitment and its alternatives: questions yet to be answered. *Psychiatric Services*, **65**:812–815.

Moser LL, Bond GR (2009). Scope of agency control: assertive community treatment teams' supervision of consumers. *Psychiatric Services*, **60**:922–928.

Nakhost A, Perry JC, Frank D (2012). Assessing the outcome of community treatment orders on management of psychiatric patients at 2 McGill University-affiliated hospitals. *Canadian Journal of Psychiatry*, **57**:359–365.

Newfoundland and Labrador Centre for Health Information (2012). *Newfoundland and Labrador Mental Health Care and Treatment Act evaluation. Final report*. St Johns, NL: Newfoundland and Labrador Centre for Health Information. Available at: http://www.health.gov.nl.ca/health/mentalhealth/MHCTA_Final_EVALUATION_Report.PDF (accessed 11 August 2014).

O'Brien AM, Farrell SJ (2005). Community treatment orders: profile of a Canadian experience. *Canadian Journal of Psychiatry*, **50**:27–30.

O'Reilly RL (2001). Seven deadly sins of mental health reform. *Canadian Psychiatric Association Bulletin*, **33**(3):17–20.

O'Reilly RL, Gray JE (2014). Canada's mental health legislation. *International Psychiatry*, **11**(3):65–67.

O'Reilly R, Dawson J, Burns T (2012). Best practices in the use of involuntary outpatient treatment. *Psychiatric Services*, **63**:421–423.

Poythress N, Petrila J, McGaha A, Boothroyd R (2002). Perceived coercion and procedural justice in the Broward Mental Health Court. *International Journal of Law and Psychiatry*, **25**:1–17.

RA Malatest and Associates (2012). *The legislated review of community treatment orders (final report)*. Toronto, ON: Ministry of Health and Long-Term Care. Available at: http://www.health.gov.on.ca/en/common/ministry/publications/reports/mental_health/cto_review_report.pdf (accessed 11 August 2014).

Rondon MB (2009). Peru: mental health in a complex country. *International Psychiatry*, **6**(1):12–14.

Sealy P, Whitehead PC (2004). Forty years of deinstitutionalization of psychiatric services in Canada: an empirical assessment. *Canadian Journal of Psychiatry*, **49**:249–257.

Stettin B, Geller J, Ragosta K, et al. (2014). *Mental health commitment laws a survey of the states*. Arlington, VA: Treatment Advocacy Centre. Available at: http://tacreports.org/storage/documents/2014-state-survey-abridged.pdf (accessed 25 November 2014).

Statistics Canada (2014). Website. URL: http://www.statcan.gc.ca/start-debut-eng.html (accessed 22 August 2014).

Strachan JG (2009). Compulsory treatment in the community: considerations for legislation in Europe. *International Psychiatry*, **6**(3):55–56.

Steadman HJ, Gounis K, Dennis D, et al. (2001). Assessing the New York City involuntary outpatient commitment pilot program. *Psychiatric Services*, **52**:330–336.

Stein LI, Test MA (1980). Alternative to mental hospital treatment. I. Conceptual model, treatment program, and clinical evaluation. *Archives of General Psychiatry*, **37**:392–397.

Swanson JW, Swartz MS (2014). Why the evidence for outpatient commitment is good enough. *Psychiatric Services*, **65**:808–811.

Swartz MS, Swanson JW, **Wagner HR**, et al. (1999). Can involuntary outpatient commitment reduce hospital recidivism?: Findings from a randomized trial with severely mentally ill individuals. *American Journal of Psychiatry*, **156**:1968–1975.

Swartz MS, **Wagner HR**, Swanson JW, et al. (2002). The perceived coerciveness of involuntary outpatient commitment: findings from an experimental study. *Journal of the American Academy of Psychiatry and Law*, **30**:207–17.

Taborda JGC (2013). Mental health law in Brazil. *International Psychiatry*, **10**(1):13–15.

Thompson M, Osher F, Tomasini-Joshi D (2007). *Improving responses to people with mental illnesses. The essential elements of a mental health court*. New York: Council of State Governments Justice Center. Available at: https://www.bja.gov/Publications/MHC_Essential_Elements.pdf (accessed 25 August 2014).

Torrey EF (1997). *Out of the shadows: confronting America's mental illness crisis*. New York: John Wiley and Sons Inc.

Torrey EF (2011). History of outpatient committal sought. *Psychiatric News*, **46**(7):23.

Wikipedia. *Americas*. URL: http://en.wikipedia.org/wiki/Americas (accessed 15 August 2014).

Wikipedia. *Brazil*. URL: http://en.wikipedia.org/wiki/Brazil (accessed 15 August 2014).

Winick B (2003). Outpatient commitment. A therapeutic jurisprudence analysis. *Psychology, Public Policy, and Law*, **9**:107–144.

World Health Organization (2007). *WHO-AIMS report on mental health system in Brazil*. Brasilia: WHO and Ministry of Health Brazil. Available at: http://www.who.int/mental_health/evidence/who_aims_report_brazil.pdf (accessed 11 August 2014).

World Health Organization (2011a). *Mental health atlas*. Geneva: World Health Organization. Available at: http://www.who.int/mental_health/publications/mental_health_atlas_2011/en/ (accessed 25 August 2014).

World Health Organization, Argentina [country profile]: http://www.who.int/mental_health/evidence/atlas/profiles/arg_mh_profile.pdf (accessed 25 August 2014).

World Health Organization, Brazil [country profile]: http://www.who.int/mental_health/evidence/atlas/profiles/bra_mh_profile.pdf?ua=1 (accessed 25 August 2014).

World Health Organization, Canada [country profile]: http://www.who.int/mental_health/evidence/atlas/profiles/can_mh_profile.pdf (accessed 25 August 2014).

World Health Organization, Jamaica [country profile]: http://www.who.int/mental_health/evidence/atlas/profiles/jam_mh_profile.pdf (accessed 25 August 2014).

World Health Organization, Mexico [country profile]: http://www.who.int/mental_health/evidence/atlas/profiles/mex_mh_profile.pdf (accessed 25 August 2014).

World Health Organization, USA [country profile]: http://www.who.int/mental_health/evidence/atlas/profiles/usa_mh_profile.pdf?ua=1 (accessed 25 August 2014).

World Health Organization (2011b). *WHO-AIMS report on mental health systems in the Caribbean region*. Available at: http://www.who.int/mental_health/evidence/mh_systems_caribbeans_en.pdf (accessed 11 August 2014).

World Population Review (2014a). United States population 2014. URL: http://worldpopulationreview.com/countries/united-states-population/ (accessed 15 August 2014).

World Population Review (2014b). Brazil population 2014. URL: http://worldpopulationreview.com/countries/brazil-population/ (accessed 11 August 2014).

Xavier M (2008). Mexico: the Hidalgo experience a new approach to mental health care. In: *Innovative mental health programs in Latin America and the Caribbean* (ed. JM Caldas de Almeida, A Cohen), pp. 93–111. Washington, DC: Pan American Health Organization. Available at: http://www.gulbenkianmhplatform.com/conteudos/00/83/00/01/Innovative-programms_6775.pdf (accessed 28 August 2014).

Chapter 16

Coercion and mental health services in the Indian subcontinent and the Middle East

B. N. Raveesh, Swaran P. Singh,
and Soumitra Pathare

Introduction

Coercive practices are relatively common in mental health care, but coercion is ethically problematic because it involves acting against an individual's autonomy (Sjöstrand and Helgesson 2008). Ethical, legal, and clinical considerations become more complex when mental incapacity is temporary and coercive measures aim to restore autonomy (Prinsen and Van Delden 2009). It is contentious whether coercive actions are acceptable for the protection of others, since medical treatment is primarily meant for the individual. Coercive treatment may be required in order to promote the patient's health interests, but health interests have to be balanced against autonomy (O'Brien and Golding 2003). As elsewhere, coercive measures are controversial in India: while some have suggested that it may be acceptable if patients are a danger to others or to themselves, others are committed to eliminating it (Shah and Basu 2010).

Mental health law in the Indian subcontinent and the Middle East has been evolving over the past few decades, in keeping with improved delivery of care, societal changes, and the demand for enhanced accountability from a population that is increasingly aware of its rights (Lepping and Raveesh 2013). There have been rapid socio-economic, cultural, and psychosocial changes in the traditional, rurally oriented, and family centred societies of the Middle East and Asia. Despite the fact that family and friends are often intimately involved in patient care and often resort to coercion, criteria for coercion and restraint have not been defined. With a lack of international comparisons, it is even more important to be aware of patients' rights and preferences regarding the necessity, mode, and place of psychiatric treatment while also recognizing the legitimate interests of family members. Many people with mental illness are abandoned by their families (Poreddi et al. 2013) and their outcome is both unknown and a matter of grave concern.

In this chapter we review the provision of mental health care, including the relevant legislative developments, where available, in this region and present the very limited research data on coercion. There are common problems of limited resources and training and inadequate service provision across the entire region. Anecdotal evidence suggests that coercion, restraint, and seclusion are common, both in mental health facilities and within homes, but robust data are lacking.

India

During British colonial rule mentally ill patients were kept under custodial care in prisons and asylums. The Lunatic Asylum Act of 1856 was modified to form the Indian Lunacy Act (ILA) of 1912. The enactment of the ILA resulted in the opening of new asylums and improvements in the condition of asylums. The name 'lunatic asylum' was changed to 'mental hospital' in 1920, and the control of mental hospitals was shifted from prison authorities to civil surgeons. Before Indian independence, the Bhore Committee was asked to survey mental hospitals in India. The committee recommended that the 1912 ILA was out-dated and had outlived its usefulness (Mills 2001). The terminologies used were obsolete. A draft Mental Health Act was prepared by the Indian Psychiatry Society in 1949, but it took nearly 40 years for this Act to be passed by parliament. The Act finally got presidential assent on 22 May 1987. The central and state mental health rules were framed in 1990, and with effect from 1 April 1993 the Mental Health Act (MHA) 1987 came into force. Even then, the real implementation of this act only occurred after the 'Erwadi tragedy' (Sharma and Chadda 1996) in which 28 shackled inmates of a faith-based mental home burned to death (see Figure 16.1). It became public that these inmates had been tied to trees during the day and then to beds at night and offered little if anything in the way of 'therapy'.

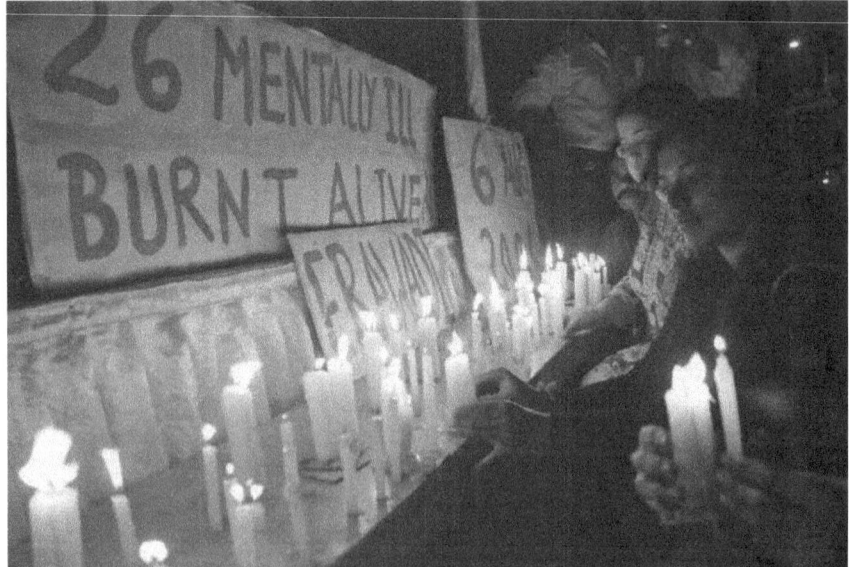

Figure 16.1 Candlelit vigil marking the ninth anniversary of the Erwadi tragedy in which 28 people died following a fire in a faith-based mental health facility.

The development of community psychiatry resulted in the integration of mental health care in the community under the National Mental Health Programme (NHMP) in 1982. The NMHP was developed with the objective of ensuring the availability and accessibility of effective mental health care for all sections of the population. A very important development has been the recognition by the National Human Rights Commission (NHRC) of the human rights of the mentally ill. The NHRC carried out two systematic examinations of mental hospitals in India in 1998 (National Human Rights Commission 1999) and 2008 (Nagaraja and Murthy 2008). Following these reports, funds were provided to upgrade facilities. This has resulted in positive changes over the past 10 years, as shown by the 2008 NHRC report (Nagaraja and Murthy 2008): the percentage of admissions through courts has decreased from about 70% in 1996 to around 20% in 2008; long-stay patients have decreased from 80–90% to about 35%; and custodial care indicators such as staff wearing compulsory uniforms have decreased. While 20 hospitals used prison-like cells for seclusion in 1999, this had decreased to 8 in 2008. Recreation facilities increased and were present in 29 institutions in 2008 compared with 8 in 1999. Rehabilitation facilities were present in 23 institutions rather than the previously recorded 10. The budget had doubled in nine institutions, increased two to four times in thirteen, four to eight times in four and more than eight times in three institutions. The overall use of electroconvulsive therapy (ECT) had reduced and the use of modified ECT increased from 9 to 27 institutions. There were more changes in the 10 years between 1998 and 2008 than in the preceding 50 years. A persistent problem has been inadequate staffing, despite the creation of new positions (Murthy 2011).

The recent Mental Health Care Bill (2013) shifted the focus to a rights-based approach to the protection of people with mental illness. The 2013 bill fills an important requirement of the UN Convention on the Rights of Persons with Disabilities (UNCRPD) by the right:

- to access to mental health care (including shelter homes, supported accommodation, community-based rehabilitation)
- to community living
- to live with dignity and protection against cruel, degrading, and inhuman treatment
- to equality and non-discrimination
- to information, confidentiality, and access to medical records
- to personal communication, legal aid, and to make complaints about deficiencies in provision of services.

The Bill restricts and regulates the use of seclusion and restraints, and the parliamentary standing committee has suggested that the Bill be amended to ban seclusion completely on the grounds that it has no therapeutic purpose. The government has agreed to make this amendment. It is the first time that a law in India has guaranteed such rights to equality and non-discrimination and enshrined positive rights of access to basic services to people with mental illness. However, the recent draft proposal to amend the Indian MHA has not brought certainty to issues of coercion (Shah and Basu 2010).

Coercion in India

Very little is known about the use and utility of coercive measures in psychiatry and other medical specialties in India. The existing evidence supports the view that informal coercion is widely used, although patterns of its use may differ. Some evidence suggests relatively high levels of cooperation between family members and clinicians in the use of coercive measures (Srinivasan and Thara 2002). Covert medication is the practice of hiding medication in food or beverages so that it goes undetected, while covert prescribing is the practice of supplying a prescription to a family member or a health-care worker, knowing fully well that the medication is going to be used for an unwilling patient. The terms 'surreptitious medication/surreptitious prescribing' are sometimes used interchangeably with covert medication, but this may often indicate negative intent. Covert medication is commonly used in the context of patients with schizophrenia or bipolar disorder who refuse to take medication (Kala 2012). Srinivasan and Thara (2002) reported that Indian families administered covert treatment under the supervision of a psychiatrist in half the cases of non-adherent patients studied. The treatment helped many patients to recover sufficiently from the illness to participate in further treatment voluntarily, with few reported negative effects and at a low cost. Delays in seeking treatment are often attributed to the choice of the caregivers, who may also make major decisions about treatments for patients who lack capacity (Rajkumar et al. 2007). The family in India plays a major role in health-seeking for its members. Any intervention planned for the patient should take into account the family's considerable influence over many aspects of patient management, including outpatient consultation and continuing care. There are many barriers standing in the way of achieving the desired levels of care for people with mental disorder, such as lack of awareness, prejudice, lack of resources, and lack of adequate advocacy.

A study conducted by Rajkumar et al. (2007) showed that all relatives signed consent for the administration of ECT. Many reported that the details of ECT were discussed with them and alternative treatments offered and they were happy with the outcome. However, many relatives also perceived that they were forced to provide their consent. Even the minority of patients who signed the consent form could not recall the details of the procedure. Many patients also reported coercion. Complete understanding and true voluntary acceptance of ECT are rarely attained in actual practice. A power differential between doctor and patient is often seen in Indian society and health care. In the context of a dependent therapeutic relationship, informed consent almost always contains an element of coercion. In India, the process is complicated by a reduced emphasis on personal autonomy and a lack of awareness of human rights. This may be compounded by illiteracy and poverty. In this situation the patient submissively yields to the physician's authority: informed consent becomes a mere formality, given in order to maintain harmony in the doctor–patient relationship. In *S.P. Sathe vs. State of Maharashtra*[1] the Bombay High Court regulated the prescription of indiscriminate electric shocks to people with mental illness. The directions included that reports must be made whenever electric shocks are given by a prison psychiatrist. A case in the High

---

[1] High Court of Bombay petition no. 1537 of 1984.

Court of Bombay challenged the practice of administering ECT without anaesthesia and without informed consent at the Institute of Psychiatry and Human Behaviour (IPHB), Panaji, Goa.[2] The petitioner acted on behalf of patients and their relatives, since patients were in no position to approach the court and relatives were reluctant to come forward, given the stigma attached to mental illness. The court opined that the practice was barbaric, inhuman, and hence in violation of Article 21 of the Indian Constitution.

Mysore declaration

In February 2013 experts from India and Europe came together in Mysore, India, for an international symposium on coercion. A declaration was drafted, discussed, and ratified which defined coercive measures in the Indian context and outlined aims and possible ways to minimize coercion in medical settings in India. The declaration asserted that:

> there is an urgent need for the recognition and implementation of the rights of persons with mental illness, following principles with regard to equality, security, liberty, health, integrity and dignity of all people, with a mental illness or not . . . All parties responsible for the care and treatment of mental illness should work towards the elimination of all forms of discrimination, stigmatisation and violence, cruel, inhumane or degrading treatment. We affirm that disproportionate, unsafe or prolonged coercion or violence against persons with mental illness constitutes the violation of the human rights and fundamental freedoms and impairs or nullifies their enjoyment of those rights and freedoms.

The declaration recognizes the potential tension between the rights of patients who refuse medication and the benefits of potential restoration to normal functioning through involuntary treatment, as well as the wishes of family members, who often play an important role in the treatment of mental illness in India (Lepping and Raveesh 2013).

Sri Lanka

Mental health services in Sri Lanka are integrated with primary care services in a bid to achieve equal standards. People with mental health problems are one of the most marginalized groups in Sri Lanka. The country has high suicide rates, increasing substance misuse, and many psychosocial problems (Weerasundera 2011). After years of civil conflict, the 2004 tsunami, and with an estimated 2% of the population suffering from serious mental illness, the need for an effective policy has never been greater. Mental health services operate within a policy framework where services are community based, client centred, holistic, focused on rehabilitation, and sensitive to gender and age (Weerasundera 2011). The education of health professionals and support workers in at least two institutions promotes a 'rights-based approach' to caring for people with mental health problems (De Silva 2002).

---

[2] High Court of Bombay petition no. 357 of 1998.

Sri Lanka has some archaic legislation dating back to the Lunacy Ordinance of 1873 when the country was a British colony. These laws still operate with minor amendments, most recently in 1956. The mental health policy sanctions involuntary treatment only at the country's premier mental health facility, the National Institute of Mental Health. However, people with mental disorder are often treated at regional centres. Due to social stigma, lack of awareness, and financial constraints involuntary admissions are mostly unchallenged. Mental health services continue to grow and services are moving towards greater, if not comprehensive, coverage (Weerasundera 2011).

Bangladesh

Bangladesh's mental health policy, strategy, and plan were approved in 2006 as a part of an action plan for surveillance and prevention of non-communicable diseases. Community-based mental health care is the main approach of the policy. According to the national mental health survey of 2003–5 about 16% of the adult population in the country suffer from a mental disorder. Many fewer than this attend for treatment, however. Mental disorders are not covered by any social insurance schemes and there is no human rights review body in the country to inspect mental health facilities (World Health Organization 2009a).

Bangladesh does not have a specific mental health authority. There are 50 outpatient mental health facilities but none provide follow-up care in the community. There are also no day treatment mental health facilities in the country. There are 31 community-based psychiatric inpatient units giving a total of 0.58 beds per 100,000 population, and on average patients spend 29 days in the facility. There are 11 community residential facilities in the country: 55% of the beds in these facilities are for children and adolescents, 81% of admitted patients are female, and 73% are children. There are no legislative or financial provisions to protect and provide support for mental health service users in respect of employment and rights. The spectrum of community mental health facilities is increasing, but the existing provision is inadequate. There are no mechanisms for supervision or protection of the human rights of mental patients in the country and no available data concerning coercion in mental health services. Special efforts are needed to make mental health services more accessible to the poor, tribal minorities, and the vulnerable (World Health Organization 2005).

Essential psychotropic medicines are available in mental hospitals and the National Institute of Mental Health, but are not widely available in general hospital psychiatry units. There is only one small family association in the country and no consumers' association. There is a lack of interaction between the family association and mental health service facilities. Initiatives have been taken around the capital city to develop community mental health services (Jacob et al. 2007).

Pakistan

Pakistan's mental health policy was last revised in 2003 and mental health legislation was enacted in 2001. It focuses on access to mental health care including access to the least restrictive care, rights, family, capacity, and guardianship issues for people with mental illness. It also considers voluntary and involuntary treatment, the accreditation of professionals and facilities, mechanisms to oversee involuntary admission and treatment, and mechanisms to implement the provisions of mental health legislation (World Health Organization 2009a).

A national mental health authority exists which advises the government on mental health policies and legislation. This authority is also involved in service planning, service management and coordination, and in monitoring and quality assessment of mental health services. Five mental hospitals are available in the country and are organizationally integrated with mental health outpatient facilities. In the last 5 years the number of beds in mental hospitals has risen by 4% (Karim et al. 2004).

Policy and legislation, however, are not uniformly implemented (World Health Organization 2009a). The health system is not well established and lacks sufficient resources. Community services are limited to a few tertiary-care hospitals and only in big cities such as Lahore, Islamabad, and Karachi, and there are no community-based residential facilities or day treatment facilities. The density of psychiatrists in or around the largest city is over twice that outside it. None of the mental disorders are covered by social insurance schemes and only 0.4% of health-care expenditure by the government health department is devoted to mental health. The following legislative and financial provisions exist to protect and provide support for users: (1) provisions concerning a legal obligation for employers to hire a certain percentage of employees who are disabled; (2) provisions concerning protection from discrimination (dismissal, lower wages) solely on account of mental disorder; (3) provisions concerning priority in state housing and in subsidized housing schemes for people with severe mental disorders; and (4) provisions concerning protection from discrimination in allocation of housing for people with severe mental disorders. However, none of these provisions are enforced (World Health Organization 2005). There are no mechanisms for monitoring coercive measures in the mental health services (Mubbashar and Saeed 2001).

Patients in Pakistan are mostly looked after by their families. It is therefore important that training is focused on community-based psychiatry. Drug misuse is increasing and is generally treated by non-psychiatric doctors. Psychological therapies are not readily available in Pakistan and there are currently no psychotherapists working in the national health system in Pakistan. Family is an important resource, and psychotherapies in this area could be used to improve patient care (Gadit 2006).

Nepal

Nepal's mental health policy was formulated in 1996. Key components include:

(1) to ensure the availability and accessibility of minimum mental health services for the whole population of Nepal;

(2) to prepare human resources in the area of mental health;

(3) to protect the fundamental human rights of the mentally ill;

(4) to improve awareness about mental health.

Less than 1% of government health-care expenditure is directed towards mental health. There is no human rights review body with the authority to inspect mental health facilities and impose sanctions on those facilities that persistently violate patients' rights (Upadhyaya 2009). Nepal has no community-based psychiatric inpatient units as such. Physician-based primary health care and non-physician-based primary health-care clinics are organized in the country. There is an unequal distribution of human resources between urban and rural areas (IASC Reference Group 2012).

Whenever necessary, patients with medico-legal issues are admitted to mental hospital inpatient units for evaluation, court report, and treatment. There are no data on how many patients are detained or secluded each year in community-based psychiatric inpatient units, but 6–10% of the patients in mental hospitals had been detained or secluded (Jha and Adhikari 2009).

Bhutan

The needs of people with mental illness who require care are increasing in Bhutan. The organization of mental health services in Bhutan is difficult due to a scattered population with diverse cultural practices, limited financial resources, a scarcity of mental health personnel, lack of a comprehensive mental health policy, and the presence of conflicting healing systems and stigma (Nirola 2010).

A National Mental Health Programme (NMHP) was started in July 1997 with the objective of ensuring the availability and accessibility of primary mental health care for all sectors of the population by integrating mental health into general health care. The NMHP integrates mental health care with the primary health-care system by training personnel in mental health at primary health-care centres. The integration of mental health into primary health care has helped to create an awareness of mental health in the community and reduce stigma. Patient admission may be voluntary or involuntary. None of the community mental health facilities have trained psychiatrists (Pelzang 2012). The majority of patients are brought to the hospital by families and relatives. Only a few are referred from the criminal justice system or from prison. Bhutan does not have any mental health legislation to protect the rights of people with mental illness and there are no clear policies to prevent unlawful institutionalization, coercive medications/therapies, and/or inappropriate detention for psychiatric evaluation (Saxena et al. 2007).

Afghanistan

The last mental health legislation in Afghanistan was enacted in 1997. The Ministry of Public Health is planning to revise the current mental health policy and legislation and to formulate a new national mental health programme. However, there is no regular budget allocation for mental health (World Health Organization 2006). A national human rights review body exists (the Independent Human Rights Commission) which has the authority to inspect mental health hospitals. Only one review has occurred, in 2004, in response to a complaint by a family member (World Health Organization 2005). Female users account for 47% of the population in all mental health facilities in the country. The proportion of female users is highest in day treatment and outpatient facilities. Less than 1% of medical doctors' training is devoted to mental health compared with 2% of nurses' training. Four per cent of primary-care doctors and 1% of nurses received at least 2 days of refresher training in mental health in 2004. There is no financial or legislative support for people with psychiatric problems (World Health Organization 2006).

Although there have been efforts to promote equity of access to mental health services, these efforts have been inadequate. Limited resources are available for mental health and many of these resources are directed towards mental hospitals, leaving outpatient facilities under-funded. Most of the resources are spent on the training of primary-care staff and no supervision and monitoring systems have been established (Saraceno et al. 2007).

Iraq

Iraq and Iraqi society have been devastated by violence following the two Gulf wars. Many years of political and social repression, punctuated by wars, followed by a post-war period characterized by interrupted and insufficient basic services have taken their toll on the Iraqi people. According to the World Health Organization (WHO), mental health disorders are the fourth leading cause of ill-health in Iraqis over the age of 5 years and many studies have repeatedly shown a high prevalence of mental health problems in the Iraqi population (Hicks et al. 2011)

In 2009, Médecins sans Frontières in collaboration with the Iraqi Ministry of Health launched a programme aimed at opening up access to psychological counselling and catalysing the integration of mental health care as a crucial component of the Iraqi health system. Iraq's first national mental health survey in collaboration with the WHO in 2007 assessed the prevalence of common mental health disorders (such as anxiety, depressive, post-traumatic stress disorder, behavioural conditions, substance abuse) in the general population. It revealed significantly high levels of psychological distress in the population: one in five women and one in seven men were likely to suffer a mental disorder in their lifetime, with higher rates in those exposed to trauma. Almost 70% of those with any mental disorder reported experiencing suicidal thoughts. Fewer than 10% of these people, however, reported receiving care (Sadik et al. 2010).

As with many countries in the region, the main component of Iraq's mental health service has been institutionalized care for those suffering chronic psychiatric disorders such as schizophrenia. There are currently only four psychiatrists per million population, far below what is needed. Even fewer people are trained in the related mental health professions, including psychological counselling. As a result there is a significant gap for those experiencing conditions that are better resolved without hospitalization or medication, such as the commonly occurring anxiety and depressive disorders. While the security circumstances of Iraq have often complicated implementation, the challenges have also brought out innovative solutions which may help sustain services in future. For example, video conference links were trialled and then used extensively for training and technical support through case discussions and clinical supervision. When face-to-face visits have not been possible, this has also been used for 'intervision'—the personal support that all counsellors need to remain effective. While circumstances in Iraq may be considered to have improved to some extent since these surveys (at least until recent incursions and violence by ISIS), there is little reason to believe that the burden of mental ill-health has reduced and access to appropriate mental health care is still a critical issue (Tarantino et al. 2009)

Iran

A mental health policy and programme was initially formulated in 1986. Its main components are advocacy, promotion, prevention, treatment, and rehabilitation. The strategy aims to integrate the mental health programme within the primary health-care system. From 1988 to 1990 successful pilot studies were implemented in Shahr-e-Kord and Shahreza in central Iran, resulting in significantly increased knowledge in health workers. There have been immense improvements in the provision of mental health services in rural areas over the last 15 years (World Health Organization 2005).

A national mental health authority is involved in service planning, service management, coordination and monitoring, and quality assessment. In rural areas there is better implementation of the national guidelines compared with large urban areas. Residential facilities in Iran are run by the Social Welfare Organization (Noorbala et al. 2004).

A lack of comprehensive and coherent mental health legislation is evident. Although available laws cover some areas such as competency, capacity, and guardianship, and despite the ratification of progressive laws in 1997 that provided legislative support for employment, many areas including involuntary hospitalization are not addressed (Patel, 2009). There is an urgent need to implement existing legislation as well as to monitor human rights. Outpatient services are available, and lack of medication is not an issue. The number of patients in community residential facilities providing long-term hospitalization and in mental hospitals is large and growing. Recently launched mobile services (a home visits initiative) are still essentially pilots and provide little coverage.

Jordan

Mental health services and activities in Jordan are provided by a range of stakeholders. There are four major providers (government, military, private, and non-governmental/international), each with its own separate financing and delivery system. Jordan's mental health system relies strongly on medical treatment, with few resources dedicated to recovery or bio-psychosocial treatment modalities. This is reflected in the high number of psychiatric versus psychosocial and allied medical staff in Jordan's mental health system and the fact that the majority of mental health services are delivered through tertiary-level facilities, with virtually no primary, community-based, or self-care (World Health Organization 2011).

Recent years have seen a growing commitment to improving mental health in Jordan. In 2010, Jordan was selected as one of six countries for the implementation of the WHO's Mental Health Gap Action Program. Mental health is poorly integrated within general health structures, and until late 2011 there was no single policy-making and budget-holding mental health authority. The new authority will be responsible for service development, developing legislation and establishing mechanisms to protect and promote human rights and advocacy (Hijiawi et al. 2013).

There are no coordinating bodies overseeing any public education and awareness campaigns on mental health and mental disorders, although there have been limited and infrequent campaigns led by non-governmental organizations and professional associations. There are very few formal community mental health-care services in Jordan. Three Ministry of Health facilities have been transformed into community mental health centres, with the support of the WHO. One is a standalone mental health centre in the capital city Amman, and the other two are situated in comprehensive health centres in Amman and in Irbid. In Jordan there is a relationship between traditional healers and physicians which remains informal and disorganized (World Health Organization 2011).

Saudi Arabia

Saudi Arabia had no psychiatric hospitals until the 1950s. In 1989, primary health-care centres were established throughout the country in order to improve the diagnosis and treatment of medical problems in the community (Okasha and Karam 1998). Primary care is regarded as the foundation of the health service and most patients are seen at this level—about 83% of public sector attendances occur in primary-care clinics (World Health Organization 2009a).

Mental health law exists and helps to protect patient rights at local and national levels. Although mental health services are expanding, much of the care for those with mental illness continues to take place in family settings. The family is sacred in Saudi Arabia, and caring for family members is considered a religious obligation. Children do not leave home until they are married, and elders are usually cared for within the family unit, not sent to a nursing home as in Western countries. This results in large extended families living together. Mental health care also takes place within the nuclear and extended family, and problems of mental ill-health are often kept secret. Due to guilt and shame, family members often refuse to discuss mental health problems with non-family members, including medical physicians and mental health professionals. Traditional healers constitute part of the household staff, using religious texts and recitation in management (Farooqi 2006).

The United Arab Emirates (UAE)

There is no official mental health policy in the UAE, but mental health is specifically mentioned in the general health policy. A mental health plan exists and was approved or most recently revised in 2010. It includes a shift of services and resources from mental hospitals to community mental health facilities and the integration of mental health services into primary care. Dedicated mental health legislation exists and legal provisions concerning mental health are also covered in other laws (e.g. welfare, disability, general health legislation, etc.) (World Health Organization 2011).

Despite recent improvements, mental health infrastructure and services are grossly insufficient for the large and growing needs. Prescription regulations authorize doctors in primary health care to prescribe and/or to continue prescription of psychotherapeutic medicines, but with restrictions. The Department of Health does not authorize nurses in primary health care to prescribe and/or to continue prescription of psychotherapeutic medicines and official policy does not permit them to independently diagnose and treat mental disorders within the primary-care system (World Health Organization 2011).

There has been remarkable progress in the UAE in the recognition and treatment of mental health disorders, especially in the last 20 years. The UAE's mental health system is making huge strides toward addressing the mental health needs of its people.

Egypt

Egypt has a mental health policy, legislation, and plan. All mental disorders and all mental health problems of clinical concern are covered in social insurance schemes. At least 80% of the population has free access to essential psychotropic medicines. There is a national human rights review body and a national mental health authority, which provides advice to the government on mental health policies and legislation (World Health Organization 2009b). Most mental health facilities are in or near large cities. There is significantly more provision in urban areas but some areas have no mental health facilities. In order to promote equity of access to mental health services, Egypt is encouraging the development of community-based psychiatric units and outpatient facilities in each area throughout the country. Funding is insufficient to cover the costs of mental health services. Non-governmental organizations and community leaders share in the support and the improvement of mental health services. Resources from international organizations like the WHO and from other countries also help to support the mental health system in Egypt (World Health Organization 2009a).

A national mental health authority is involved in service planning and coordination, monitoring and quality assessment of mental health services. However, residents in those areas that are not covered by basic mental health services have access to services in adjoining regions. It is difficult to gather accurate data regarding the length of stay of patients in mental hospitals due to a large patient population and high patient turnover (Okasha and Okasha 2000). There are no consumer or family associations for people with mental disorders. There is a coordinating body, the General Secretariat of Mental Health, that oversees public education and awareness campaigns on mental health and mental disorders but there are no community residential facilities for patients with mental disorders—the reasons for this include stigma, lack of trained personnel and lack of funding (Okasha 2004).

Conclusions

People with mental disorders are amongst the most vulnerable in society. They are often isolated, stigmatized, discriminated against, humiliated, and marginalized. They often end up in unhealthy or even inhumane living conditions either in the community or in mental hospitals, and experience an increased likelihood of human rights violations. Lack of understanding and poor management of mental illness by health professionals and people in the community may contribute to neglect. Allocation of resources to mental health care and particularly community services, is grossly inadequate in many of the countries considered in this chapter, beyond that which might be expected from general health budgets.

There is, however, an increasing awareness of mental health in the general population, and the number of people seeking treatment is increasing. To ensure the availability and accessibility of mental health services for all of the population, and in particular for the most vulnerable and under-privileged groups, mental health services have to be integrated into the general health system of the region. Mental health resources have to be distributed in accordance with mental health policy and an adequate supply of essential psychotropic drugs should be maintained.

Improved training of workers and greater education of populations may help to reduce stigma and discrimination and eliminate damaging practices. Existing legislation first needs to be enforced and then improved upon to increase protection for those in need, both in hospitals and in the community. In this region there is little research evidence or detailed reports of formal or informal coercion conducted by services. It seems clear that coercion related to ways in which families attempt to help patients, covert medication, and widespread lack of resources is common and damaging. It is imperative that we work to improve our understanding of these issues and push for adequate treatment resources and good-quality basic legislation to protect the most vulnerable amongst us.

References

De Silva D (2002). Psychiatric service delivery in an Asian country: the experience of Sri Lanka. *International Review of Psychiatry*, 14:66–70.

Farooqi YN (2006). Traditional healing practices sought by Muslim psychiatric patients in Lahore, Pakistan. *International Journal of Disability, Development and Education*, 53:401–415.

Gadit AM (2006). Mental health in Pakistan: where do we stand? *Journal of Pakistan Medical Association*, 56:198–199.

Hicks MH-R, Dardagan H, Bagnall PM, et al. (2011). Casualties in civilians and coalition soldiers from suicide bombings in Iraq, 2003: a descriptive study. *The Lancet*, 378:906–914.

Hijiawi B, Elzein Elmousaad H, Marini A, et al. (2013). *WHO proMIND profiles on mental health in development. Hashemite Kingdom of Jordan*. Geneva: World Health Organization. Available at: http://apps.who.int/iris/bitstream/10665/92504/1/9789241505666_eng.pdf

IASC Reference Group for Mental Health and Psychosocial Support in Emergency Settings (2012). *Who is where, when, doing what (4Ws) in mental health and psychosocial support: manual with activity codes (field test-version)*. Geneva. Available at: http://www.who.int/mental_health/publications/iasc_4ws.pdf

Jacob KS, Sharan P, Mirza I (2007). Mental health systems in countries: where are we now? *The Lancet*, 370:1061–1077.

Jha A, Adhikari SR (2009). Mental health services in New Nepal—observations, objections and outlooks for the future. *JNMA: Journal of the Nepal Medical Association*, 48:185–190.

Kala AK (2012). Covert medication; the last option: a case for taking it out of the closet and using it selectively. *Indian Journal of Psychiatry*, 54:257–265.

Karim S, Saeed K, Rana MH, et al. (2004). Pakistan mental health: country profile. *International Review of Psychiatry*, 16:83–92.

Lepping P, Raveesh BN (2013). The Mysore declaration. *International Psychiatry*, 10:98–99.

Mills J (2001). The history of modern psychiatry in India 1858–1947. *History of Psychiatry*, 12:431–458.

Mubbashar MH, Saeed K (2001). Development of mental health services in Pakistan. *Eastern Mediterranean Health Journal*, 7:392–396.

Murthy RS (2011). Mental health initiatives in India (1947–2010). *The National Medical Journal of India*, 24:98–107.

Nagaraja D, Murthy P (eds) (2008). *Mental healthcare and human rights*. New Delhi: National Human Rights Commission.

National Human Rights Commission (1999). *Quality assurance in mental health*. New Delhi: National Human Rights Commission.

Nirola DK (2010). Where psychiatrists are scarce: Bhutan. *Asia-Pacific Psychiatry*, 2:126.

Noorbala AA, Bagheri Yazdi SA, Yasamy MT, et al. (2004). Mental health survey of the adult population in Iran. *British Journal of Psychiatry*, 184:70–73.

O'Brien AJ, Golding CG (2003). Coercion in mental healthcare: the principle of least coercive care. *Journal of Psychiatric and Mental Health Nursing*, 10:167–173.

Okasha A (2004). Focus on psychiatry in Egypt. *British Journal of Psychiatry*, 185:266–272.

Okasha A, Karam E (1998). Mental health services and research in the Arab world. *Acta Psychiatrica Scandinavica*, 98:406–413.

Okasha A, Okasha T (2000). Mental health in Cairo (Al-Qahira). *International Journal of Mental Health*, 28:62–68.

Patel V (2009). The future of psychiatry in low- and middle-income countries. *Psychological Medicine*, 39:1759–1762.

Pelzang R (2012). Mental health care in Bhutan: policy and issues. *WHO South-East Asia Journal of Public Health*, 1:339–346.

Poreddi V, Ramachandra, Reddemma K, et al. (2013). People with mental illness and human rights: a developing countries perspective. *Indian Journal of Psychiatry*, 55:117–124.

Prinsen EJ, van Delden JJ (2009). Can we justify eliminating coercive measures in psychiatry? *Journal of Medical Ethics*, 35:69–73.

Rajkumar AP, Saravanan B, Jacob KS (2007). Voices of people who have received ECT. *Indian Journal of Medical Ethics*, 4:157–164.

Sadik S, Bradley M, Al-Hasoon S, Jenkins R (2010). Public perception of mental health in Iraq. *International Journal of Mental Health Systems*, 4:26.

Saraceno B, van Ommeren M, Batniji R (2007). Barriers to improvement of mental health services in low-income and middle-income countries. *The Lancet*, 370:1164–1174.

Saxena S, Thornicroft G, Knapp M, et al. (2007). Resources for mental health: scarcity, inequity, and inefficiency. *The Lancet*, 370:878–889.

Shah R, Basu D (2010). Coercion in psychiatric care: global and Indian perspective. *Indian Journal of Psychiatry*, 52:203–206.

Sharma S, Chadda RK (ed.) (1996). *Indian Mental Health Act, 1987—a critique*, pp. 101–112. Delhi: Institute of Human Behavior and Allied Sciences.

Sjöstrand M, Helgesson G (2008). Coercive treatment and autonomy in psychiatry. *Bioethics*, 22:113–120.

Srinivasan TN, Thara R (2002). Management of medication noncompliance in schizophrenia by families in India. *Schizophrenia Bulletin*, 28:531–535.

Tarantino DAJ, Morton MJ, Kosaraju A, et al. (2009). Health system reconstruction in Iraq—the way ahead: a report from the Iraq Health Symposium, May 20–21, 2008. *World Medical and Health Policy*, 1:125–142.

Upadhyaya KD (2009). Policy, strategy and plan of action to improve the mental health service in Nepal. *Journal of Gandaki Medical College—Nepal*, 2(4):1–4.

Weerasundera R (2011). Mental health legislation in Sri Lanka: the time for change is now. *Sri Lankan Journal of Psychiatry*, **2**(2):43–44.

World Health Organization (2005). *World Health Organization assessment instrument for mental health systems*. WHO-AIMS, Version 2.2. Geneva: World Health Organization. Available at: http://www.who.int/mental_health/evidence/AIMS_WHO_2_2.pdf.

World Health Organization (2006). *WHO-AIMS report on mental health system in Afghanistan*. Kabul, Afghanistan: World Health Organisation and Ministry of Public Health. Available at: http://www.who.int/mental_health/evidence/Afghanistan_WHO_AIMS_Report.pdf.

World Health Organization (2009a). *Mental health systems in selected low-and middle-income countries: a WHO-AIMS cross-national analysis*. Geneva: World Health Organization. Available at: http://apps.who.int/iris/bitstream/10665/44151/1/9789241547741_eng.pdf.

World Health Organization (2009b). *The work of WHO in the Eastern Mediterranean Region. Annual report of the regional director*. Cairo: WHO Regional Office for the Eastern Mediterranean.

World Health Organization (2011). *WHO-AIMS report on mental health system in Jordan*. Amman, Jordan: WHO and Ministry of Health. Available at: http://www.who.int/mental_health/evidence/mh_aims_report_jordan_jan_2011_en.pdf.

Chapter 17

Southeast Asia

Hui Ching Wu, Frank Huang-Chih Chou,
Mariam Ali, and Andrew Molodynski

Introduction

The population of Southeast Asia is over 2 billion, more than in Europe and Africa combined. The term 'Southeast Asia' is in common use but often is often hazily understood. It is a recognizable group of 20 countries on the west of the Pacific Ocean and the east of the Indian Ocean. The largest, most populous, and most economically important country is China, with an area of almost 10 million square kilometres and a population estimated at 1.3 billion. Its major religions are Confucianism, Buddhism, and Taoism and its main language is Mandarin. China has the world's second largest economy, closely followed in third place by its neighbour Japan. Japan has a much smaller population of 126 million. Its main religions are Buddhism and Shinto and its main language Japanese. Indonesia, with a population of 250 million, is the largest Muslim country in the world. Its inhabitants mostly speak Indonesian. Taiwan consists of a group of islands off the east coast of mainland China; it is home to 23 million people. Its geographical and historical uniqueness has given rise to a diversity of ethnic groups, cultures, and languages. Given the complexities of covering the whole region Taiwan will be used as a detailed example.

The objective of this chapter is to explore how coercion is used in community mental health care across the four countries stated above, as a broadly representative sample of Southeast Asia. There is great variety in the region with regards to the financing of mental health care and overall economic resources. Unfortunately there is little literature regarding coercion in mental health care.

Coercion and collectivist cultures

It is common to make a broad brush distinction between cultural traditions that have an individualistic orientation (found in many Western countries) and those that have a collectivist orientation (found in many in Eastern countries, including many in Southeast Asia). In collectivist traditions, filial piety is enormously important and respect for and subservience to one's parents or authority figures is expected and valued (perhaps not dissimilar to the concept of paternalism often used to describe some aspects of Western health-care systems). These values are reflected in Confucian thinking, which emphasizes subservience of one's self for the good of the family and community. The individual is considered as an interdependent part of the family and community (Chen 1994). As a result, there is more acceptance that the autonomy of the mentally ill can be limited by their caregivers' desire to prevent relapse or to adhere to socially acceptable behaviour. Caregivers tend to be protective of the family as a unit (Chu et al. 2010). Often motivated by fear, caregivers may overlook the possibility that their relative could live independently within the community. Therefore they may inadvertently remove the opportunity for that family member to learn from experience and develop life skills, and this could potentially slow down the rehabilitation process.

The role of mental health professionals is attributed a degree of authority. This can be reinforced by cultural beliefs and is often associated with high social status (Wang 2008). Given their education and specialized knowledge, doctors have traditionally assumed the right to make paternalistic judgements based on what they think is best for their patients. As Harris (1985) points out, paternalism makes it possible for someone to expect another to follow their orders, irrespective of that person's own wishes or judgements. This approach has certainly been challenged in the West, where today patient advocate groups contribute to a greater emphasis on patient involvement in treatment decisions and service delivery more widely. In collectivist traditions, just as people are expected to follow the directions set by their parents or teachers, it has traditionally been expected that patients accept decisions made by their doctor and health-care workers. Indeed, the views of psychiatric patients have traditionally been secondary to those of both caregivers and doctors.

Mental health legislation often reflects how an individual society perceives and responds to mental illness. The concepts of mental health and mental illness are constructed within contexts that include historical, political, social, economic, and cultural dimensions (Butler 1992), and mental health legislation often needs to encompass conflicting values and ethical perspectives (Rogers and Pilgrim 2001). Public opinion or stigma may potentially have more influence in collective societies where communal as opposed to individual concerns are prioritized (Werner et al. 2008). Lee et al. (2005) concluded that living in a collectivist culture does not protect people with severe mental illness against stigma. The level of stigma and discrimination reported from, for example, Taiwan may therefore not be surprising (Lin et al. 2008).

The differences between Western and Eastern perceptions of individual autonomy are reflected in differing interpretations of human rights. Even so, in Eastern countries there is also discussion and controversy as to what extent caregivers and professionals should respect the patient's autonomy and when it is right for mental health professionals to intervene to prevent people with severe mental illnesses from harming themselves or others. Many argue that unless decision-making capacity is impaired, the patient's autonomy should be respected, as is the case in many Western legislation and policies (Department of Health, Executive Yuan 1999). According to Reichert (2007), the principles of economic, social, and cultural human rights should permeate mental health ethics, values, and principles.

In Taiwan, the 2007 amendment to the mental health legislation aimed to protect human rights. The subsequent high rate of compulsory admissions (approximately 94.73% were authorized in 2009; Department of Health, Executive Yuan 2010), however, may indicate that there remains a lack of respect for patient autonomy and human rights. Alternatively it may reflect greater concern for public safety or caregiver burden alongside inadequate community support. During a similar time period the rate of compulsory admissions in several European countries was approximately one in ten (Salize and Dressing 2004). Such a discrepancy is striking given the broadly similar legal criteria. It might reflect different cultural orientations, such as individualistic versus collectivist ones.

The legislative changes towards placing more emphasis on patient autonomy in the region have not been supported financially or practically by administrations. In contrast to some other countries, increased rights for the mentally ill in Taiwan may remain an ideological priority rather than a reality. It has been suggested that psychiatrists facing unpredictable and risky behaviour tend to overestimate risk and consider the needs of the family, as a result pursuing more coercive interventions (Liu et al. 2010).

The relative scarcity of mental health professionals and resources is a problem in many Asian countries. Meagre financial resources and an inadequate workforce and infrastructure cause significant limitations in mental health-care systems. There is a shortage of community rehabilitation services to follow up, support, and empower vulnerable and isolated individuals. This may fuel the so-called 'revolving door' of repeated admissions, often involving coercion. In Taiwan, the number of compulsory admission requests has decreased since the 2007 legislation (Chou 2014), though the reasons for this are unclear. Great strides have also been made in talking openly about, and respecting the rights of, vulnerable minorities in Taiwan in recent decades (Taiwan Association for Human Rights 1990; Lee et al. 2005; Yeh 2009). However, much remains to be done.

Taiwan

Taiwan has a population of 24 million and the vast majority of people live in the lowlands near the western coast of the main island. Taiwan, officially the 'Republic of China', consists of the island of Taiwan (an island 160 km off the Asian mainland in the Pacific), three off-shore islands, and the nearby islets of the Pescadores chain. Taiwan's overall area is 35,883 km² and the island is highly urbanized, with almost 9 million people living in the Taipei–Keelung–Taoyuan metropolitan area and over 2.5 million each in the urban areas of Kaohsiung and Taichung. Han Chinese (including Hakka people) make up over 95% of the population. Aboriginal Taiwanese comprise approximately 2% of the population and now mostly live in the mountainous eastern part of the island. Taiwan is a democratic country with relatively low levels of crime and unrest. It has considerable ethnic and cultural diversity: 380,000 people belong to 12 officially recognized indigenous tribes, each with their own social structure, language, and cultural traditions (https://en.wikipedia.org/wiki/Geography_of_Taiwan). The average per capita income is USD 18,373 (Directorate-General of Budget, Accounting and Statistics 2014). Sixty-two per cent of residents profess 'Eastern religions', such as Buddhism, Taoism, and Yi Guan Dao, and 38% practice Catholicism, Protestantism, or Islam (https://en.wikipedia.org/wiki/Geography_of_Taiwan). There are 1,125,000 registered disabled people in Taiwan, of whom 10% are diagnosed with severe mental disorders (SMI) (Ministry of Health and Welfare 2014). The vast majority (83%) of people with SMI live with their family and 53% are unmarried (Department of Statistics 2013). The number of people receiving outpatient treatment for mental disorders rose from 1,667,000 in 2001 to 2,292,000 in 2012 (Department of Statistics 2014). The prevalence of schizophrenia and affective psychosis in Taiwan has been measured at 0.27% and 0.17%, respectively (Yang et al. 2012).

Prior to the latter part of the twentieth century psychiatric patients were either in the community not receiving care or locked in a prison-like institution. In 1970, Master Shi Kaifeng founded the Hall of Dragon Metamorphoses in a thatched building in Kaohsiung County for Buddhist practices. Shi took in the mentally ill and created his own folk therapy. Shi Kaifeng first tied a rope to the patient and stabilized their condition through the teaching of traditional aphoristic literature (sutras). The rope used was referred to as the 'emotional chain' and was later replaced with the 'metal chain'. This understandably raised serious human rights concerns. In the 1980s, these abuses by the Hall of Dragon Metamorphoses attracted the attention of the press and the public along with two significant events involving violence by mentally ill people in the community. A substance misuser with severe psychotic symptoms threw sulphuric acid over 42 students and teachers and then committed suicide in front of them. In a separate incident, a customs administration secretary was killed by his mentally ill wife. In 1981, the mental health association was entrusted to draft the Mental Health Act (MHA). The Act was designed to protect the public and reduce the level of risk from psychiatric patients. It highlighted the need to balance the rights of the individual and of society. In 2014 this conflict was heightened by a brutal knife attack on the Taipei metro system. This event caused mass media outcry and public concern regarding safety.

Stigma is a significant problem in Taiwan, with the mentally ill often being labelled as risky and uncontrollable. It was previously common to apply compulsory restraint on this vulnerable population. Over recent decades there has been increasing attention in Europe and North America on coercion in mental health care, and the majority of research has come from these places. In Taiwan, an Eastern collectivist culture and prevailing respect for those in authority generate a different emphasis upon public safety and the use of paternalistic decision making.

The mentally ill are often stigmatized as being incapable of making decisions and may be ignored or disrespected (Bindman et al. 2003; Szmukler 2004). Spandler and Calton (2009) argued that the diagnosis of 'psychosis' might be conceived of as a human rights issue, especially as it pertains to enforced treatment and choice. Human rights activism in Taiwan has tried to prevent coercive treatment and develop alternative support strategies (Spandler and Calton, 2009). Patients have been granted the right to seek non-medical alternatives to compulsory treatment (Gottstein 2007) and the right to receive written justification for the compulsory treatments they receive (Thomas and Thomas 2004).

The conflict between individualism and collectivism is embedded in Taiwanese culture and this issue remains controversial. Clinical decisions need to integrate such cultural and social factors.

Mental health-care provision

Hospitals are the main source of care for the mentally ill in Taiwan. There are 378 psychiatric clinics and 103 hospitals/clinics providing outpatient appointments and home visits for the mentally ill. Like Japan (which has a similar shared collectivist culture) bed use is high. Bed numbers have increased by 50% from 15,116 in 2001 to 22,686 in 2013 (National Health Insurance Administration, Ministry of Health and Welfare 2013). This is a rate of approximately 94 beds per 100,000 population. Community rehabilitation centres provide additional and respite care. In 2013 there were 3442 places in 72 day-care rehabilitation institutions, 4784 beds in 106 full-day accommodated hospitals, and 3467 beds in 33 psychiatric nursing homes, 5 clubhouses, and 48 non-governmental organizations providing psychiatric rehabilitation.

Prior to 2013 two bodies were responsible for the treatment and welfare of Taiwan's disabled citizens: the Ministry of Interior and the Department of Health. Legislation for the disabled started in 1980 with the enactment of the 'Handicapped Welfare Law', designed to protect people with disabilities and provide them with social services. Chang (2007) has proposed that this law was passed for the sake of political stability, suggesting that the government, which was controlling the island state under martial law in the early 1980s, could show some beneficence and win approval. The law, however, did not bring disability rights into practice (Chang 2007) and did not even include mental illnesses until 1995. Until the 1980s, the general public and the government had no clear understanding of mental health and chronic mental illness (Tang 1997). People who were thought by the public or their family to exhibit mentally unstable and uncontrollable behaviours were often involuntarily admitted to asylums without psychiatric evaluation upon the request of their family or the police. In 1990, the MHA was introduced to provide legislative recognition that people with mental illness have a right to reasonable treatment (Wang 1997). The initial purpose of the MHA is explained in its introduction: prevention and treatment of mental illness, protection of patient rights, promoting wellbeing, enhancing the mental health of the population, and maintaining society's harmony and peace. It does attempt to balance rights, but there are many sections requiring compliance with medication with few alternatives. The Act also stipulated that compulsory admissions of psychiatric patients must be decided by two licensed psychiatrists. The Act was heavily based upon the risk to self and the community and used an explicit medical model to justify lawful detention. The Act was amended in 2007 to ensure that human rights were also respected. For example, the new Act requires that a panel consisting of several professionals (i.e. psychiatrists, registered psychiatric nurses, occupational therapists, psychologists, psychiatric social workers, lawyers) and a patient representative be formed to determine whether someone should be hospitalized against their will (Wu et al. 2013).

The 2007 People with Disability Rights Protection Act is considered a civil rights landmark for Taiwan as it states that the dignity, legal rights, and the interests of people with disabilities must be respected and guaranteed. The 2007 amendment of the MHA in Taiwan also stipulated that involuntary hospitalization of these patients be based on review by a Psychiatric Disease Mandatory Assessment and Community Care Review Committee (or Review Committee). These consist of several specialists who check and ensure that the criteria for involuntary hospitalization are met. The decision must be made within 5 days and the maximum length of an order is 60 days. In July 2013, the Ministry of Health and Welfare was created to promote the health and wellbeing of all Taiwanese citizens. Its vision is to assure quality, increase efficiency, distribute resources equally, care for vulnerable groups, and establish a welfare state.

As can be seen, in the past three decades there has been a gradual transition from exclusion to inclusion and greater protection of rights. These changes have led to discussion and disagreement on several matters, most importantly the issue of the so-called 'quasi-patient' or someone who may or may not be mentally ill but requires assessment (Legislative Yuan Gazette 2007). The criteria for admission were the critical aspect in this debate. The president of the Taiwanese Society of Psychiatry, Dr Chou, proposed a comprehensive evaluation for these circumstances using standardized criteria for admission based upon level of illness and level of risk. However, it can be difficult to clearly define either the level of illness severity or the level of risk. There has also been heated debate regarding the criteria for using community treatment orders (CTOs), an important new provision in the 2007 amendment. The initial proposal was 'when a severely ill patient does not comply with medical instructions so that his/her personal functioning may deteriorate' (Executive Yuan 2007, p. 30). This was challenged by legislators because of the poor definition of so-called 'personal functioning' and its ambiguity. The Department of Health defended the clause on the basis that preventive treatment slows down the speed of deterioration of personal functioning and also reduces the possibility of a relapse (Executive Yuan 2007). The psychiatrist who attended the review committee did not support the stance of the Department of Health (Legislative Yuan Gazette 2007). A compromise was eventually reached that 'when a severe patient does not comply with medical instructions so that their illness condition is unstable or their personal functioning may deteriorate' (Legislative Yuan Gazette 2007). These debates confirm that rights are more clearly respected (Tamiroc 2007) and community care and rehabilitation are increasingly being emphasized.

China

China is the largest country in the region, both in land mass and population, as well as the strongest economic power. China spends 2.35% of its total health budget on mental health. It has 0.87 psychiatric beds in mental health hospitals and 0.1 in general hospitals per 10,000 of the population. The number of psychiatrists per 100,000 population is 1.29. China's first mental hospital, now known as the Guangzhou Brain Hospital, was established by the American missionary John Kerr in 1898 (Liu et al. 2011). The number of mental hospitals gradually rose following this. In 1949, following the founding of the People's Republic of China, a mental hospital was built in every province. The National Five-Year Plan of 1958 published by the Ministry of Health encouraged local authorities to provide greater outpatient services, and community mental health services were set up in five provinces, including Beijing and Shanghai. The plan focused largely on the protection of society and its order, and psychiatry was closely linked with the security system, setting the conditions for the later politicization of mental health care. The three main outcomes of the 5-year plan were (Pearson 1995, p. 18):

(1) Three types of resource; a medical base, a preventive unit, and a sanatorium (for chronic care).

(2) Caring for people in their homes or sending them to rural areas where there was a need for labour.

(3) Four kinds of cure: Chinese and Western medicines and physical therapy; labour therapy; organized sports and cultural amusements; systematic educational therapy.

The First National Conference of Psychiatrists took place at Nanjing in 1959 and was organized by the Ministry of Health. Both the 5-year plan and the specialist conference concluded that physical restraints were no longer to be used and that wards were to be kept unlocked. The degree of implementation of these plans is unclear and it is reported that during the Cultural Revolution (1966–76), these community mental health programmes almost ceased (Andrews and Brown Bullock 2014). During the Cultural Revolution, an individual's family or workplace could make the recommendation for them to be institutionalized. According to Brown (1980), there was no involuntary admission procedure at the time, although persuasion or even coercion was often necessary before hospitalization would be accepted.

When the Cultural Revolution ended mental health services were re-examined at the Second National Meeting on Mental Health Services in Shanghai in 1986. This recommended general improvement in treatment facilities, increased training of staff, and better understanding of the importance of mental health at a national level (Yip 2005). Since then, mental health care has continued to improve.

The first national mental health law of the People's Republic of China was approved and adopted in 2012. Under Article 27, 'Except when laws specify otherwise, it is prohibited to force persons against their will to undergo a medical examination to determine whether or not they have a mental disorder'. However, this will not be the case when a patient's safety is at risk. Article 30 states that inpatient treatment of mental disorders shall generally be voluntary. However, if the result of the psychiatric evaluation indicates that a person has a severe mental disorder, the medical facility may impose inpatient treatment if the individual meets either of the following conditions:

(1) self-harm in the immediate past or current risk of self-harm;

(2) behaviour that harmed others or endangered the safety of others in the immediate past or current risk to the safety of others.

There are provisions for an independent second opinion but none for legal hearings of the appropriateness of compulsory treatment (Chen et al. 2012). However, these independent assessments do not need to be approved by a court hearing (Gou et al. 2014).

China has been influenced by Confucianism in which the submissiveness of individuals is stressed in order to achieve the harmony of the collective (Yip 2003). Historically, psychiatry has been used as political tool to detain individuals who did not conform to Communist ideology. The Geneva Institute on Psychiatry found that 15% of forensic cases during the 1980s were political (Yip 2005).

China has both the highest proportion of patients and the world's largest population of patients receiving clozapine treatment, with estimates that between 25% and 60% of those with schizophrenia receive the drug. It is also often used as a first-line agent and in some other conditions. Clozapine has been found to be the most effective antipsychotic drug in terms of improving positive and negative symptoms, cognition, and reducing the risk of suicidality. However, its used in the West is restricted because of its potentially fatal risk of agranulocytosis (Meltzer 2012). The use of clozapine without the safety regimes required in other nations could be considered an example of a collectivist culture where the 'wider view' is taken, or alternatively as a breach of the human rights of the individuals concerned.

In 2004 the 686 Project was developed. This is a national community-based service delivery model which integrated resources from mental health hospitals and existing community health systems to try to improve training in mental health and further establish community-based services. It has had significant government funding and is based upon the recommended methods of the World Health Organization (WHO). It has led to a substantial increase in the number of people working with mental health patients and the number of people able to access treatment (Ma 2012).

Japan

Japan is a high-income nation formed of a group of islands to the east of China. Its inhabitants have the world's longest life expectancy. Japan spends 5% of its total health budget on mental health. It has 20.6 psychiatric beds in mental hospitals and 7.8 psychiatric beds in general hospitals per 10,000 of the population. There are 9.4 psychiatrists per 100,000 of the population. The care structure is therefore heavily institutionalized with very high bed numbers.

The *Tale of Genji* is a Japanese novel written in the eleventh century. It describes the prevailing opinion at the time that mental illness was due to either 'Mononoke' (a monster) or 'Kitsune' (a fox) entering a person's body after a curse has been placed upon them. It was thought that a priest would need to say a prayer for the monster or fox to escape, in which case the patient would completely recover.

Japan's first mental health law was the Confinement and Protection for Lunatics Act 1900 in which the traditional confinement of the mentally ill at home was upheld. Thousands of mentally ill people were being held in domestic cells. A professor of psychiatry at Tokyo University, Dr Shuzo Kure, lobbied the government for more humane conditions. This led to the passing of the 1919 Mental Hospital Act, which allowed certain groups of patients to be admitted to hospital.

The prevailing societal attitude towards mental illness through time was shame, and the mentally ill were largely kept hidden by their families. Many were thought to be dangerous and the safety of the public was prioritized over the rights of the affected individual. The Mental Hygiene Law was passed in 1950 during the Allied Occupation of Japan. This forbade the domestic confinement of patients (Totsuka 1990). However, this law was revised in 1965 after the killing of the US ambassador to Japan by a young Japanese man with a history of psychosis (Mizuno et al. undated). A review of this case concluded that there was a lack of outpatient care and treatment.

Human rights violations in Japanese hospitals were highlighted by the case of the Utsunomiya Hospital Scandal in which two hospital inpatients were murdered by nursing staff and overall death rates were disturbingly high (222/1000 in a 3-year period). This led to further revision of the law, leading to the 1987 Mental Health Law which stressed the importance of the promotion of human rights and community rehabilitation and integration for the mentally ill. Voluntary admission was introduced, as well as the right to appeal against involuntary admission. Community rehabilitation was slow to develop, possibly due to the profit-driven nature of Japan's private institutions, which provide 90% of Japan's psychiatric beds (Miyata et al. 2008; Horiguchi 2014). There have been increasing revisions of law and practice, such as the 1993 Fundamental Law for People with Disabilities in which welfare provisions were granted for the mentally ill. Further amendments were made in 1995 to produce Japan's current mental health law. This classified mental illness as a disability, and produced stricter criteria for involuntary psychiatric admission and pushed for reduced stigmatization of mental health. It also provided rights of appeal against compulsory treatment. The reduction of stigma was thought to be particularly necessary as lack of social welfare on discharge was considered to be major cause of excessive inpatient stays (Tsuchiya and Takei 2004).

Long-term inpatient care remains standard practice in Japan, with an average stay of 377 days in the year 2000 (Ministry of Health, Labour and Welfare 2002). Contributing factors are thought to include lack of social care and continuing stigmatization of mental health, meaning that many families find it preferable to institutionalize unwell relatives. Cultural values may make a significant contribution to this stigmatization. A 2013 review of the stigma of mental illness in Japan showed that most Japanese people consider factors such as weakness of character to be the cause of mental health problems rather than biological factors such as genetic predisposition. Confucian principles are widely followed in Japan. One of the central doctrines of Confucianism is filial piety (obedience to one's parents). Its values also advocate a life where one's individual desires come second to that of the group to which one belongs, as the Japanese cultural view is that the 'self' is socially embedded (Young 2002). Deviation from the social norm is a cause for shame in this context. There is also a low expectation of recovery from mental illness, which contributes to an increased pressure for long hospital stays. Patients with schizophrenia in particular are thought to be dangerous and unpredictable (Ando et al. 2013). In addition the use of mechanical restraints has been found to be more widespread in Japan than in other countries (Beghi et al. 2013).

As we noted above, voluntary admissions for patients in Japan were introduced in 1987. There are four possible legal statuses for inpatient admissions:

(1) Voluntary admission with the patient's consent.

(2) Compulsory admission by order of the prefectural governor for the patient who is dangerous to himself or others.

(3) Compulsory admission at the request of the legal guardian of a patient who is not dangerous to himself or others but does not consent to admission.

(4) Emergency temporary admission by order of a certified psychiatrist when a mental disorder is suspected but time is required to make a diagnosis.

Perhaps surprisingly, a patient's hospitalization is considered to be 'with consent' if the patient's family agrees with the psychiatrist, even if the patient himself does not. This is thought to be the case in 29% of admissions.

Japanese psychiatry today has the highest number of psychiatric beds and the highest ratio of beds per capita in the world (Ng et al. 2010). The primary providers of community mental health care in Japan are its 600 local health centres. The Mental Health and Welfare Law states that each of Japan's 47 prefectures should also have at least one centre specializing in mental health care (Tsuchiya and Takei 2004). In 2002, the Ministry of Health, Labour and Welfare developed a policy to try to expedite the discharge of over 70,000 inpatients to the community with adequate social support in place upon discharge. The overall aim was to realize the transition from 'institution-based medical treatment to community-based care' (Ng et al. 2010). However, this has not yet been achieved. Since the late 1990s, community service departments of psychiatric hospitals have provided home visits to patients. More recently, multidisciplinary assertive community treatment teams for the mentally ill have been set up and have attracted increased funding (Taplin and Lawman 2012). This is known as the Japanese Outreach Model Project and aims to prevent repeated hospitalizations. There is a continued move towards finding a balance between institutional and community care in Japan in order to improve mental health services overall.

Indonesia

Indonesia is an archipelago comprising over 17,000 islands. It has the world's fourth largest population, a mix of racial groups, and the world's largest Muslim population. Indonesia is a middle-income group country and spends 1% of its total health budget on mental health. There are 0.38 psychiatric beds in mental hospitals and 0.02 psychiatric beds in general hospitals per 10,000 of the population. There are 0.21 psychiatrists per 100,000 of the population.

The first mental hospital in Indonesia was opened in the 1830s when the country was under Dutch rule. It was largely designated for the care of visiting or expatriate Europeans but also cared for any indigenous people who were found to have caused a social disturbance. By the time Indonesia had gained independence in 1949, there were four such hospitals and the number continued to grow with increased spending on mental health care. In 1966, a national meeting of psychiatrists was organized by the Ministry of Health and this led to the creation of mental health laws separate from general health laws. Around the same time psychiatric hospitals officially became part of community mental health programs, with the provision of both inpatient and out-patient services. In 1993, the 1966 mental health law was re-incorporated into general health law, and the feeling is that since then standards in mental health care have been poor (Pols 2006). The 1966 law included clauses that aimed to protect the rights of the mentally ill, particularly the right to treatment and rehabilitation. However, in the new law there are just four articles concerning mental health (Irmansyah et al. 2009). Article 26 permits individuals to be taken to a mental health hospital by family members, a guardian, local state officials, or others. It can be interpreted as promoting fear of the mentally ill. The four mental health articles are shown in Table 17.1.

Human rights violations are commonplace in Indonesia. The practise of *pasung*, in which the mentally ill individual is physically restrained, often by the use of wooden stocks, is still rife despite having been banned in 1977 (Minas and Diatri 2008). It is usually the case that the individual, who will often have a diagnosis of schizophrenia, has been restrained by their family because of lack of access to mental health services

Table 17.1 Extracts from the 1993 Indonesian legislation

Chapter 7, Law #23 (Health)	
Article 24	1. Mental health care should aim to achieve optimal intellectual and emotional mental health state
	2. Mental health activities include maintaining and improving mental health, prevention and management of psychosocial problems and mental disorders, treatment and rehabilitation of mental disorders
	3. Activities on mental health are carried out by individual, family, school, work place, community members, and are supported by mental health services and other facilities
Article 25	1. Government provides treatment and hospitalization, and gives support to the person who has recovered to return to the community
	2. Government encourages, supports, and supervises community activities on the prevention and intervention of psychosocial problems and mental disorders, and recovery process of the person with mental disorder to return to the community
Article 26	1. Persons with mental disorder who are considered dangerous and disturb the community have to be treated and hospitalized in the mental health service facilities or in other health services
	2. Treatment and hospitalization of person with mental health problems could be requested by husband or wife or the guardian or other family members or by person who is responsible for local security, or by court if the detainee has mental disorder
Article 27	1. Government will provide a presidential decree for other regulations and the management of mental health

in rural areas and concerns about potential harm to the individual or others around them. The death rate from over-crowding, malnutrition, and diarrhoea in mental hospitals is high (Irmansyah et al. 2009).

Community mental health treatment did not exist in Indonesia before the 2004 tsunami. Following this, local general practitioners in Aceh, the worst hit area, were given training in psychiatry and significant resources were made available to develop capable community resources for the mentally ill for the first time.

Conclusions

The picture in Southeast Asia is undoubtedly complex. There is much coercion. This largely results from a lack of resources for 'medical' health care resulting in an inability for many to make a positive choice to accept treatment and support. The widespread shackling in Indonesia appears to generally result from lack of resources and is much more common in isolated rural areas than in cities. Undoubtedly, shame and stigma play a part. In Japan, the practice of keeping the mentally ill 'hidden' is becoming less prevalent and community services are now being developed. Here the high rate of detained admissions and lack of community integration can in no way be related to finance as Japan is one of the wealthiest countries in the world. It is likely that it arises from the shame culture described in detail above.

The world's most populous country, China, has a varied past regarding mental health care. There is no doubt that psychiatry and the coercion associated with it has been used for political purposes in the past. At the same time most patients with schizophrenia in China receive clozapine, generally accepted as the best treatment available, albeit without the safeguards normally provided. This lack of safeguards appears to reflect a collectivist culture in which the most good can be done overall with the harm limited to a few. From the standpoint of an outside observer it appears to eliminate choice and thus be coercive.

Taiwan, China, and the other nations described in this chapter appear to be adopting strategies, at some pace in Indonesia's case especially, to improve the care of the mentally ill and at the same time reduce stigma and coercion, both from families and from the state. There is little evidence upon which to base change and still limited data on routine care. What evidence exists from elsewhere is of limited relevance because of the very different cultural, religious, and financial contexts.

References

Ando S, Yamaguchi S, Aoki Y, et al. (2013). Review of mental-health-related stigma in Japan. *Psychiatry and Clinical Neurosciences*, **67**:471–482.

Beghi M, Peroni F, Gabola P, et al. (2013). Prevalence and risk factors for the use of restraint in psychiatry: a systematic review. *Rivista di Psichiatria* **48**(1):10–22.

Bindman J, Maingay S, Szmukler G (2003). The Human Rights Act and mental health legislation. *British Journal of Psychiatry*, **182**:91–94.

Brown LB (1980). A psychologist's perspective on psychiatry in China. *Australian and New Zealand Journal of Psychiatry*, **14**:21–35.

Brown Bullock M, Andrews B (eds) (2014). *Medical transitions in twentieth-century China*. Bloomington, IN: Indiana University Press.

Butler RN (1992). Quality of life: can it be an endpoint? How can it be measured? *American Journal of Clinical Nutrition*, **55**:1267S–1270S.

Butts JB, Rich K (2005). *Nursing ethics: across the curriculum and into practice*. London: Jones and Bartlett.

Chang HH (2007). Social change and the disability rights movement in Taiwan: 1980–2002. *Review of Disability Studies: an International Journal*, **3**(1,2):3–19.

Chen S (1994). Investment in education and human resource development in postwar Taiwan. In: *Cultural Change in Postwar Taiwan* (ed. S Harrell, H. Chun-Chieh), pp. 91–110. Chicago, IL: University of Chicago Press.

Chen HH, Phillips MR, Cheng H, et al. (2012). Mental health law of the People's Republic of China [English translation with annotations]. *Shanghai Archives of Psychiatry*, **24**:305–321.

Chou SH (2014). Preliminary study of brief community counseling services at a disaster rescued location: mental health interventions for typhoon Morakot. *Bulletin of Educational Psychology*, **45**:517–537.

Chu TY, Lee SC, Wang TC, et al. (2010). A qualitative study of burden among female caregivers. *Taipei City Medical Journal*, **7**:144–153.

Department of Health, Executive Yuan (1999). http://www.mohw.gov.tw/EN/Ministry/Index. aspx (accessed 16 July 2014).

Department of Health, Executive Yuan (2010). http://www.mohw.gov.tw/EN/Ministry/Index. aspx (accessed 16 July 2014).

Department of Statistics [Ministry of the Interior] (2013). Physically and mentally disabled population by classification. Available at: http://sowf.moi.gov.tw/stat/year/list.htm (accessed 20 July 2014).

Department of Statistics [Ministry of Health and Welfare] (2014). Physically and mentally disabled population by classification. Available at: http://sowf.moi.gov.tw/stat/year/list.htm (accessed 20 July 2014).

Directorate-General of Budget, Accounting and Statistics (2014). [Statistical tables.] http:// eng.stat.gov.tw/ct.asp?xItem=37408&CtNode=5347&mp=5 (accessed 20 July 2014).

Executive Yuan (2007). The explanatory notes to the Mental Health Bill.

Gottstein J (2007). Money, rights and alternatives: enforcing legal rights as mechanism for creating non-medical alternatives. In *Alternatives beyond psychiatry* (ed. P Stastny, P Lehmann), pp. 308–317. Berlin: Peter Lehmann Publishing.

Gou L, Zhou JS, Xiang YT, et al. (2014). Frequency of involuntary admissions and its associations with demographic and clinical characteristics in China. *Archives of Psychiatric Nursing*, **28**:272–276.

Harris J (1985). *The value of life*. London: Routledge.

Horiguchi S (2014). Mental health and therapy in Japan: conceptions, practices, and challenges. In: *Critical issues in contemporary Japan* (ed. J Kingston). London: Routledge.

Irmansyah I, Prasetyo YA, Minas H (2009). Human rights of persons with mental illness in Indonesia: more than legislation is needed. *International Journal of Mental Health Systems*, **3**:14.

Lee CY, Chou FHC (2003). The exploration of ambiguity of Mental Health Act on the compulsory admission: the case of psychiatric patient hospitalization *Journal of Law and Medicine*, **10**(3):42–49.

Lee S, Lee MT, Chiu MY, et al. (2005). Experience of social stigma by people with schizophrenia in Hong Kong. *British Journal of Psychiatry*, **186**:153–157.

Legislative Yuan Gazette (2007). *The Legislative Yuan Gazette*, **96**(32) [in Chinese]. URL: http://lci.ly.gov.tw/ (accessed 20 July 2014).

Lelliott P, Audini B (2003). Trends in the use of Part II of the Mental Health Act 1983 in seven English local authority areas. *British Journal of Psychiatry*, **182**:68–70.

Lin CLE, Kopelowicz A, Chan CH, et al. (2008). A qualitative inquiry into the Taiwanese mentally ill persons' difficulties living in the community. *Archives of Psychiatric Nursing*, **22**:266–276.

Liu RY, Tsai KY, Chou FHC, et al. (2010). The characteristics of severe mentally Ill patients who need forced hospitalization before and after the amended mental health act in Taiwan. *Taiwanese Journal of Psychiatry (Taipei)*, **24**:131–139.

Liu J, Ma H, He Y-L, et al. (2011). Mental health system in China: history, recent service reform and future challenges. *World Psychiatry*, **10**:210–216.

Lorant V, Depuydt C, Gillain B, et al. (2007). Involuntary commitment in psychiatric care: what drives the decision? *Social Psychiatry and Psychiatric Epidemiology*, **42**:360–365.

Ma H (2012). Integration of hospital and community services—the '686 Project'—is a crucial component in the reform of China's mental health services. *Shanghai Archives of Psychiatry*, **24**:172–174.

Macer DRJ (1992). *Attitudes to genetic engineering: Japanese and international comparisons.* Christchurch, New Zealand: Eubios Ethics Institute.

Mackelprang RW, Salsgiver RO (2009). *Disability: a diversity model approach in human service practice,* 3rd edn. Chicago, IL: Lyceum Books.

Meltzer HY (2012). Clozapine: balancing safety with superior antipsychotic efficacy. *Clinical Schizophrenia and Related Psychoses,* 6:134–144.

Mental Health Alliance (2007). Get the latest information on the Mental Health Bill. URL: http://www.mentalhealthalliance.org.uk/ (accessed 18 July 2014).

Minas H, Diatri H (2008). *Pasung:* physical restraint and confinement of the mentally ill in the community. *International Journal of Mental health Systems,* 2:8.

Ministry of Health, Labour and Welfare (2002). *Data on mental health and welfare* [in Japanese]. Ichikawa: National Institute of Mental Health in Japan.

Miyata H, Tachimori H, Takeshima T (2008). Providing support to psychiatric patients living in the community in Japan: patient needs and care providers perceptions. *International Journal of Mental Health Systems,* 2:5.

Mizuno M, Murakami M, Rizzoli AA (undated).The mental health and welfare system and its related laws in Japan. *Psychiatry Online Italia.* Available at: http://www.psychiatryonline.it/node/4200

National Health Insurance Administration, Ministry of Health and Welfare (2013). URL: http://www.nhi.gov.tw/English/webdata/webdata.aspx?menu=11&menu_id=296&WD_ID=296&webdata_id=4456 (accessed 31 July 2014).

Ng C, Setoya Y, Koyama A, et al. (2010). The ongoing development of community mental health services in Japan: utilizing strengths and opportunities. *Australasian Psychiatry,* 18:57–62.

Pols H (2006). The development of psychiatry in Indonesia: from colonial to modern times. *International Review of Psychiatry,* 18: 363–370.

Reichert E (2007). *Challenges in human rights: a social work perspective.* New York: Columbia University Press,

Rogers A, Pilgrim D (2001). *Mental health policy in Britain.* Basingstoke: Palgrave.

Salize HJ, Dressing H (2004). Epidemiology of involuntary placement of mentally ill people across the European Union. *British Journal of Psychiatry,* 184:163–168.

Spandler H, Calton T (2009). Psychosis and human rights: conflicts in mental health policy and practice. *Social Policy and Society,* 8:245–256.

Szmukler G (2004). Mental health legislation in the era of community psychiatry. *Psychiatry,* 3(3):16–19.

Taiwan Association for Human Rights (1990). *Taiwan human rights reports, 1987–1990.* Taipei: Taiwan Association for Human Rights.

Taplin R, Lawman SJ (eds) (2012). *Mental health care in Japan.* London: Routledge.

Thomas S, Thomas T (2004). The impact of the Human Rights Act 1998 on mental health care. *Psychiatry,* 3(3):20–22.

Totsuka E (1990). The history of Japanese psychiatry and the rights of mental patients. *Psychiatric Bulletin,* 14:193–200.

Tsuchiya KJ, Takei N (2004). Focus on psychiatry in Japan. *British Journal of Psychiatry,* 184:88–92.

Wang JY (2008). Amendments to the Mental Health Act in Taiwan and England. *Social Policy and Social Work,* 12:189–218.

Wang KY (1997). A review of mental health policy in Taiwan: types of elite and the decision-making process. *Chinese Journal of Mental Health*, 10:29–47.

Werner P, Aviv A, Barak Y (2008). Self-stigma, self-esteem and age in persons with schizophrenia. *International Psychogeriatrics*, 20:174–187.

Wu HC, Tang IC, Lin WI, et al. (2013). Professional values and attitude of psychiatric social workers toward involuntary hospitalization of psychiatric patients. *Journal of Social Work*, 13:419–434.

Yang YH, Yeh EK, Hwu HG (2012). Prevalences of schizophrenia, bipolar disorder, and depressive disorders in community between Taiwan and other countries. *Taiwanese Journal of Psychiatry*, 26:77–87.

Yeh CC (2009). *Introduction to social work*. Taipei: Yang-Chih Book.

Yip KS (2003). Traditional Confucian concepts of mental health: its implications to social work practice with Chinese communities. *Asia Pacific Journal of Social Work and Development*, 13:65–89.

Yip KS (2005). An historical review of the mental health services in the People's Republic of China. *International Journal of Social Psychiatry*, 51:106–118.

Young J (2002). Morals, suicide, and psychiatry: a view from Japan. *Bioethics*, 16:412–424.

Chapter 18

Coercion in Europe

Angelo Fioritti and Thomas Marcacci

Introduction

Modern psychiatry was born in Europe with Philippe Pinel in the Age of Enlightenment: the concept of human rights was first conceived and the first laws to protect citizens' rights in psychiatry were introduced. All psychiatrists like to present themselves as disciples of Pinel, who is said to have freed the mentally ill from their chains in Parisian prisons. For the past 200 years much international legislation has been based on the original French law, *Loi sur les aliénés no. 7443 du 30 juin 1838*, approved in order to protect free citizens from the risk of abuse through unnecessary coercive treatments.

However, Europe is also where the worst violations of human rights in psychiatry have taken place. One cannot forget the abominable killing of the mentally ill by the Nazi regime (Lifton 1986; Friedlander 1995) and the political use of psychiatry by the fascist regime in Italy (Babini 2014) and in the Soviet Union (Richard and Bonnie 2002), and also the fact that an eminent psychiatrist from the former Yugoslavia is currently being prosecuted for war crimes by the International Criminal Tribunal (Dekleva and Post 1997).

Europe has developed several international institutions such as the European Council, the European Union (EU), and the European Court of Human Rights. Their covenants, along with those from the United Nations (UN), have repeatedly attempted to address the issue of freedom and coercion in medicine and in psychiatry. The World Health Organization (WHO) Regional Office for Europe has paid extensive attention to coercion and human rights in psychiatry.

After World War II the movement for human rights has steadily increased in importance and has produced many groups of stakeholders relevant to the field of psychiatry. The Geneva Initiative and the Open Society, for example, have been successful in orientating national and EU policies and in keeping alive the debate about coercion in psychiatry. Scholars and researchers have carried out extensive research on the clinical, social, and epidemiological aspects of coercion.

This chapter addresses all these issues, with particular attention to coercion in the community. This is a relatively recent development, so most references will cover coercion in general and examine its consequences for coercion in the community.

Values, declarations, and internationally binding documents

The madness of the British king George III in the eighteenth century (Peters and Beveridge 2010) is probably the clearest representation of the relationship between freedom and coercion at the beginning of psychiatry. The French philosopher Michel Foucault (1972) considers the act of taking possession of the king's body to treat his insanity in 1788 to be the actual birth of modern psychiatry, with its immense power and responsibility for having human lives at its disposal. The problem of regulating this power soon led to national legislation in a number of countries, which generally replicated the structure of the French law of 1838, a law that was only eventually repealed in 1990. All these laws defined the criteria for involuntary admissions (usually dangerousness against the patient or others, risk of deterioration, public scandal). They also determined procedures to be followed, authorities responsible for the decision, and the proper places of treatment. The patient's legal status during involuntary admission and issues of legal guardianship during admission were also covered. This is how the balance between freedom and coercion has been regulated in Europe for almost two centuries.

After the horrors of the concentration camps and the many tragedies of World War II, issues of individual freedom and human rights acquired unprecedented importance. The Universal Declaration of Human Rights (UDHR) (United Nations 1948) still exerts its influence on how the balance between freedom and coercion is conceived and managed in psychiatry today. Since the approval of the UDHR the gap between its principles and much existing psychiatric legislation has become evident. The International Covenant on Civil and Political Rights (ICCPR) (United Nations 1966) did not contain any specific provision for psychiatry, but Article 7 on the prevention of torture and inhumane or degrading treatments in medical and psychiatric care generated much debate. Eventually, in 1991, the UN released the Principles for the Protection of Persons with Mental Illness and the Improvement of Mental Health Care (better known as the MI Principles; United Nations 1991). This led to a reform of some European legislation on involuntary treatment (e.g. in Hungary and Portugal). It also constituted the basis for the WHO Checklist of Mental Health Legislation (World Health Organization 2005a), an instrument to assess the extent to which national legislation respected the principles of human rights. Although more human rights-orientated, the MI Principles and the WHO Checklist still contain specific exceptions to the universality of human rights acceptable in psychiatry, particularly around coercion.

The UN Convention on the Rights of Persons with Disabilities (UNCRPD) (United Nations 2006) challenges this assumption. It is a binding document ratified by all European nations and it substitutes all previous provisions regarding physical, intellectual, and/or psychiatric disability. All national legislation in the ratifying states must conform to its standards. It promotes changes in the balance between freedom and coercion, both in the legislation (Szmukler et al. 2014) and in clinical practice. In particular Article 12 (legal capacity), Article 14 (personal freedom and safety), Article 17 (physical and mental integrity), and Article 18 (freedom of movement) appear to leave all European legislation in need of revision. The International Disability Alliance, for example, argue for a revision of the case *Herczegfalvy vs. Austria* (European Court on Human Rights 1992), which upheld the validity of delegating to medical authorities the use of force to administer treatment to persons unable to take decisions for themselves.

It is difficult to foresee what the UNCRPD earthquake will produce in the near future. We are probably moving towards a new balance between freedom and coercion in Europe. This may involve more room for supported decision-making procedures rather than coercive measures and, at the same time, a shift from dangerousness criteria to impaired decision-making capacity as a broader category for involuntary treatments. The recent Capacity Bill in Northern Ireland is an example of a generic 'fusion' law covering everyone with impaired capacity, whatever the cause (Griffith 2014). Most likely more negotiation will take place in the process of imposing coercion, with the involvement of several stakeholders.

Mental health policies in Europe and the issue of coercion

The most important trend in European mental health policies in the last 40 years has been the shift from a hospital-based to a community-based mental health system. Mental health reforms in Italy in 1978 (Fioritti and Amaddeo 2014), the United Kingdom in 1984 (Killaspy et al. 2006), and Spain in 1986 (Bobes et al. 2012) showed that deinstitutionalization is possible, that comprehensive community mental health services can be more effective than a hospital-based system, and that it is not more expensive. However, it requires strong political commitment, careful planning, and intensive training of professionals.

Several countries (but by no means all) have adopted policies that are consistent with this trend, and several international bodies and commissions are monitoring the transition locally and globally (World Health Organization 2005b; European Commission 2009; European Commission Expert Group 2012; Samele et al. 2013; OECD 2014). One of the five thematic areas of the Joint Action on Mental Health and Wellbeing (http://www.mentalhealthandwellbeing.eu), a strategic programme by the European Commission, is 'Managing the evolution towards community-based and socially inclusive approaches to mental health'.

Wide differences exist between EU member states, with different levels of implementation of the principles of community psychiatry. A review of the scientific and grey literature (Amaddeo et al. 2007) showed that the psychiatric beds available in each country ranged from 1.7 per 10,000 population in Italy to 25 per 10,000 in Belgium. Seven countries had more than 10 beds per 10,000 population: Belgium, Denmark, France, Ireland, Luxembourg, Netherlands, and Finland. Only four countries (Spain, Italy, Austria, and the UK) had fewer than 6 beds per 10,000 population. In Italy and Finland there were no psychiatric beds remaining in mental hospitals, only those in general hospitals.

Mental Health Europe (2008, 2012) found that nine countries have a deinstitutionalization strategy or programme in social care (Bulgaria, Croatia, the Czech Republic,

Estonia, Hungary, Slovakia, Moldova, Romania, and Ireland) with Lithuania preparing their strategy. Four countries (Hungary, Romania, Latvia, and Slovenia) are currently investing in psychiatric hospitals rather than community care. The European landscape of deinstitutionalization remains patchy and confused.

Deinstitutionalization comes with the assumption that moving care into the community brings less coercion and promotes less-repressive practices. This is possible, but cannot be taken for granted. Many countries that have switched to a community-based mental health system (e.g. the UK) or have incorporated substantial community services in a hospital-based system (e.g. the Netherlands, Portugal, some *Länder* in Germany) have a high number of psychiatric beds. There may also be less visible processes of 'reinstitutionalization'. This can involve relabelling old mental hospitals, transferring patients to asylum-like nursing homes, increasing the size of forensic hospitals, or developing large supported housing systems with heavy institutional features. They may also include the adoption of radical 'no dropout policies' within assertive community treatment schemes that make extensive use of informal coercion (Priebe et al. 2005). These developments make the investigation and monitoring of coercion in the community even more important than in traditional institutional settings.

Mental health legislation

The current state of EU mental health legislation still reflects the traditional approach to balancing the protection of society and individual freedoms rather than the active promotion of citizens' rights as envisaged by the UNCRPD, as stated above. It is possible that an era of radical revision of most EU legislation is coming, perhaps very soon.

A comparison of the texts of laws from all EU member states (Fioritti 2002) allowed for an outline of models regulating this complex issue. Mental health laws came under scrutiny in most countries in the 1990s. The most recent acts at that time were the British (1983) and Italian (1978). Today they are the oldest. Most other countries changed their legislation in the 1990s and some have changed them more than once (e.g. the Netherlands). These changes may reflect the impact of shifts in public attitudes and treatment practices that have called for debate and remodelling of the legal framework for care. In the 1970s the mean lifespan of a law was 30 years; it is now just 15.

The distinction between the functions of a general/federal law (encompassing provisions for general principles, patient rights, and procedures for involuntary care) and of a local/regional law (covering organization of services and provision of standards for staff and care) has become more routine. This is logical given the significant differences that can exist within large nations. Standards for staffing may depend on local needs and the availability of resources, especially given the broader political trend towards devolution.

Current legislation has completely abolished most terms that were at the basis of national legislation only 30 years ago. Words such as *alienè* in French have been amended and terms such as *citizen, user,* or *patient* have taken their place. *Asylum* or *mental hospital* have been replaced by mental health departments. These changes, which may seem merely cosmetic, can be seen as a result of changes happening independently in the professional/institutional field and also as a conscious strategy to promote change in countries that have not yet started this process.

Current laws generally emphasize patients' rights to protection rather than the protection of society from disturbing or criminal behaviour by the mentally ill. Dangerousness is no longer the unique basis for compulsory treatment (the *dangerousness criterion*); most legislation contains provisions which allow for the treatment of patients solely for their benefit (the *health benefit criterion*) and on the basis of the clinical judgement of a one or more physicians (the *need for care criterion*).

Direct involvement of the judicial authorities in the procedures for compulsory admission is much less common, and is usually provided only for appeals. The administrative authority (Italy, Ireland, UK) is responsible for the whole process comprising assessment, decision, and enactment of decisions in the procedures for obligatory treatment. However, France has recently changed its mental health law— in 2011 and again in 2013—to introduce a judicial hearing after 12 days in hospital. This reflects a significant shift in public attitudes and in health philosophy in this area.

Places where care can be delivered (voluntarily or involuntarily) are much more differentiated and so are the procedures for commitment: emergency commitment, inpatient commitment, outpatient mandated care, medium- and long-term commitment. This reflects the search for modulated responses in terms of protection and coercion, while respecting the primary goal of protecting patients' rights.

The role of the medical profession in the process of compulsory treatment is split into two major models: the medical model and the legal model.

In *medical model* thinking it is emphasized that compulsory treatment is always treatment, only skilled clinicians know what is in their patients' best interests, and that this decision is part of their professional activity. A broad criterion (*need for treatment*) is usually preferred, and doctors can either admit based upon their assessments or after their request has been formally validated by an administrative authority. Controls for preventing abuses are enacted in forms of revisions and involvement of judicial authorities.

In the *legal model* it is emphasized that compulsory treatment is always a limitation of personal freedom and therefore can only be determined upon the decision of a legal authority, either administrative or judicial. Physicians can propose treatment, but their proposal must be thoroughly examined by a non-clinical authority, which must check that all the conditions are met and no alternatives exist. A behavioural criterion (dangerousness, self neglect) is often preferred and the role of the medical profession is limited to the input phase.

Finally, a few countries have introduced into their laws some provisions which mandate for future trends and developments These include implementation of clinical governance and quality management, involvement of users and carers in the planning and evaluation of services, adaptation of procedures for emerging clinical profiles (personality disorders, learning disabilities, drug abuse), health promotion, and the prevention of stigma.

Mental health legislation must be viewed as a process. It reflects changes and can also promote them. As a result it is destined to be at the core of the debate about any country's mental health system, more so in the era of implementation of UNCRPD principles.

Empirical research

Research on formal and informal coercion is gaining momentum internationally, under the convergent stimuli provided by human rights advocacy, legislative changes, and professional attempts to improve treatment outcomes. Initially it developed across the Atlantic as a UK/US debate about what is more ethically sound and what works better for patients. However, during the last decade several contributions have also appeared from Scandinavia and Germany and one large European collaborative project (EUNOMIA).

Coercion as an object of empirical research is mostly viewed as a spectrum of *treatment pressures* (Szmukler and Applebaum, 2008). These range from persuasion to compulsion, passing through leverage, inducement, and threats. Objective and subjective elements of each of these stages have been outlined, both during admission to hospital and in community programmes. Areas of research comprise refinement of research instruments (mainly scales and interviews), epidemiology of different levels of coercion, effects on clinical outcome (especially through engagement and treatment adherence), and clinical and environmental factors associated with coercion. Lastly we are beginning to see trials comparing the outcomes of inpatient and community compulsion.

A review conducted by Newton-Howes (2011) shows that European research is probably more orientated to balancing the study of both objective and subjective elements of coercion than research in the USA. Most thematic articles on coercion and themes relating to patients' experiences of coercion come from Europe, particularly from the Nordic countries.

The MacArthur Perceived Coercion Scale (Gardner et al. 1993), developed in the USA, is still the most widely used instrument in this field of research, but European researchers have developed measurement tools combining quantitative and qualitative methodologies that consider the perspectives of both patients and staff (Killaspy et al. 2012).

In terms of the epidemiology of coercion in Europe there are strikingly different rates of compulsory inpatient treatment between countries, from 12 per 100,000 population/year in Italy to 213 in Finland (Fiorillo et al. 2011). Some authors have also explored the differences in the use of seclusion and restraint in European countries, finding four-fold differences between Scandinavian countries (Bak and Aggernæs 2012) and an even higher prevalence and duration in other countries (Steinert et al. 2010). Seclusion and restraint are forbidden in some countries, and some of these studies stemmed from the activity of the European Committee for the Prevention of Torture and Inhuman or Degrading Treatment. This body regularly visits psychiatric and other institutions and releases accurate reports with requirements for change. Another ethical issue highlighted by empirical research is the excess use of coercion among first- and second-generation immigrants compared with the native population (Norredam et al. 2010).

European research into inpatient treatment has concentrated on clinical and environmental factors associated with coercion and on clinical and subjective outcomes. Diagnosis of psychosis and emergency admissions (Myklebust 2012) are generally associated with higher rates of formal compulsion. Analysis of the large dataset from the EU EUNOMIA project involving 11 countries showed that involuntary admission, female gender, lower Global Assessment of Functioning score, and positive symptoms were significantly associated with higher perceived coercion (Fiorillo et al. 2012). However, perceived coercion decreased over time, mostly related to improvements in global functioning and positive symptoms.

Staff attitudes have been widely investigated as one of the environmental elements related to coercive measures following hospitalization. A Norwegian group failed to find relevant differences among inpatient units in decision-making processes about seclusion and restraint. They found that physical violence was the predominant factor leading to their use, but also that male staff and unskilled staff were more prone to choose highly restrictive interventions (Wynn et al. 2011). In a study of 33 Norwegian inpatient units using the Staff Attitude to Coercion Scale (Husum et al. 2010) the authors found an 8–11% variance between wards, mostly attributable to the personality characteristics of individual members of staff (Husum et al. 2011). These studies underline the importance of training and also the development of special intervention programmes for specific population groups (migrants, women, violent, and intellectually disabled patients).

Research on the consequences of inpatient coercion has been reasonably extensive in Europe during the last decade. Another study from EUNOMIA showed that, independent of legal status and perceived coercion, unemployment, number of previous hospitalizations, and dissatisfaction at intake predicted poorer final outcome (Kallert et al. 2011). However, a 1-year follow-up of 778 patients admitted involuntarily to 22 wards in England showed a correlation between the subjective experience of high perceived coercion at intake and better objective measures of social functioning 1 year later (Priebe et al. 2011). Even more important is the finding that 1 year later only 40% of involuntary patients reported that detention was justified, regardless of how much the treatment helped, but with a significant association with patient satisfaction during the first week of admission (Priebe et al. 2009). A German study of voluntary and involuntary admissions 2 years after discharge found that formal compulsion had little influence on later adherence to medication and engagement in inpatient and outpatient treatment. However, it was significantly associated with higher perceived coercion in all subsequent treatments (Jaeger et al. 2013).

Some studies have explored the psychological dimensions related to coercion in more depth. Rüsch et al. (2014), in a semi-quantitative study of 186 patients with a history of recent involuntary hospitalization, described a cascade of psychological consequences of high levels of coercion and compulsion. These ranged from shame to reduced self-esteem through self-contempt and self-stigma, and were independent of diagnosis, age, gender, and number of hospitalizations. These emotional and cognitive reactions have also been described by researchers investigating the issue of procedural justice, i.e. the perception by the patient of whether their compulsion or coercion was right or wrong. Two studies (O'Donoughue et al. 2010, 2011) investigated separately formal coercion, perceived coercion, and procedural justice. They concluded that they may independently affect future compliance and engagement in treatment. They highlighted the importance of working actively with the patient to acknowledge and explore the experience and the sense of coercion. Another Irish study (Smith et al. 2014) showed a strong correlation between perceived procedural injustice and less satisfaction and engagement at follow-up. Procedural justice has also been investigated by a British study in 22 hospitals. This has similarly highlighted the importance of working collaboratively with patients who experience procedural injustice and those who are ambivalent about their treatment (Katsakou et al. 2012) In a separate analysis from the EUNOMIA dataset the authors found that subjective experience of coercion in voluntary patients predicted poorer clinical outcomes when compared with involuntary patients (Kallert et al. 2011).

These studies on the psychological aspects of coercion together suggest that coercion is a phenomenon with a significant and enduring psychological impact on patients. It can lead to poorer clinical outcomes associated with poor engagement and with poorer social outcomes related to self-stigma and disempowerment. These effects may be reduced by a full awareness of the consequences of coercion among professionals and by timely cognitive and emotional work with patients.

Finally the issue of coercion in the community has been widely investigated, both in assertive community treatment programmes in different countries (Thøgersen et al. 2010) and with regard to the debated issue of community treatment orders (CTOs), now provided in more than 70 legislations worldwide (Maughan et al. 2013). In the OCTET trial the imposition of compulsory supervision on community treatment did not reduce the rate of readmission or produce any other improvements in clinical progress (Burns et al. 2013). A recent update by Maughan et al. (2013) of Churchill et al.'s (2006) comprehensive review has called for caution and reflection about this form of coercion. There are only three published randomized controlled trials, two from the USA (Swartz et al, 1999; Steadman et al. 2001) and one from the UK (Burns 2013), and none of them found any evidence that CTOs affect admission rates or number of inpatient days. These studies are extensively reported and discussed elsewhere in this book.

Conclusions

Although modern psychiatry was born in Europe more than two centuries ago, the issue of human rights and the limitation of coercive measures achieved an international dimension only after World War II. Even more recently the development of European political and administrative bodies has brought these issues to a prominent position in the political agenda of most European states. The approval and ratification of the UNCRPD is an important step to further study and better legislate about coercion in psychiatry. Its use is now monitored on a continental scale and this gives the opportunity to better understand its dynamics and its consequences. Awareness is growing in the professions and in public opinion about the importance of limiting coercion and implementing practices that are more respectful of personal rights. A new, less coercive framework for psychiatric practice is emerging in the twenty-first century.

References

Amaddeo F, Becker T, Fioritti A, et al. (2007). Reforms in community care: the balance between hospital and community-based mental health care. In: *Mental health policy and practice across Europe. The future direction of mental health care* (ed. M Knapp, D McDaid, E Mossialos, et al.), pp. 235–249. Maidenhead: McGraw-Hill.

Babini VP (2014). Looking back: Italian psychiatry from its origins to law 180 of 1978. *Journal of Nervous and Mental Disease*, 202:428–431.

Bak J, Aggernæs H (2012). Coercion within Danish psychiatry compared with 10 other European countries. *Nordic Journal of Psychiatry*, 66:297–302.

Bobes J, Garcia-Portilla MP, Bobes-Bascaran MT, et al. (2012). The state of psychiatry in Spain. *International Review of Psychiatry*, 24:347–355.

Burns T, Rugkåsa J, Molodynski A, et al. (2013). Community treatment orders for patients with psychosis (OCTET): a randomised controlled trial. *The Lancet*, 381:1627–1633.

Dekleva KB, Post J (1997). Genocide in Bosnia: the case of Dr. Radovan Karadzic. *Journal of American Academy of Psychiatry and Law*, 25:485–496.

European Commission (2009). *Report of the ad hoc Expert Group on the transition from institutional to community-based care.* Available at: http://ec.europa.eu/social/BlobServlet?d ocId=3992&langId=en

European Commission Expert Group (2012). *Common European guidelines on the transition from institutional to community-based care.* Available at: http:// deinstitutionalisationguide.eu/

European Court of Human Rights (1992). *Case of Herczegfalvy v. Austria.* Available at: http:// hudoc.echr.coe.int/eng?i=001-57781

Fiorillo A, De Rosa C, Del Vecchio V, et al. (2011). How to improve clinical practice on involuntary hospital admissions of psychiatric patients: suggestions from the EUNOMIA study. *European Psychiatry*, 26:201–207.

Fiorillo A, Giacco D, De Rosa C, et al. (2012). Patient characteristics and symptoms associated with perceived coercion during hospital treatment. *Acta Psychiatrica Scandinavica*, 125:460–467.

Fioritti A (2002). *Leggi e salute mentale: panorama europeo delle legislazioni di interesse psichiatrico* Torino: Centro Scientifico Editore.

Fioritti A, Amaddeo F (2014). Community mental health in Italy today. *Journal of Nervous and Mental Disease*, 202:425–427.

Foucault M (1972). *Histoire de la folie à l'âge classique.* Paris: Gallimard.

Friedlander H (1995). *The origins of Nazi genocide: from euthanasia to the Final Solution.* Chapel Hill, NC: University of North Carolina Press.

Gardner W, Hoge SK, Bennet NB, et al. (1993). Two scales for measuring patients' perception for coercion during mental hospital admission. *Behavioral Sciences and the Law*, 11:307–321.

Griffith R (2014). Mental capacity and mental health act part 4: a new framework. *British Journal of Nursing*, 23:1090–1091.

Husum TL, Bjørngaard JH, Finset A, et al. (2010). A cross-sectional prospective study of seclusion, restraint and involuntary medication in acute psychiatric wards: patient, staff and ward characteristics. *BMC Health Services Research*, 10:89.

Husum T, Bjørngaard J, Finset A, et al. (2011). Staff attitudes and thoughts about the use of coercion in acute psychiatric wards. *Social Psychiatry and Psychiatric Epidemiology*, 46:893–901.

Jaeger S, Pfiffner C, Weiser P, et al. (2013). Long-term effects of involuntary hospitalization on medication adherence, treatment engagement and perception of coercion. *Social Psychiatry and Psychiatric Epidemiology*, **48**:1787–1796.

Kallert TW, Katsakou C, Adamowski T, et al. (2011). Coerced hospital admission and symptom change. a prospective observational multi-centre study. *PLoS ONE*, **6**(11):e28191.

Katsakou C, Rose D, Amos T, et al. (2012). Psychiatric patients' views on why their involuntary hospitalisation was right or wrong: a qualitative study. *Social Psychiatry and Psychiatric Epidemiology*, **47**:1169–1179.

Killaspy H, Bebbington P, Blizard R, et al. (2006). The REACT study: randomised evaluation of assertive community treatment in north London. *British Medical Journal*, **332**:815.

Killaspy H, White S, Wright C, et al. (2012). Quality of longer term mental health facilities in Europe: validation of the quality indicator for rehabilitative care against service users' views. *PLoS ONE*, **7**(6):e38070.

Lifton RJ (1986). The Nazi doctors: medical killing and the psychology of genocide. *Journal of Medicine and Philosophy*, **12**:305–307.

Maughan D, Molodynski A, Rugkåsa J, et al. (2013). A systematic review of the effect of community treatment orders on service use. *Social Psychiatry and Psychiatric Epidemiology*, **49**:651–663.

Mental Health Europe (2008). *From exclusion to inclusion—the way forward to promoting social inclusion of people with mental health problems in Europe*. Available at: http://ec.europa.eu/health/ph_determinants/life_style/mental/docs/conf_co17_en.pdf

Mental Health Europe (2012). *Mapping exclusion. Institutional and community-based services in the mental health field in Europe*. Available at: http://www.epha.org/spip.php?article5449

Myklebust LH, Sørgaard K, Røtvold K, et al. (2012). Factors of importance to involuntary admission. *Nordic Journal of Psychiatry*, **66**:178–182.

Newton-Howes G, Mullen R (2011). Coercion in psychiatric care: systematic review of correlates and themes. *Psychiatric Services*, **62**:465–470.

Norredam M, Garcia-Lopez A, Keiding N, et al. (2010). Excess use of coercive measures in psychiatry among migrants compared with native Danes. *Acta Psychiatrica Scandinavica*, **121**:143–151.

O'Donoghue B, Lyne J, Hill M, et al. (2010). Involuntary admission from patients' perspective. *Social Psychiatry and Psychiatric Epidemiology*, **45**:631–638.

O'Donoghue B, Lyne J, Hill M, et al. (2011). Perception of involuntary admission and risk of subsequent readmission at one-year follow-up: the influence of insight and recovery style. *Journal of Mental Health*, **20**:249–259.

OECD (2014). *Making mental health count: the social and economic costs of neglecting mental health care*. OECD Health Policy Studies. Paris: OECD Publishing.

Peters TJ, Beveridge A (2010). The madness of King George III: a psychiatric re-assessment. *History of Psychiatry*, **21**:20–37.

Priebe S, Badesconyi A, Fioritti A, et al. (2005). Reinstitutionalisation in mental health care: comparison of data on service provision from six European countries. *British Medical Journal*, **330**:123–126.

Priebe S, Katsokou C, Amos T, et al. (2009). Patients view and readmission one year after involuntary hospitalisation. *British Journal of Psychiatry*, **194**:49–54.

Priebe S, Katsakou C, Yeeles K, et al. (2011). Predictors of clinical and social outcomes following involuntary hospital admission: a prospective observational study. *European Archives of Psychiatry and Clinical Neuroscience*, **261**:377–386.

Richard J, Bonnie LLB (2002). Political abuse of psychiatry in the Soviet Union and in China: complexities and controversies. *Journal of the American Academy of Psychiatry and Law*, 30:136–144.

Rüsch N, Müller M, Lay B, et al. (2014). Emotional reactions to involuntary psychiatric hospitalization and stigma-related stress among people with mental illness. *European Archives of Psychiatry and Clinical Neuroscience*, 264:35–43.

Samele C, Frew S, Urquía N (2013). *Mental health systems in the European Union Member States, status of mental health in populations and benefits to be expected from investments into mental health.* A report prepared on behalf of the Institute of Mental Health, Nottingham for the EU Executive Agency for Health and Consumers. Available at: http://ec.europa.eu/health/mental_health/docs/europopp_full_en.pdf

Smith D, Roche E, O'Loughlin K, et al. (2014). Satisfaction with services following voluntary and involuntary admission. *Journal of Mental Health*, 23:38–45.

Steadman HJ, Gounis K, Dennis D, et al. (2001). Assessing the New York City involuntary outpatient commitment pilot program. *Psychiatric Services*, 52:330–336.

Steinert T, Lepping P, Bernhardsgrütter R, et al. (2010). Incidence of seclusion and restraint in psychiatric hospitals: a literature review and survey of international trends. *Social Psychiatry and Psychiatric Epidemiology*, 45:889–897.

Swartz MS, Swanson JW, Wagner HR, et al. (1999). Can involuntary outpatient commitment reduce hospital recidivism? Findings from a randomized trial with severely mentally ill individuals. *American Journal of Psychiatry*, 156:1968–1975.

Szmukler G, Applebaum PS (2008). Treatment pressures, leverage, coercion, and compulsion in mental health care. *Journal of Mental Health*, 17:233–244.

Szmukler G, Daw R, Callard F (2014). Mental health law and the UN Convention on the Rights of Persons with Disabilities. *International Journal of Law and Psychiatry*, 37:245–252.

Thøgersen MH, Morthorst B, Nordentoft M (2010). Perceptions of coercion in the community: a qualitative study of patients in a Danish assertive community treatment team. *Psychiatric Quarterly*, 81:35–47.

United Nations (1948). *Universal Declaration of Human Rights.* URL: http://www.un.org/en/universal-declaration-human-rights/index.html

United Nations (1966). *The International Covenant on Civil and Political Rights.* URL: http://www.ohchr.org/en/professionalinterest/pages/ccpr.aspx

United Nations (1991). Principles for the protection of persons with mental illness and the improvement of mental health care. *UN Resolution 46/119.* URL: http://www.un.org/en/ga/search/view_doc.asp?symbol=A/RES/46/119

United Nations (2006). *Convention on the Rights of Persons with Disabilities.* URL: http://www.un.org/disabilities/convention/conventionfull.shtml

World Health Organization (2005a). *WHO resource book on mental health, human rights and legislation.* Geneva: World Health Organization.

World Health Organization (2005b). *Mental health action plan for Europe: facing the challenges, building solutions.* Copenhagen: World Health Organization.

Wynn R, Kvalvik A-M, Hynnekleiv T (2011). Attitudes to coercion at two Norwegian psychiatric units. *Nordic Journal of Psychiatry*, 65:133–137.

Chapter 19

Coercion in community mental health care: African perspectives

Atalay Alem and Catherine Manning

Africa is the second largest and second most populous continent in the world after Asia. According to the latest available data the population of Africa is around 1.2 billion (World Population Review 2015). In most countries of the continent population growth is over 2.5% per annum. The continent has 54 recognized sovereign states and countries, nine territories, and two de facto independent states (World Population Statistics 2014). Africa is sometimes called the 'mother continent' because it is believed to be the first continent on earth to be inhabited by humans (National Geographic Society 2014).

The Sahara Desert bisects the continent from the Atlantic Ocean to the Red Sea. Countries to the north of the Sahara Desert form the North African region and those to the south the Sub-Saharan region. Sub-Saharan Africa has a majority black population with traditional African cultures while North Africa is predominantly inhabited by non-black peoples with an Arab language and culture. The North African countries except Algeria belong to the Eastern Mediterranean Region of the World Health Organization (WHO) while the Sub-Saharan countries make up the African Region. Descriptions in this chapter mainly focus on Sub-Saharan countries or the African Region of the WHO.

Political and social problems are common in Africa. Protracted civil wars, border conflicts, poverty, economic inequality, violence, and human rights violations are frequent. Civil wars span decades, resulting in the loss of millions of lives and the displacement of many more. The abduction of small girls and the forcing of young boys to become so-called 'freedom fighters' are among common social ills witnessed by civilians in those countries where there is civil war. Current conflicts in the Sudan, South Sudan, Democratic Republic of Congo, and the Central African Republic are highly likely to include such acts.

Health status of the continent

With their enormous populations, African countries have a clear need to match health resources in terms of budget, qualified health personnel, facilities, and necessary supplies to ensure the wellbeing of their people. However, a lack of essential resources is common in Africa because of its low economic and infrastructural development. Up to 62% of the African population live in slum conditions (World Health Organization

2014a). Ongoing conflicts resulting in displacement and poverty compound the problems. In 2011 Africa had the highest adult mortality rate (339 per 1000 population), maternal mortality (480 per 100,000 live births in 2010), child mortality, and malnutrition worldwide (World Health Organization 2014b). The adult literacy rate in Africa, at 63%, is the lowest in the world (World Health Organization 2014b).

In 2011, average life expectancy at birth in the African region was 56 years (World Health Organization 2014b). The corresponding figures worldwide are 67 years for Southeast Asia, 68 for the Eastern Mediterranean, and 76 years for the European, Western Pacific, and Americas regions. Mortality rates in general decreased between 1990 and 2011, but in some countries they increased during this period. Much of this is attributed to the HIV/AIDS epidemic, the resurgence of malaria and tuberculosis, the steady increase in non-communicable diseases, and increasing poverty.

Mental health services

History

The history of mental health services in Africa has been divided into four phases (Kigozi 2003):

(1) The time when dealing with the mentally ill was mostly dependent on traditional and spiritual healers.

(2) The rise of asylums mainly focusing on custodial confinement.

(3) Modern asylums like large hospitals during and soon after the colonial period.

(4) Most recently, decentralization and integration of mental health services into existing general health services which were initiated following WHO recommendations over three decades ago.

Pre-colonialism

Prior to the arrival of Europeans in Sub-Saharan Africa, the responsibility for people with mental illness lay with families, communities, and traditional healers. Often the only option available was to physically restrain the affected person. By contrast, in North Africa institutionalized mental health care existed before colonization. The mentally ill in Algeria, Tunisia, and Morocco were housed in Maristans, which had originated in Baghdad in the ninth century. In their early form they embodied many of the positive aspects of Islamic medicine, offering water therapy and utilizing soothing aromas and music. By the late nineteenth century they had become merely places to confine the insane, feared by the local population who would do everything they could to avoid sending their relatives there (Keller 2005).

Colonialism and psychiatric reform in Africa

Missionaries were the first to bring hospitals to East and West Africa, followed by the conversion of military hospitals into public hospitals with the influx of colonialists (Mahone 2006; Oyebode 2006). Asylums were built in Sierra Leone, Kenya, Uganda, Zanzibar, Nigeria, and Ghana from 1847 onwards, though many were extensions or annexes of prisons. Few offered any treatment.

In the early twentieth century the French raised a humanitarian 'call to arms' to modernize the Maristans in French North Africa, importing the asylum model that was already failing in Europe. Unfortunately this resulted in a different kind of restraint and containment. Some asylums became sites of extreme maltreatment, such as by psychiatrists in Algeria who experimented in dangerous practices on their patients and assisted the regime in interrogation and torture. In Tunisia, Mareschal allowed his patients to be used as test subjects in typhus experiments (Keller 2005).

Decolonization

In the aftermath of World War II the European nations began to slowly remove their administrations from the African continent. The newly liberated states were left with a scattering of outdated asylums and minimal mental health legislation. As Africa followed the rest of the world in the move to care in the community, new challenges emerged.

The current situation

Mental healthcare in resource-poor regions

Until the 1990s, when the concept of disability adjusted life years (DALYs) was introduced, the traditional measures of health such as morbidity and mortality had failed to show the contribution of mental disorders to the global burden of disease (GBD). Now we know that mental illnesses contribute 14% to the GBD (Prince et al. 2007). In the African Region, the contribution of neuropsychiatric disorders is estimated at 5.15% (World Health Organization 2014b). The median percentage of health budget allocated for mental health in the African Region is 0.62% while it is 5.0% in the European Region.

Policy makers and health planners remain reluctant to give mental illness parity in resource allocation. This may be for a number of reasons:

(1) Lack of awareness about the magnitude of the socio-economic burden that mental illness can bring to a country.

(2) Where survival is an uphill struggle for many, it may be difficult to place value on quality of life.

(3) Ignorance about the availability of effective interventions for mental illnesses.

(4) The attribution given to mental illnesses both by policy makers and the general public—many believe that mental illnesses are afflictions caused by supernatural forces and cannot be dealt with by modern interventions.

(5) Lack of acceptance that health is a human rights issue and that mental health is an integral part of health and wellbeing.

The WHO launched Project Atlas in 2000 to map mental health resources in the world. The latest version of the *Mental health atlas* was published in 2011. Forty-five out of the 46 African Member States that comprise the WHO African Region participated in the survey. Of these, 66% were low-income countries, 18% were lower middle-income countries, and 16% were upper middle-income countries at the time of the survey (World Health Organization 2011).

The *Mental health atlas* reported that the region has the lowest allocation of resources compared with the other WHO regions. This can be partly explained by the higher proportion of low-income countries in the region, as mental health expenditure in high-income countries was 200 times higher than that of low-income countries. Income level does not fully explain the difference, however, because the gross national incomes of the high-income countries were only 76 times higher than those of the low-income countries.

Seventy-seven per cent of Africa's mental health expenditure is spent on psychiatric hospitals. Day-care facilities, follow-up community care, and community residential facilities are scarce. Only 56% of African countries have reported that they have community mental health services (World Health Organization 2011). Even in those countries, achieving adequate population coverage has been problematic and has resulted in significant treatment gaps (Hanlon et al. 2010).

There is an extreme shortage of trained mental health workers. The global median rate of health workers in mental health is 10.7 per 100,000 population, while the lowest rate is found in the African Region, at 1.7 per 100,000 population. The number of nurses working in mental health in Sub-Saharan Africa is only 0.61 per 100,000 population and the median rate of psychiatrists is 0.05 per 100,000 population (World Health Organization 2011).

The status of mental health policy and legislation in Africa

Only 42% of African countries have a dedicated mental health policy, 44.4% have mental health legislation, and 67% have a mental health plan (World Health Organization 2011). Those countries that have no dedicated policy argue that mental health is part of general health and the overall health policy encompasses mental health. The same argument is often presented for the absence of mental health legislation. Many governments say that civil and criminal laws cover all that is needed for care provision and the protection of rights and have thus remained silent on the issue. However, in the absence of policy guides and legislation, prevention of the violation of the human rights of the mentally ill is extremely difficult. As a result, the United Nations (UN) has developed several conventions to protect the rights of people with disabilities.

Many African governments have ratified these conventions, which include the Universal Declaration of Human Rights (1948), the UN Convention on the Rights of Persons with Disabilities (UNCRPD; 2006), and the African Charter on Human and Peoples' Rights (ACHPR; 1981). These conventions are supposed to be translated into practice by signatories through their national constitutions and legislations. However, actions to this effect are minimal, particularly when it comes to protection of the rights of people with disabilities such as the mentally ill (Debebe 2013; Lund et al. 2012). UN conventions make little difference if ratification is not binding and if there are no consequences for governments that fail to translate them into action. However, the implementation of these conventions requires significant resources, which may be beyond the capacity of low-income countries.

Areas lacking mental health legislation

Where there is no mental health legislation, there is no legal procedure to follow to treat people with mental illness. Invariably, people with severe mental illnesses receive treatment against their will in both formal and informal traditional treatment sites. In countries such as Ethiopia, where there is no mental health law, people who are observed to show abnormal behaviour will be taken to a variety of places including the only specialized mental hospital, Amanuel Hospital, other general hospitals, holy water sites, churches, mosques, and witchcraft practitioners (Alem et al. 1996). For admission to Amanuel Hospital three conditions must be fulfilled: there must be a bed available, admission must be recommended by a medical officer, and there must be verbal consent from the caregiver. Consent from the patient is not required. Once admitted, treatment will be administered regardless of consent. Seclusion or the application of restraints requires no legal procedure. There is no legal counsel available. There is no privacy on the wards during clinical interviews or bathing and no place of safety to keep private property or money. Amanuel Hospital has been the backbone for the care of the mentally ill in Ethiopia for over 60 years. Unsurprisingly, a recent review of the care provided described basic human rights violations in the areas of liberty, privacy, freedom from abuse, refusal of treatment, and seeking legal counsel (Debebe 2013).

Legislation dating from the colonial period

Some lawyers regard the Mental Disorders Act of Zambia,[1] the Lunacy Act of Nigeria,[2] and the Mental Health Treatment Act of Uganda[3] as insensitive and incompatible with the modern concept of human rights (Mulumba 2007; Lund et al. 2012). The criticism starts with the terminology used. Terms which are widely accepted to be derogatory and stigmatizing, such as idiot, lunatic, and imbecile, are still used. The definition of mental disorders is not clear and is left to the discretion of medical officers and magistrates (Mulumba 2007).

The main focus of these acts is protection of the public from the mentally ill, with far less emphasis on the protection of the mentally ill from harm or violation of their rights. The issue of basic rights, such as rights to health and treatment, rehabilitation, liberty, privacy and security, protection against torture, cruel, inhumane and derogatory treatment, and the right to consent to/refuse treatment are very far from being a reality (Lund et al. 2012). These laws do not make a clear distinction between voluntary and involuntary treatment and do not oblige governments to provide the necessary resources for mental health services. Independent reviews of decisions or inspection of detention and treatment facilities are rare (Lund et al. 2012). This leaves the mentally ill vulnerable to various kinds of deprivations of basic care and violation of their rights.

---

[1] The Mental Disorders Act 1951. Cap. 305. Zambia.

[2] The Lunacy Act 1958. Cap. 112. Nigeria.

[3] The Mental Treatment Act (Revised Edition), 1964. Cap. 270. Uganda.

The Nigerian Act, for example, does not mention anything related to treatment but has much to say about detention and confinement. The procedure for detention requires that both the magistrate and a medical officer need to agree that the individual is a 'lunatic'. Furthermore, families who have mentally ill relatives can hand them over to prisons when they find it too difficult or expensive to care for them at home. These constitute a class of persons in the prison system known as 'civil lunatics'; they may be confined for unlimited periods without receiving any treatment (Westbrook 2011). The Ugandan mental health law gives power to medical officers to detain a suspected person with 'unsound mind' for 10 days without authorization from a magistrate.

There seems to be either a lack of understanding of the deficiencies of the existing mental health laws or a reluctance to revise them. The 2006 bill proposed to replace the 1951 Act of Zambia has still not been processed for the intended amendment (Lund et al. 2012). The attempt to repeal the Nigerian Lunatic Act has failed (Westbrook 2011). It took over 6 years to pass the bill that repealed the 1972 Mental Health Decree of Ghana and replace it with the current Mental Health Act in 2012 (Lund et al. 2012; Republic of Ghana 2012). Similar lengthy delays are occurring in Uganda and Malawi.

Introduction of modern mental health law in Africa

The 2002 Mental Health Act of South Africa (Republic of South Africa 2002) and the 2012 Mental Health Act of Ghana (Republic of Ghana 2012) can be cited as good examples of mental health laws, having clear provisions for care and protection of the rights of the mentally ill. They have avoided derogatory language, created a distinction between voluntary and involuntary patients with clear procedures to follow when administering treatment to involuntary patients, and made provision for review bodies to inspect facilities and review admissions or documentation. Review boards are to be established in different regions and districts for closer monitoring of services and to ensure that they maintain high standards of care and protection of the rights of the mentally ill individuals.

How community care is provided in practice

The role of the family

Families shoulder the biggest share of caring for the mentally ill in Africa (Alem 2000). Social services are not yet well developed in the continent. In most African countries, family ties and the social network are closely knit. When someone exhibits signs of mental illness, families, friends, workmates, neighbours, and even passers-by get involved in the care of that individual. This imposes a significant carer burden on families, even in rural areas where caring for such persons is shared among an extended family system (Shibre et al. 2003).

The care provided by the family in Africa could be equated to community mental health care in the West where the care is mainly left to social services. Although the close involvement of families in the care of the mentally ill in Africa is a great asset to be cherished, the socio-economic crisis those families face is beyond imagination, especially when a breadwinner is affected by mental illness. Carers may have to give up their jobs or other social roles and may suffer severe stress, with consequences for their own mental health. Urbanization across Africa is bringing new challenges as many families of patients are no longer available to provide full-time care. The cracks, long since visible, in the system of over-reliance on families and communities become in the urban setting wide crevasses into which patients are lost.

Coercion in the home

Families may keep the mentally ill member at home under restraint, often shackled, until he or she is considered to be no longer a danger to others. The care of the majority of the mentally ill in Africa falls in this category. Once the feared behaviour settles, such individuals will be released from their chains. If their family can no longer cope, people with severe mental illness will become homeless vagrants and, in addition to destitution, they will frequently suffer stigmatization and mockery and are at severe risk of illness and early death. The number of homeless mentally ill people who can be seen in towns and villages throughout the continent clearly demonstrates that this is not a rare outcome (Fekadu et al. 2014). It points to the fact that although the extensive care provided by families and communities is an extraordinary blessing in many African cultures it is not enough on its own.

The role of traditional healers

Traditional health practitioners such as herbalists, diviners, or faith healers are consulted about many problems such as bone setting, midwifery, mental health service, and AIDS, for example (Robertson 2006; Mhame et al. 2010). About 60–80% of African people consult traditional health practitioners for their primary health care.

Since mental health problems are regarded by many Africans as afflictions caused by supernatural forces, they do not believe that they should be dealt with by Western medicine (Alem et al. 1999). Seeking help from traditional health practitioners, especially from diviners, is consistent with their attribution of mental illness: 'Divination ... plays a significant role in the treatment of neurosis and helps re-trace a patient's life from its metaphysical past to how it interplays with the present and future' (Mhame et al. 2010). Users of the services of traditional healers seem to have greater satisfaction than those attending Western medical centres, despite the cost being ten- to a hundred-fold greater than conventional primary care (Robertson 2006). Patients tend to come to psychiatric hospitals after they have tried and failed all available traditional means (Alem 2002), though the reverse also happens.

Coercion by traditional health practitioners

Unfortunately, when it comes to such treatment centres, violation of the rights of the mentally ill who seek help is not uncommon. Examples of inhumane treatments include chaining, flogging, and some forms of exorcism. Figures 19.1 and 19.2 show some photographs by Robin Hammond that are described in the accompanying captions. The procedures described are regarded as therapeutic for seriously agitated patients and are usually sanctioned by the carers of those patients. Families will rent small huts close to the healer's practice, hire people to look after the patients, and present them to the traditional healers on a regular basis for treatment. More often than not, people who stay in such sites live in chains and are undernourished and unclean for unlimited periods of time.

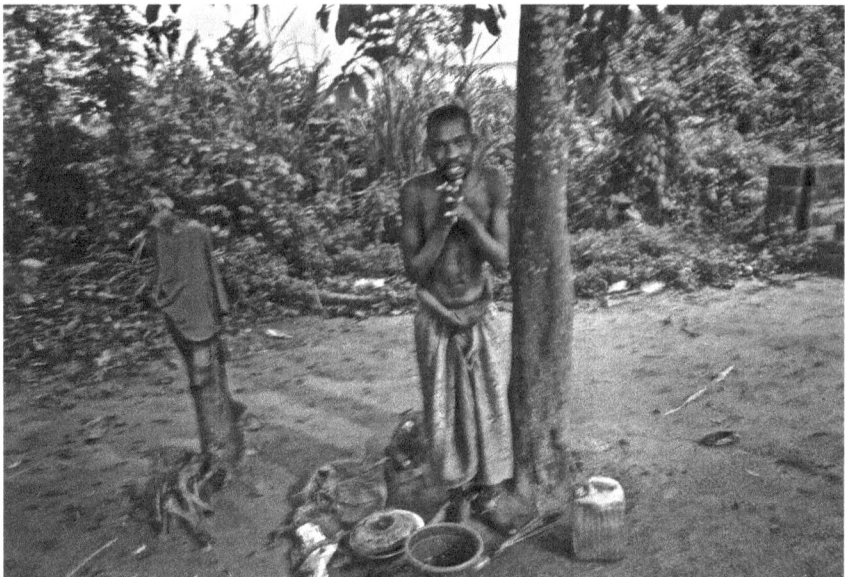

Figure 19.1 A native doctor claims to heal mental illness through the power of prayer and traditional herbal medicines. While receiving treatment, which can sometimes take months, his patients are chained to trees in his courtyard. They are not given shelter or protection from the elements. They are visibly terrified of the doctor. Away from the doctor the patients beg the photographer for food. They say they are only fed once a day, sometimes only once every 3 days. One cries and says how cold he gets and that he is attacked by mosquitoes every night. His body is covered in bites. He says they are sometimes beaten for no reason and if a piece of fruit falls from the tree and they try to eat it they are beaten. In regions where both fortune and sickness are attributed to the spirit world, mental illness is considered a curse. Spiritual remedies are often sought, and chains regularly used as restraints. The Niger Delta, Nigeria. October 2012. Photo Robin Hammond/Panos.

The WHO has been passing resolutions for almost 40 years to embrace traditional health practitioners in the health system of low- and middle-income countries. The rationale for doing this was to increase health-care coverage through partnership between the conventional health-care system and the traditional one, and also to pave the way to investigating their efficacy. Many African countries have adopted those resolutions and included them in their health legislations (Sackey and Kasilo 2010).

Community care facilities

The interpretation of the meaning of community mental health among African countries is diverse (Hanlon et al. 2010). Community mental health care akin to that seen in Western countries is probably only practised in South Africa, an upper middle-income country. For the low-income African countries, community mental health care means care provided by a non-specialist primary-care health worker. Psychiatric hospitals,

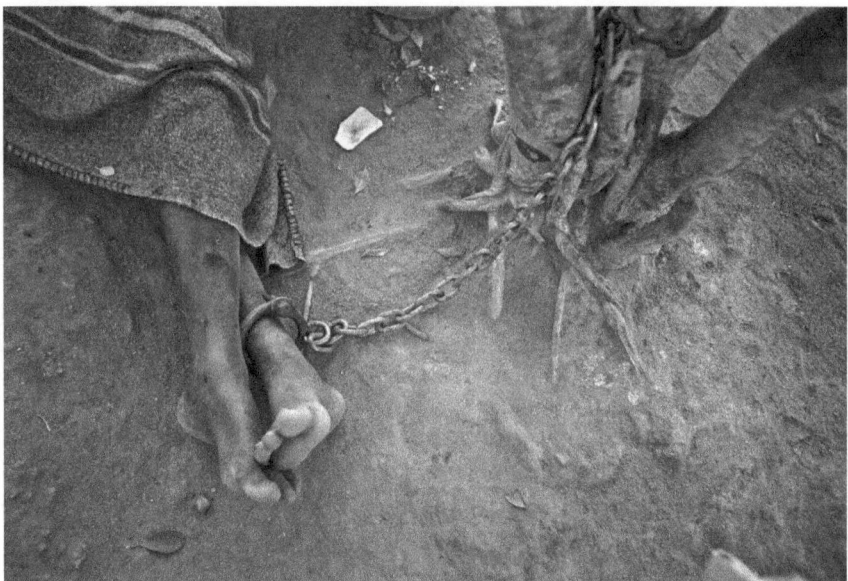

Figure 19.2 Men and women with mental illness and/or intellectual disability are shackled and locked away in Juba Central Prison for years on end. The new nation of South Sudan faces a tremendous challenge to build a modern country capable of caring for all of its citizens. Juba, Sudan. January 2011. Photo Robin Hammond/Panos.

the main care-providing facilities for the mentally ill, are not accessible to most people because of distance and the cost of transport to those cities where the hospitals are located (Alem 2002).

Coercion in the form of scarcity: lack of services

Many countries in Africa equate mental health care provided at primary-care level to a community mental health service, despite there being very little community involvement in the service provision. As a result, there is a huge treatment gap between those individuals with mental illness who need treatment and those who get it. This gap varies from 75% in South Africa to 90% in Ethiopia (Kebede et al. 2003; Lund et al. 2012). In the case of Ethiopia, a large population-based survey screening for severe mental disorders showed that 10% of people with severe mental illness had visited a psychiatric hospital at least once, but within this group of patients, only 1% were on regular treatment and follow-up (Kebede et al. 2003). It is this treatment gap that forces many families and communities into physically coercive measures as their only resort.

With inadequate training and a high case load in primary-care facilities, the health workers at some sites are limited to a biomedical model of intervention, and in some cases a negative attitude of the primary-care workers toward the mentally ill has been observed (Petersen 2000). Swartz (2002) observed the use of inappropriate medicines because of lack of competency. There is very little follow-up in the primary-care setting and a significant proportion of patients default on treatment (Freeman et al. 1999).

Some countries, like Uganda, provide free medical treatment to all patients with mental illnesses. However, since shortages of medication are common, the only option may be to buy medicines from private pharmacies, which is not affordable for many. Shortages of medicines are common in all low-income African countries.

Challenges facing mental health workers in Africa

Stigma

Stigma has dogged the development of mental health services in Africa in a variety of ways over the centuries. Many of the colonial leaders of mental health reforms in Africa were convinced of the inferiority of the African mind. This false belief allowed for the emergence of different care pathways for European settlers and indigenous populations and was used to justify ongoing occupation and harsh responses to anti-colonial rebellions (Keller 2005; Mahone 2006; Oyebode 2006).

Nowadays, the stigma comes more from within the cultures themselves. Even professionals may hold beliefs that are inconsistent with evidence-based medicine. A survey of Nigerian medical and nursing students (Iheanacho 2014) found that 65% of students at Ibadan Medical School (a regional leader in psychiatric research) believed that mental illness was God's punishment, while 21% believed it was caused by possession of by evil spirit. In Owerri Medical School, where there is far less psychiatric teaching, these figures were 84% and 47%, respectively. In countries where suicide is illegal, it is thought that there is a significant group of patients suffering in silence, afraid to consult a health-care provider because of the unacceptability of suicidal ideation. The effect of such beliefs is to raise even more barriers to people accessing the limited mental health-care facilities available.

At a societal and political level, stigma results in non-prioritizing of mental health policies, legislation, and training. For example, the Ugandan Mental Health Bill has been struggling to reach completion for 10 years (Ssebunnya et al. 2010), with the Finance Minister not convinced that it is worth the cost. Poor resources make it impossible to fund formal research to inform the new mental health law and some stakeholders do not respond at all when called upon.

Training

In the majority of low- and middle-income countries around the globe mental illnesses are not properly diagnosed or treated. Africa is no exception to this. There is a lack of knowledge about the burden of mental illness and its treatment. This is coupled with shortage of resources, a large burden of disease from preventable communicable diseases, and a growing burden of non-communicable life-threatening diseases such as hypertension and diabetes in the African continent. In the face of this, the issue of training psychiatrists is likely to remain very low on the health intervention priority list.

As a result many countries in Africa have tried to decentralize the service to regional and district hospitals by training mid-level health workers (psychiatric nurses and medical officers). This is thought by many to have brought great improvements in service provision to those countries where this has been put in place (Alem 2004; Kigozi

2007). Unfortunately, high turnover of trained workers and a lack of adequate support from the health system remain great challenges for the continuity of the service at this level.

There have been similar difficulties in rolling out a WHO package called the Mental Health Gap Action Programme (mhGAP). This was developed to help primary care workers in low- and middle-income countries to identify and treat priority mental health conditions. It has been piloted successfully in several African countries, but scaling up has not been easy because of lack of resources to train the primary-care workers and to supervise and monitor the intervention.

Economic challenges

Caring for the mentally ill and protecting their rights demands resources. Even in countries that have mental health policies and better mental health legislations, such as South Africa and Ghana, there are challenges to fully translate intentions into practice, both in the provision of the necessary care and in the protection of the rights of people with mental illness (Lund et al. 2012). In addition to the large resources needed make the necessary services available to communities, the cost of setting up mental health authorities, review boards, and tribunals to monitor the standard of care is immense (Lund et al. 2012). Thus, just putting legislation in place will not guarantee high-quality mental health service and protection of human rights.

Lack of community care facilities and pressure on families

As stated earlier, in the absence of community mental health services, many people with mental illness are kept at home and thus away from scrutiny. It is not difficult to imagine that coercive measures are being practised in those environments where there is no easy means of tranquillizing or calming disturbed cases.

In most cases this is done in good faith and to alleviate the suffering of a family member. However, it may be regarded as a violation of human rights and thus unlawful. Here comes the dilemma: families, the main and largest care-providing institutions in the continent, are going to be considered as the people who infringe the rights of the mentally ill while they are trying to help. In countries where there are limited resources and no social services to provide care and support to people with mental illness, what is the alternative? If the law tries to prohibit communities from such benevolent actions what would be the fate of that particular individual? One needs to answer this question before applying the Western concept of human rights violations. Of course it is undeniable that human rights issues are universal irrespective of colour, race, or social class. But the socio-economic realities of societies must dictate applications of conventions.

Summary

Mental health care on the African continent is plagued by a number of difficulties that range from a scarcity of resources to the stigma about and misunderstanding of mental illness itself. Some of these problems are not unique to mental health. A significant number of African countries are struggling to provide their population with adequate transport, sanitation, and communication infrastructure, to say nothing of those countries in the midst of civil war. Solutions will need comprehensive initiatives with sufficient funding from governments that have the organizational capacity to make such changes. It can therefore be expected that progress in these areas will be a slow process, affected as much by the economic situation of individual nations as by their policies.

In the meantime, advocates for sufferers of mental illness struggle to ensure that they receive the parity of care they deserve, overshadowed as they are by the physical health crises to which Africa is no stranger. While bills to replace or create adequate mental health legislation stutter through parliamentary processes, families are left shouldering the burden of caring for their mentally ill relatives with minimal support or guidance in doing so. Whilst one cannot ignore that coercion frequently occurs within the homes of carers, they are often left with impossible choices. Most people would acknowledge that none of the options available are desirable, but given that the alternative may be sending the mentally ill onto the streets or into prisons, being tied up at home may ultimately be the least restrictive option.

It is small wonder that traditional healers continue to play a central role in the treatment of mental illnesses in a continent where many countries have perhaps a handful of psychiatrists, most of whom are largely inaccessible to the majority. The sometimes harsh or brutal methods used by traditional healers, whilst perhaps less easily understood than those reported in family homes, could be seen as an extension of the community's desperation; a cry for help when other options have been exhausted.

In the few centres that providing community mental health care in Africa, the most common form of coercion is the product of scarcity: scarcity of human resources, of training, of medication, and of basic infrastructure. The result is an absence either of consistent community mental health care or of choice about what form the care will take.

There are signs of positive changes occurring: the success of the mhGAP programme, where it has been piloted, the evidence of less stigmatizing beliefs about mental illness found in health-care students who have received psychiatric training, and the introduction of modern mental health legislation in Ghana and South Africa. It remains to be seen whether the rest of the continent will be able to learn from and build on these success stories.

References

Alem A (2000). Human rights and psychiatric care in Africa with particular reference to the Ethiopian situation. *Acta Psychiatrica Scandinavica*, **101**:93–96.

Alem A (2002). Community-based vs hospital-based mental health care: the case of Africa (commentary). *World Psychiatry*, **2**:98–99.

Alem A (2004). Psychiatry in Ethiopia: country profile. *International Bulletin of the Royal College of Psychiatrists*, **4**:8–10.

Alem A, Jacobsson L, Desta M (1996). Perception of mental disorders and their treatment in central Ethiopia. *Yearbook of cross-cultural medicine and psychotherapy*, pp. 105–119. Berlin: VWB—Verlag für Wissenschaft und Bildung.

Alem A, Jacobsson L, Araya M, et al. (1999). How are mental disorders seen and where is help sought in a rural Ethiopian community? A key informant study in Butajira, Ethiopia. *Acta Psychiatrica Scandinavica*, **100**:40–47.

Debebe A (2013). Behind closed doors: the human rights conditions of persons with mental disabilities in Ethiopian psychiatric facilities. *Jimma University Journal of Law*, 5. Available at: http://ju.edu.et/jl/sites/default/files/Aytenew.pdf

Fekadu A, Hanlon C, Gebre-Eyesus E, et al. (2014). Burden of mental disorders and unmet needs among street homeless people in Addis Ababa, Ethiopia. *BMC Medicine*, **12**:138.

Freeman M, Lee T, Vivian W (1999). Evaluation of mental health services in the Free State. Part IV. Family burden and perspectives. *South African Medical Journal*, **89**:316–318.

Hanlon C, Wondimagegn D, Alem A (2010). Lessons learned in developing community mental health care in Africa. *World Psychiatry*, **9**:185–189.

Iheanacho T, Marienfeld C, Stefanovics E, et al. (2014). Attitudes toward mental illness and changes associated with a brief educational intervention for medical and nursing students in Nigeria. *Academic Psychiatry*, **38**:320–324.

Kebede D, Alem A, Shibre T, et al. (2003). Onset and clinical course of schizophrenia in Butajira, Ethiopia. *Social Psychiatry and Psychiatric Epidemiology*, **38**:625–631.

Keller RC (2005). Pinel in the Maghreb: liberation, confinement, and psychiatric reform in French North Africa. *Bulletin of the History of Medicine*, **79**:459–499.

Kigozi F (2003). Challenges to the current provision of mental health services and development of psychiatry in Africa. *South African Journal of Psychiatry*, **9**:27–29.

Kigozi F (2007). Integrating mental health into primary health care—Uganda's experience. *South African Psychiatry Review*, **10**:17–19.

Lund C, Sutcliffe T, Flisher AJ, et al. (2012). Protecting the rights of the mentally ill in poorly resourced settings: experiences from four African countries. In: *Mental health and human rights: vision, praxis and courage* (ed. M Dudley, D Silove, F Gale), pp. 527–537. Sydney: Oxford University Press.

Mahone S (2006). Psychiatry in the East African colonies: a background to confinement *International Review of Psychiatry*, **18**:327–332.

Mhame PP, Busia K, Kasilo OMJ (2010). Clinical practices of African traditional medicine. *Africa Health Monitor*, issue no. 13:33–39.

Mulumba M (2007). *Analysis of the Uganda Mental Treatment Act from a human rights and public health perspective*. Available at SSRN: http://ssrn.com/abstract=1006230 or http://dx.doi.org/10.2139/ssrn.1006230

National Geographic Society (2014). *Africa: human geography*. National Geographic Education. Available at: http://education.nationalgeographic.com/education/encyclopedia/africa-human-geography/ (accessed 24 May 2014).

Oyebode F (2006). History of psychiatry in West Africa. *International Review of Psychiatry*, **18**:319–325.

Petersen I (2000). Comprehensive integrated primary mental health care for South Africa. Pipedream or possibility? *Social Science and Medicine*, **51**:321–334.

Prince M, Patel V, Saxena S, et al. (2007). No health without mental health. *The Lancet*, **370**:859–877.

Republic of Ghana (2012). *Mental Health Act, 2012. The eight hundred and forty-sixth act of the parliament of the Republic of Ghana, 31st May, 2012.*

Republic of South Africa (2002). *Mental Health Care Act: Republic of South Africa, Vol. 449, Cape Town 6 November 2002, no. 24024.* Available at: http://www.gov.za/sites/www.gov.za/files/a17-02.pdf

Robertson BA (2006). Does the evidence support collaboration between psychiatry and traditional healers? Findings from three South African studies. *South African Psychiatry Review,* 9:87–90.

Sackey EKA, Kasilo OMJ (2010). Intellectual property approaches to the protection of traditional knowledge in the African Region. *Africa Health Monitor,* issue no. 13:89–102.

Shibre T, Kebede D, Alem A, et al. (2003). Schizophrenia: illness impact on family members in a traditional society—rural Ethiopia. *Social Psychiatry and Psychiatric Epidemiology,* 38:27–34.

Ssebunnya J, Kigozi F, Kizza D, et al. (2010). Integration of mental health into primary healthcare in a rural district in Uganda. MHaPP Research Programme Consortium. *African Journal of Psychiatry,* 13:128–131.

Swartz L (2002). Integrating services, marginalizing patients: psychiatric patients and primary health care in South Africa. *Transcultural Psychiatry,* 39:155–172.

Westbrook AH (2011). Mental health legislation and compulsory commitment in Nigeria: a call for reform. *Washington Global Studies Law Review,* 10(2):397.

World Health Organization (2011). *Mental health atlas 2011.* Geneva: World Health Organization.

World Health Organization (2014a). *Africa Heath Observatory. Analytical summary—health status and trends.* WHO Regional Office for Africa. Available at: http://www.aho.afro.who.int/profiles_information/index.php/AFRO:Analytical_summary_-_Health_Status_and_Trends/ (accessed 30 May 2014).

World Health Organization (2014b). *Atlas of African health statistics 2014.* Brazzaville, Congo: WHO Regional Office for Africa.

World Population Review (2015). *World population 2015.* Available at: http://www.worldpopulationreview.com/continents/africa-population/ (accessed 8 February 2016).

World Population Statistics (2014). *Africa population 2014.* Available at: http://www.worldpopulationstatistics.com/world-population-2014/ (accessed 24 May 2014).

Chapter 20

Compulsory community mental health care: Oceania

Anthony J. O'Brien

Introduction

This chapter covers community-based coercion in Australasia and the Oceania region. The countries covered are a grouping of convenience rather than representing a unified geopolitical entity; hence the chapter covers countries with quite diverse histories, socio-economic structures, cultures, and health systems. Eight of Oceania's 16 sovereign countries are covered to illustrate coercion in community mental health. The remaining nine countries of Oceania are dependencies administered by Australia, Britain, France, New Zealand, or the United States. Coverage of the countries of Oceania is limited by a paucity of published material.

The discussion in this chapter is centred around two aspects: (1) Australia and New Zealand, which have well-established and comprehensive mental health systems including community treatment order (CTO) regimes; and (2) countries which either have no form of compulsory community treatment or (as in the case of Fiji, Tonga, and Samoa) legislative provision but limited service provision to support it. The outline of individual countries is followed by a discussion of current issues in the use of coercion in community mental health. A major point of discussion is the variation between coercion in high-income developed countries and developing countries. High-income countries, through the provision for CTOs, place a heavy reliance on specialist mental health services and formal coercion through legislation, whereas in less developed countries there is greater reliance on providing mental health care within the primary-care sector and correspondingly less emphasis on legislation. An issue that confronts the whole Oceania region is its response to the 2007 United Nations Convention on the Rights of Persons with Disabilities (UNCRPD). The absence of an Oceania or Pacific international mental health body means that it is difficult to coordinate a regional response, which limits the potential to establish a tribunal to hear cases of alleged inappropriate coercion (Perlin 2012, 2013).

Data sources

Data for each country have been obtained from the following sources: population, gross domestic product (GDP) and country income status (World Bank); proportion of GDP spent on health (World Health Organization, WHO); geography, politics, and social data from various sources. Data on service availability are taken from the WHO *Mental health atlas* (World Health Organization 2011). Dollar figures for economic data are given in US dollars (USD).

The Oceania region

The Oceania region covers a vast area of ocean and includes numerous island states, some of which themselves comprise large numbers of islands. Populations of the countries of Oceania vary from 1600 (Niue) to 23 million (Australia), with the total population of the region estimated at 37 million. Almost all countries of Oceania are low or low to middle income, with only Australia and New Zealand being classified by the World Bank as high-income countries. The health budget across Oceania countries is highly variable. Of those countries included in the WHO's 2013 survey of health spending, the proportion of GDP spent on health varies from 4.2% (Fiji) to 17.6% (Marshall Islands), with the industrialized countries of Australia and New Zealand devoting 9.0% and 10.1%, respectively, of their GDP to health (World Health Organization 2013). There is also significant variation across the region in the availability of psychiatric hospital beds, community services, psychiatrists and other health professionals, and medicines (World Health Organization 2011). Australia and New Zealand established national networks of psychiatric hospitals in the nineteenth century, and in the twentieth century pursued policies of deinstitutionalization and the development of community mental health services (MacKinnon and Coleborne 2003). Under colonial rule some of the smaller countries of Oceania also established psychiatric hospitals in the nineteenth century. In several cases these hospitals continue to provide a significant component of the mental health service (Mahone and Vaughan 2007).

In Oceania most mental health care is provided in the government sector, although Australia also has significant private mental health services. Australian mental health legislation is enacted in the eight states and territories, whereas in New Zealand and all other Oceania countries that have legislation there is a single mental health act for the entire country. CTOs have been part of the mental health landscape in Australia and New Zealand since the late 1980s (McIvor 1998) and several Australian jurisdictions have recently revised their legislation to include new CTO provisions. Fiji also makes provision for CTOs, and Samoa and Tonga have recently adopted new mental health legislation that includes CTOs (Fadgen 2013).

Australia and New Zealand

Australia and New Zealand are Oceania's two most developed countries. Both are classified by the World Bank as high-income countries, and are ranked by the Organisation for Economic Cooperation and Development at sixth and twentieth, respectively, in rankings of GDP per capita (http://www.oecd.org/). Both countries have a dedicated mental health sector (including statutory and non-statutory services) and a large mental health workforce, including specialist addiction, age-related, and other services. In addition there is a relatively high, if variable, capacity for mental health response within the primary-care sector, including mental health specialists. Both countries have seen several iterations of national mental health plans, as well as dedicated plans for areas such as mental health promotion, indigenous mental health, suicide prevention, and addictions. Australia and New Zealand also provide programmes of mental health awareness and stigma reduction. Australia has a Mental Health Commission, while New Zealand's Mental Health Commission has been absorbed into a wider Disability Rights Office. Leverage of the type commonly used in the USA (Monahan 2011), for example having a representative payee to manage benefit payments, landlord's requirement for treatment compliance, and a court requirement to comply with psychiatric treatment as an alternative to imprisonment, is not commonly practised in Australia and New Zealand, although mental health courts are available in some Australian settings and are in the early stages of implementation in New Zealand.

The most significant difference between the two countries is that Australia has a dual private and public health-care system, while New Zealand's health-care system is substantially government funded.

Australia

Australia is the most populous country in the Oceania region, with a population of 23 million in 2015 and a GDP of USD 1.6 trillion. The country has a federal system of government, with the eight states and territories exercising considerable autonomy in political governance. Australia devotes 9.0% of GDP to health, and 7.6% of its health budget to mental health. There are 39 mental health beds and 4.65 mental health outpatient facilities per 100,000 population. Deinstitutionalization is well advanced in Australia, with a large proportion of beds in general rather than psychiatric hospitals.

Each state or territory provides its own mental health legislation, and three jurisdictions have revised their legislation in the past 3 years. CTOs are provided for in each Mental Health Act. A recent survey reported that rates of CTOs varied between 30.2 per 100,000 population (Tasmania) to 98.8 per 100,000 population (Victoria) (Light et al. 2011). Rates are among the highest in the world and are rising, creating human rights concerns for mental health stakeholders (Light et al. 2011). Despite the high rate of use of CTOs in Australia they are not prominent in mental health policy documents (Light et al. 2012), indicating that they are considered as a clinical tool rather than a policy initiative.

The high use of CTOs in Australia is interesting in light of the imperative of evidence-based medicine. Consistent with international experience, evaluation of CTOs in Australia has yielded mixed results. A study examining the impact of CTOs on readmission rates in Western Australia (Preston et al. 2002) found increased rates for both treatment and control groups, with those on CTOs also showing increased outpatient contacts. A subsequent study found CTOs to be associated with increased admissions (Kisely et al. 2004). A later study in the same state found reduced hospital stays when CTOs were used as a form of conditional release (Segal et al. 2009). The same study concluded that any effect on readmission was dependent on services provided and on patient selection. In the state of Victoria, a matched comparison study (Segal and Burgess 2006) found a reduction in admissions associated with increased outpatient service use for those on CTOs. The most recent study, conducted in Queensland, compared matched voluntary and involuntary samples using the Health of the Nations Outcome Scale to measure outcomes, and found no difference between the groups (Kisely et al. 2014).

Australians subject to mental health legislation have the right of appeal to a review tribunal or similar body (Carney 2012), although there are concerns about the length of time taken for appeals to be heard (Ryan et al. 2010). Powers of review tribunals vary across jurisdictions, as does the time required for scheduling hearings. Mental health courts have been established in several Australian jurisdictions where they are reported to have been effective in diverting people with mental illness from the criminal justice system and into the health-care system (Richardson and McSherry 2010). Judges in Australian mental health courts show a greater focus on procedural rights and are more solution-focused than their US counterparts (Richardson et al. 2013). Australian observers note the need for more a comprehensive evaluation of mental health courts (Richardson and McSherry 2010). Australia has a range of related legislation, different from one region to another, covering aspects of health and rights, such as guardianship, human rights, and health-care rights.

New Zealand

New Zealand, with a population of 4.5 million, is a country comprising two major islands and is situated 2100 km from its nearest neighbour Australia, with which it shares a similar experience of colonization as well as a recent history of agricultural and industrial development. The GDP of New Zealand is USD 185 billion, of which 10.1% is spent on health. New Zealand spends 10% of its health budget on mental health. All former psychiatric hospitals in New Zealand have been closed, and the services are now predominantly community focused, with 21 inpatient beds per 100,000 population. WHO data on outpatient facilities are not available, but a recent report indicates that 64% of mental health contacts take place in community settings (Ministry of Health 2014a).

New Zealand's current mental health legislation was passed in 1992, with a minor revision in 1999. There is currently no political initiative to revise the legislation. New Zealand's legislation provides for CTOs (Dawson 2005) and they are used in every health district in New Zealand. Official reports indicate wide regional variation in the use of CTOs, with rates varying between 46 and 177 per 100,000 (Ministry of Health 2014b). Rates have increased rapidly since 2009 (O'Brien 2014) and recent data suggest that much of this increase is due to increased use of CTOs with the indigenous Maori population (Ministry of Health 2014b). A body of research into CTOs is developing (see Dawson 2005; O'Brien et al. 2011; Newton-Howes et al. 2014), although so far there has been no systematic evaluation of the clinical outcomes of CTOs. An analysis of New Zealand's mental health legislation by legal, clinical, policy, and service user experts covers issues from the definition of mental disorder to capacity, review processes, use of legislation with Maori, and human rights (Dawson and Gledhill 2013). As in Australia, CTOs receive little comment in mental health policy documents despite apparently being a mainstay of community treatment. No data are available on the length of time patients spend on CTOs.

Patients subject to New Zealand mental health legislation have access to legal representation and to a review tribunal which has power to order release from compulsory treatment. An analysis of tribunal decisions from 1992 to 2011 found that only 7% of cases resulted in the patient's release, while 45% of applications were withdrawn prior to the hearing (Thom 2014). Applications from patients under CTOs were underrepresented, indicating either that patients were not dissatisfied with their legal status or that access to review is limited in community settings.

Mental health courts are an emerging policy innovation in New Zealand, with two alcohol and drug courts established in 2012 and currently undergoing evaluation (Richardson and McSherry, 2010). In addition to mental health legislation, other legal provisions include guardianship for those lacking capacity, rights under a health and disability code, and a bill of rights.

The developing nations of Oceania

The Oceania region contains many countries which received independence from colonial and post-colonial governments in the second half of the twentieth century. The developing nations of Oceania are typically small, with relatively small land areas dispersed over vast areas of ocean. These geographical features, combined with limited financial resources, make for major difficulties in communication, travel, and service delivery. In some countries language is an additional issue, especially in the Melanesian countries where it is not uncommon for there to be up to a hundred different languages. Under colonial rule, mental health was typically a low priority, with provision limited to hospital services. This situation has been slow to change following independence. In recent years the WHO has supported the development of mental health services in the Oceania region through its agency PIMHNet (World Health Organization/University of Auckland 2005), programmes of professional volunteers, and through policy advice. Countries such as Samoa and Vanuatu have developed mental health policies for the first time, although their implementation is constrained by the small numbers of specialist mental health professionals. Literature on mental health in the island states of Oceania countries is extremely limited and most information comes from official reports from monitoring bodies such as the WHO.

Fiji

The Republic of Fiji is a former British colony made up of over 300 islands dispersed over 18,000 km^2 of ocean. Fiji is an upper middle-income country, rich in natural resources, with a GDP of USD 3.8 billion. The country spends 4% of GDP on health. Fiji's population of 887,000 is 49% Melanesian (with some Polynesian ancestry), with a 46% ethnic Indian population as a consequence of the country's nineteenth-century history of indentured labour. The population is concentrated on Fiji's two main islands, which are home to 87% of the Fijian people. Fiji is subject to natural disasters such as floods, storms, and the threat of tsunamis.

Fiji has experienced considerable political instability in the past 30 years. Four coups have taken place, the most recent in 2006, which led to its suspension from the Commonwealth, international sanctions, and concerns about human rights. In 2014 the country held its first democratic elections since 1987.

Mental health services were first established in Fiji when a lunatic asylum opened its doors in 1884 (Leckie 2007). This asylum later became the St Giles hospital and still provides services for 136 inpatients. This equates to 15 beds per 100,000 population.

Services are centralized around St Giles, with community follow-up through public health services (Chang 2011). Some patients are admitted to general hospitals where they are managed on medical wards. A national mental health and suicide prevention policy was released in 2015. Fiji has limited mental health personnel, with few psychiatrists and small numbers of mental health nurses. Primary-care staff have little mental health training, but are able to make referrals to specialist services. Fijians make use of traditional health practitioners, often on the basis of beliefs that mental illness is caused by failure to fulfil customary obligations, curses, or demonic possession (Chang 2011).

Fiji has a recent mental health statute, the Mental Health Decree (2010). The Decree makes extensive provision for compulsory mental health care, including CTOs. The legislation is quite innovative, including provisions for advance directives, anti-discrimination clauses, a set of principles, and a review board with powers to end a period of compulsory treatment.

Papua New Guinea

The Independent State of Papua New Guinea is the Pacific's largest nation, with a population of 7.5 million and a total land area of over 485,000 km². The country is part of the Melanesian Archipelago and comprises 600 islands lying 160 km south of the Equator, and stretching from Indonesia in the west to Fiji in the east. Papua New Guinea is culturally and linguistically diverse, with over 800 languages and many distinct cultural and ethnic groups. Administratively the country is divided into four regions and 20 provinces. More than 80% of the population live in rural districts, some of which are extremely remote. Papua New Guinea is vulnerable to natural disasters such as volcanoes, earthquakes, and landslides. Following independence from Australia in 1975, Papua New Guinea has seen considerable civil unrest, including an attempt by the Bougainville region to gain independence, followed by an Australian police presence. With a GDP of USD 15.3 billion, Papua New Guinea is classified as a lower middle-income country. Health spending accounts for 5% of GDP.

A WHO report paints a bleak picture of mental health in Papua New Guinea (Adu Krow et al. 2013). There is a limited mental health service, especially in remote rural areas, and problems of substance use and sexual violence are endemic. The Laloki Psychiatric Hospital, which opened in 1967, is Papua New Guinea's only psychiatric inpatient facility. The hospital provides for 60 patients, but there are few specialist mental health clinicians to staff the hospital and conditions are often overcrowded. The Port Moresby General Hospital provides an additional 13 beds, but it too is overcrowded. Outpatient services are provided from the general hospital, but there are no formal community mental health services. Traditional practitioners provide some response to mental health problems, but the extent and quality of these services is not well known. Legislation in the form of sections of the Public Health Act (1973) refers to persons of unsound mind but makes little explicit provision for treatment or protection of rights. The WHO *Mental health atlas* (World Health Organization 2011) notes that a new Mental Health Act has been submitted to the Papua New Guinea Legislative Council for approval. A national mental health plan is in place and was most recently revised in 2010. Mental health is not specifically referenced in the health policy of Papua New Guinea.

In the absence of a robust mental health service or policy, heavy reliance is placed on traditional beliefs, which in Papua New Guinea include sorcery. The Sorcery Act (1971), which provided a defence against criminal charges, including murder, was repealed in 2013. Despite this, sorcery is widely practised, especially on people suspected to be mentally ill (Chappell 2010). Sorcery is also believed to be a cause of mental illness (Koka et al. 2004). Another source of mental health response is the primary-care sector. However, a survey of health workers found a low level of confidence in their diagnostic and treatment skills, including their knowledge of sorcery (Koka et al. 2004).

Samoa

Samoa is a tropical island state comprising the western Samoan Islands, with a population of 192,000 and a GDP of USD 802 million. Classified as a lower middle-income country, Samoa has a history since colonization of overtly coercive mental health care and custodial treatment. However Samoa also has well-developed family, community, and social networks. A hospital ward built in 1970 is considered inappropriately sited to provide mental health care but remains an important part of the mental health service system of Samoa, especially when the preferred practice of family-based care is not sufficient. Mental health care is accorded low priority in Samoa, with the annual mental health budget being barely adequate to cover mental health services.

Two main areas of reform characterize current mental health care in Samoa. They are the re-emergence in the 1980s of family-focused mental health care which gives priority to Samoan cultural values, and in the early twenty-first century the development of a national mental health policy and revised mental health legislation, including CTOs (Enoka et al. 2013). The service is led by mental health nurses and follows a partnership (*Aiga*) model in which the nurse and family share cultural observances, storytelling aimed at understanding the family's beliefs and values, and development of a family-focused plan of care (Enoka et al. 2013). In more remote villages non-specialist community nurses are the first point of contact for mental health issues, with quarterly visits to all islands by a mental health nurse. A national mental health policy developed in 2006 provides the policy direction for mental health services (Government of Samoa 2006), although resources to implement that policy are scarce (Tone 2007). Following adoption of the national mental health policy, and in pursuit of its objective of community-focused care, Samoa passed new mental health legislation in 2007, including a provision for CTOs (Fadgen 2013). The 2007 legislation was based on the legislation of South Australia. Anecdotal evidence suggests that CTOs are little used in practice, although the inpatient provisions of the same Act are used to provide compulsory treatment in Samoa's mental health unit (Enoka et al. 2013). There is no literature available on formal or informal coercion in community mental health care, but in light of the family focus of mental health care it is likely that any coercion is family mediated, with professional support from the small specialist and non-specialist nursing workforce.

Tonga

The Kingdom of Tonga is a constitutional monarchy comprising 176 islands with a total land area of 750 km^2 scattered over 700,000 km^2 of ocean. The country is an upper middle-income country with a population of 106,000, and a GDP of USD 466 million. The dispersed nature of the Tongan Islands make for difficulties in providing health and mental services, a problem Tonga has in common with its Pacific neighbours. Tonga is heavily reliant on overseas aid and experiences shortages of most health professionals. A recent democracy movement has altered the balance of the Tongan legislature and has the potential to provide greater support for human rights in Tonga, including for people with mental illness. Tonga has no written mental health policy and mental health is not generally accorded a high priority in Tongan health policy.

Early mental health response in Tonga was mainly the responsibility of the police, with a health ministry adopting a formal role during the 1970s (Fadgen 2013). A mental health unit was established in 1977; earlier reference to a 'lunatic asylum' is likely to have been to places at either the general hospital or the prison for people with mental illness.

A 1948 Lunatics Detention Act provided Tonga's first formal mental health framework and provided for people with mental illness to be detained in any premises as designated by the Privy Council. In practice, the prison was the default option. The Act was replaced with the 1992 Mental Health Act which introduced changes in terminology and extended the range of legislation to include drug addiction. Fadgen (2013) noted that the law was unworkable and was little used. Against a background of general health policy reform, the legislation was further updated in 2001, with a statute, the Mental Health Act (2001) based on the 1986 Victorian (Australia) legislation that includes CTOs. However, protective exclusions, such as promiscuity and political beliefs, are not included in the Tongan legislation. Anecdotal evidence suggests that the CTO provision is rarely used even though most mental health care in Tonga is primarily provided in a community setting. The Mental Health Act establishes a review tribunal with powers to discharge a patient from compulsory status.

Mental health response in Tonga begins at the community level where care is usually provided by family members and traditional healers. The next level of care is that provided by the general hospital which provides a small number of mental health beds. There are 22 inpatient mental health beds, but minimal community mental health services. A sole psychiatrist and a small staff provide specialist mental health care. A small non-government sector provides some mental health promotion services and policy advocacy.

Solomon Islands

The Solomon Islands is one of the larger island nations of the South Pacific with a population of 573,000 and a GDP of USD 1 billion. In recent years the Solomon Islands has been beset by civil unrest that has brought the country to the brink of collapse. The conflict led to large-scale population displacement and resulted in an Australian-brokered peace deal following a military presence (Jeffery 2013). The country shares with other Pacific countries the challenges of providing mental health services to a dispersed, mainly rural population, with limited financial and professional resources.

Professional mental health services are provided by a single psychiatrist and 11 specialist mental health nurses (Singh and Orataloa, 2011). Some informal mental health care is provided through churches and traditional healers. Hospital services date from the establishment of an asylum in 1950, and more recently have been provided from a 20-bed psychiatric unit and a four-bed acute unit. Outpatient services are provided from this hospital base, but Singh and Orataloa (2011) report that there is little in the way of community services. Families are involved in care following discharge of patients from hospital, and there is some outreach into provincial areas from the outpatient clinics. Mental health legislation dates from 1970, although it was amended in 1995 to include community and primary-care services. There is no provision for CTOs.

Vanuatu

Vanuatu is an island state of 258,000 people situated in the South Pacific. The GDP of Vanuatu is USD 828 million. The country consists of 83 islands spread over 200,000 km² of ocean, with 75% of the population living in rural areas. Vanuatu is a lower middle-income country with an economy based on subsistence and small-scale agriculture. It has a limited health infrastructure, spending just 3.6% of GDP on health. Mental health care is provided by non-specialist staff working at a primary-care level, and it has only recently received significant attention from government. In 2010 there were only four mental health inpatient beds in the country (George 2010). The first ever national mental health plan was launched in 2009 (Blignault et al. 2011) following support from PIMHNet (Benson et al. 2011). Since that time four mental health clinics have been established at regional hospitals and education has been provided for the primary-care staff who provide most mental health care (Benson et al. 2011). Traditional beliefs about the cause of mental illness are prevalent, and include weak faith, sin, curses, and demonic possession (George 2010). For most people, attendance at a traditional healer is the first response to symptoms of mental illness, followed by consultation with a church leader. Mental health legislation in Vanuatu is rudimentary and reflects a coercive and controlling model of care. The 2006 Mental Hospital Act establishes criteria for involuntary hospitalization. There is no statutory limit to the period of hospitalization and no provision for compulsory outpatient treatment. The Mental Hospital Act contains no provisions aimed at ensuring patients' access to legal advice or clinical review. Efforts to improve access to mental health care in Vanuatu focus on the primary-care workforce, rather than on establishing a workforce of mental health professionals (Benson et al. 2011). A recent initiative has been the establishment of a fellowship aimed at providing a senior nurse with advanced education and clinical experience through an Australian university nursing programme (Webster et al. 2013). This programme resulted in the nurse returning to Vanuatu and applying his new knowledge in the country's hospital and community outreach programme, and through teaching in the Vanuatu Centre for Nurse Education.

Discussion

There are clearly wide differences in mental health practice between countries in the Oceania region. Differences in mental health services between the two most developed countries, Australia and New Zealand, and their Oceania neighbours, illustrate that provision of mental health care reflects the macro-economic context of each country, as well as its social and political infrastructure. The less developed countries of Oceania place a much greater reliance on the role of family and community in mental health care, partly out of economic necessity and partly out of a recognition that family and community are critical resources in protecting, promoting, and restoring mental health. Similarly, much of the mental health care in less developed countries is provided in the primary-care sector, usually by non-specialists with varying degrees of knowledge, training, and confidence in managing mental health issues.

The concept of 'coercion' in mental health care derives from a large corpus of Western scholarship and is embedded in Western notions of rationalism and the primacy of the individual. Such notions may not be applicable in developing countries which are frequently family oriented and with enduring adherence to traditional cultural values, even under the colonial legacy (Poltorak 2013). Like other Western concepts, coercion requires interpretation in specific cultural contexts. It may also be the case that where it is culturally more acceptable to use informal coercion by families and communities there is less need for, or willingness to use, formal measures such as CTOs.

Formal models of coercion are not the only means by which people may be subjected to interpersonal pressures which limit their autonomy (Burns et al. 2011). Although community coercion is often associated with formal measures such as CTOs, people with mental illness have traditionally been subjected to various forms of pressure or leverage by families and communities (Suzuki 2006). Informal coercion may include verbal pressure from family members, threats of committal or withdrawal of emotional support, and legal proceedings in respect of property. A mental health system which places reliance on family caregivers, may be as much or more coercive than legally mandated coercion in the form of CTOs.

The international policy direction towards community-based care has much in common with the community focus of mental health care in less developed countries. However, mental illness often involves complexities and difficulties that are not readily amenable to untrained family and community caregivers. Agencies such as PIMHNet are attempting to bridge a divide between primary and community-based models of care, and extending the skills and expertise of practitioners in responding to mental illness. A related issue is that in some countries of Oceania there are high levels of stigma about mental illness, which is resistant to traditional understandings of mental distress.

Despite the need, expressed by developing countries themselves, for better understanding of mental illness and for policies and education aimed at improving care of people with mental illness, developed countries need to be cautious in providing policy advice and clinical training in less developed countries. Mental health policies, models of care, and legal frameworks that work in one country will not necessarily work in another. This is clearly demonstrated in the case of mental health legislation in Tonga and Samoa, where Western models of legislation, which assume the availability of a range of services, appear to have little impact on practice.

The most recent policy direction of the WHO continues the twentieth century's emphasis on community-focused care, but also reflects the international growth of the recovery movement in mental health and recent concerns for human rights (Saxena et al. 2013). Related to this, recent analysis of mental health legislation has questioned the long-accepted standard of danger to self and others due to mental illness as an acceptable criterion for compulsion in mental health care (Szmukler et al. 2014). Interpretation of the 2007 UNCRPD has held that legislation based on membership of a category (such as people with mental illness) is discriminatory. It is likely that no Oceania countries have mental health legislation that is non-discriminatory under the requirements of the UNCRPD. The UNCRPD also establishes rights for people with mental illness that are a significant extension of rights currently provided under most countries' codes of health rights and mental health legislation. The Australian states that have recently referenced the UNCRPD in revising their legislation (Callaghan and Ryan 2012) have not gone so far as to adopt the 'fusion' model of legislation (Dawson and Szmukler 2006) that would avoid discrimination.

Some of the real force of the UNCRPD lies in the Optional Protocol, an additional agreement that allows the Committee on the Rights of Persons with Disabilities to examine complaints from individual citizens of signatory countries. All but three of the Oceania countries have signed the UNCRPD, although only one, Australia, has signed the Optional Protocol (United Nations 2014). For individuals with mental illness, in countries with little in the way of formal legal protection, or where those protections are not realized in practice, the UNCRPD offers the possibility of legal redress outside the country in which the breach of rights occurred. However, this form of redress can only occur if the region has a disability rights tribunal under the UNCRPD (Perlin 2012, 2013). Currently, unlike other regions of the world, the Asia-Pacific Region does not have such a tribunal and so the realization of rights under the UNCRPD is at the whim of governments. The establishment of an Asia-Pacific disability rights tribunal would make a considerable contribution to protecting the human rights of people with mental illness in the region.

Conclusion

Community mental health care in the Oceania region is characterized by a wide divergence between developed and less developed countries. While the developed countries can claim well-developed mental health services with a high level of provision, they also show the world's highest rates of use of formal coercion in the form of CTOs. In the less-developed countries individuals may struggle to access intervention as many of those countries lack mental health infrastructure. New rights instruments such as the UNCRPD offer extensions of human rights to people with mental illness, and most Oceania countries have signed it. However, absence of a regional rights tribunal potentially limits the realization of those rights.

References

Adu Krow W, Funk, M, Nad P, et al. (2013). *WHO profile on mental health in development (WHO proMIND): Papua New Guinea*. Geneva: World Health Organization.

Benson J, Pond D, Funk M, et al. (2011). A new era in mental health care in Vanuatu. *International Journal of Family Medicine*, **2011**:590492.

Blignault I, Iaurel J, Nampon R, et al. (2011). Establishing mental health policy and services in Vanuatu. *Asia-Pacific Psychiatry*, 3:76–79.

Burns T, Yeeles K, Molodynski A, et al. (2011). Pressures to adhere to treatment ('leverage') in English mental healthcare. *British Journal of Psychiatry*, 199:145–150.

Callaghan S, Ryan CJ (2012). Rising to the human rights challenge in compulsory treatment– new approaches to mental health law in Australia. *Australian and New Zealand Journal of Psychiatry*, 46:611–620.

Carney T (2012). Australian mental health tribunals—'space' for rights, protection, treatment and governance? *International Journal of Law and Psychiatry*, 35:1–10.

Chang O (2011). Mental health care in Fiji. *Asia-Pacific Psychiatry*, 3:73–75.

Chappell D (2010). From sorcery to stun guns and suicide: the eclectic and global challenges of policing and the mentally ill. *Police Practice and Research: an International Journal*, 11:289–300.

Dawson J (2005). *Community treatment orders: international comparisons.* Dunedin: Otago University Print.

Dawson J, Gledhill K (ed.). (2013). *New Zealand's Mental Health Act in practice.* Wellington: Victoria University Press.

Dawson J, Szmukler G (2006). Fusion of mental health and incapacity legislation. *British Journal of Psychiatry*, 188:504–509.

Enoka MIS, Tenari A, Sili T, et al. (2013). Developing a culturally appropriate mental health care service for Samoa. *Asia-Pacific Psychiatry*, 5:108–111.

Fadgen T (2013). *Mental health policy transfer and localisation in Samoa and Tonga: International organisations, professionals and indigenous cultures.* Unpublished doctoral thesis, University of Auckland.

George K (2010). Vanuatu: happiest nation on earth, mental health and the Church. *Australasian Psychiatry*, 18:63–65.

Government of Samoa (2006). *Samoa mental health policy.* Apia: Government of Samoa. Available at: http://www.health.gov.ws/Portals/189/Final%20Mental%20Health%20Policy.pdf

Jeffery R (2013). Enduring tensions: transitional justice in the Solomon Islands. *The Pacific Review*, 26:153–175.

Kisely SR, Xiao J, Preston NJ (2004). Impact of compulsory community treatment on admission rates: survival analysis using linked mental health and offender databases. *British Journal of Psychiatry*, 184:432–438.

Kisely S, Xiao J, Crowe E, et al. (2014). The effect of community treatment orders on outcome as assessed by the Health of the Nation Outcome Scales. *Psychiatry Research*, 215:574–578.

Koka BE, Deane FP, Lambert G (2004). Health worker confidence in diagnosing and treating mental health problems in Papua New Guinea. *South Pacific Journal of Psychology*, 15:29–42.

Leckie J (2007). Unsettled minds: gender and settling madness in Fiji. In: *Psychiatry and empire* (ed. S. Mahone, M. Vaughan), pp. 99–123. Basingstoke: Palgrave Macmillan.

Light E, Kerridge I, Ryan C, et al. (2011). Community treatment orders in Australia: rates and patterns of use. *Australasian Psychiatry*, 20:478–482.

Light EM, Kerridge IH, Ryan CJ, et al. (2012). Out of sight, out of mind: making involuntary community treatment visible in the mental health system. *Medical Journal of Australia*, 196:591–593.

MacKinnon D, Coleborne C (2003). Deinstitutionalisation in Australia and New Zealand. *Health and History: Journal of the Australian and New Zealand Society of the History of Medicine*, 5(2): 1–16.

Mahone S, Vaughan M (ed.) (2007). *Psychiatry and empire*. Basingstoke: Palgrave Macmillan.

McIvor R (1998). The community treatment order: clinical and ethical issues. *Australian and New Zealand Journal of Psychiatry*, 32:223–228.

Ministry of Health (2014a). *Mental health and addiction: service use 2011/12*. Wellington: Ministry of Health.

Ministry of Health (2014b). *Office of the Director of Mental Health. Annual report 2013*. Wellington: Ministry of Health.

Monahan J (2011). Mandated psychiatric treatment in the community—forms, prevalence outcomes and controversies. In: *Coercive treatment in psychiatry. Clinical, legal and ethical aspects* (ed. TW Kallert, JE Mezzich, J Monahon), pp. 33–48. Chichester: John Wiley and Sons.

Newton-Howes G, Lacey C, Banks D (2014). Community treatment orders: the experiences of Non-Maori and Maori within mainstream and Maori mental health services. *Social Psychiatry and Psychiatric Epidemiology*, 49:267–273.

O'Brien AJ (2014). Community treatment orders in New Zealand: regional variability and international comparisons. *Australasian Psychiatry*, 22:352–356.

O'Brien AJ, Kydd RR, Frampton C (2011). Social deprivation and use of mental health legislation in New Zealand. *International Journal of Social Psychiatry*, 58:581–586.

Perlin ML (2012). Promoting social change in Asia and the Pacific: the need for a disability rights tribunal to give life to the UN Convention on the Rights of Persons with Disabilities. *George Washington International Law Review*, 44:1.

Perlin ML (2013). Human rights law for persons with disabilities in Asia and the Pacific: the need for a disability rights tribunal. *Journal of Policy and Practice in Intellectual Disabilities*, 10:96–98.

Poltorak M (2013). The efficacy and self-efficacy of treatment. *Medical Anthropology Quarterly*, 27:272–291.

Preston NJ, Kisely S, Xiao J (2002). Assessing the outcome of compulsory psychiatric assessment in the community: epidemiological study in Western Australia. *British Medical Journal*, 324:1244.

Richardson E, McSherry B (2010). Diversion down under—programs for offenders with mental illnesses in Australia. *International Journal of Law and Psychiatry*, 33:249–257.

Richardson E, Thom K, McKenna B (2013). The evolution of problem-solving courts in Australia and New Zealand: a trans-Tasman comparative perspective. In: *Problem solving courts* (ed. RL Weiner, EM Branks), pp. 185–210. New York: Springer.

Ryan CJ, Callaghan S, Large M (2010). Long time, no see-Australians with mental illnesses wait too long before independent review of detention. *Alternative Law Journal*, 35:147–148.

Saxena S, Funk M, Chisholm D (2013). World Health Assembly adopts comprehensive mental health action plan 2013–2020. *The Lancet*, 381:1970–1971.

Segal SP, Burgess PB (2006). Extended outpatient civil commitment and treatment utilization. *Social Work in Health Care*, 43(2/3):37–51.

Segal SP, Preston N, Kisely S, Xiao J (2009). Conditional release in Western Australia: effect on hospital length of stay. *Psychiatric Services*, 60:94–99.

Singh AN, Orotaloa P (2011). Psychiatry in paradise–the Solomon Islands. *International Psychiatry*, 8:38–40.

Suzuki A (2006). *Madness at home. The psychiatrist, the patient, and the family in England, 1820–1860*. Berkeley, CA: University of California Press.

Szmukler G, Daw R, Callard F (2014). Mental health law and the UN Convention on the Rights of Persons with Disabilities. *International Journal of Law and Psychiatry*, 37:245–252.

Tone C (2007). Samoa's mental health sector in need of attention. *New Zealand Herald*, 14 June. Available at: http://www.nzherald.co.nz/world/news/article.cfm?c_id=2&objectid=10445676

Thom K (2014). New Zealand Mental Health Review Tribunal characteristics and outcomes 1993–2011. *Australasian Psychiatry*, **22**:341–344.

United Nations (2014). United Nations Enable. Convention and optional protocol signatures and ratifications. Available at: http://www.un.org/disabilities/countries.asp?navid=12&pid=166 (accessed 12 December 2014).

Webster S, Allnutt J, Boss P (2013). Implementation and evaluation of a mental health program for Ni Vanuatu nurses. *Journal of Nursing Education and Practice*, 3:177–186.

World Health Organization (2011). *Mental health atlas*. Geneva: World Health Organization.

World Health Organization (2013). *World health statistics 2013*. Geneva: World Health Organization.

World Health Organization/University of Auckland (2005). *Situational analysis of mental health needs and resources in Pacific Island countries*. Report to WHO on a Technical Support Programme for mental health services organization in the Western Pacific. Geneva: World Health Organization. Available at: http://www.who.int/mental_health/policy/Pacific_islands_needs_assessments.pdf

Chapter 21

Regional themes

Andrew Molodynski

Introduction

The preceding six chapters have highlighted a range of issues regarding coercion in community mental health care, and indeed regarding health care in its widest sense. This chapter considers some of these issues and attempts to draw them together under a number of recurrent themes. To get an overview, United Nations population and country data for 2010 are shown in Table 21.1.

The enormity of the task of collecting information and the amount of variety forced us to depart from our initial idea of covering each continent in a separate chapter. Asia is so large and diverse it would have been impossible to give it any more than super-ficial consideration in one chapter. All authors battled with the dilemma of achieving geographical spread while commenting in sufficient detail to move beyond simply a roll call of places, laws, and concerns. The paucity of available information regarding mental health care was apparent throughout.

The key emergent themes appear to be as follows:

(1) The increasingly coercive nature of (relatively) well financed mental health ser-vices in high-income group countries with the increasing focus of legislation on public protection and the widening of those potentially subject to it.

(2) The central role of the family and other 'non-statutory' carers in providing care for people with severe mental illness in the community in low- and middle-income group countries.

(3) The absolute coerciveness of a lack of available treatment for those with mental illnesses in many poorer countries in an age of sustained global inequality (see Figure 21.1). The same may also be said for those in poorer areas of wealthier coun-tries, with income gaps widening over recent decades (Wilkinson and Pickett 2009).

(4) The lack of evidence on the prevalence and outcomes of coercion outside a small number of well-established centres. This is compounded by the fact that most of the available evidence is irrelevant for the majority of the world's population as it is reliant upon services, models of care, and societal structures and beliefs that either do not exist or would not be locally acceptable.

(5) Legislation that has the potential to support change may not be feasible in many countries because of a lack of resources, and is ignored by others. These are often the countries where coercion is most clearly visible within communities.

(6) Stigma and its enabling role in both 'statutory coercion' and that practised by fam-ilies and communities.

Table 21.1 United Nations population and country data from 2010

	Population (millions)	**Number of countries/important areas (UN designated)**
Africa	1,031,084	58
Americas	942,692	53
Asia	4,165,440	50
Europe	740,308	48
Oceania	36,659	23

These broad themes and their causes and implications will be considered in turn after brief summaries of each region.

Africa

In terms of coercion the most striking issues identified in Africa relate to lack of resources, attitudes, stigma, and the role of the family and traditional healers. As Chapter 19 describes, life expectancy is significantly lower than elsewhere (only

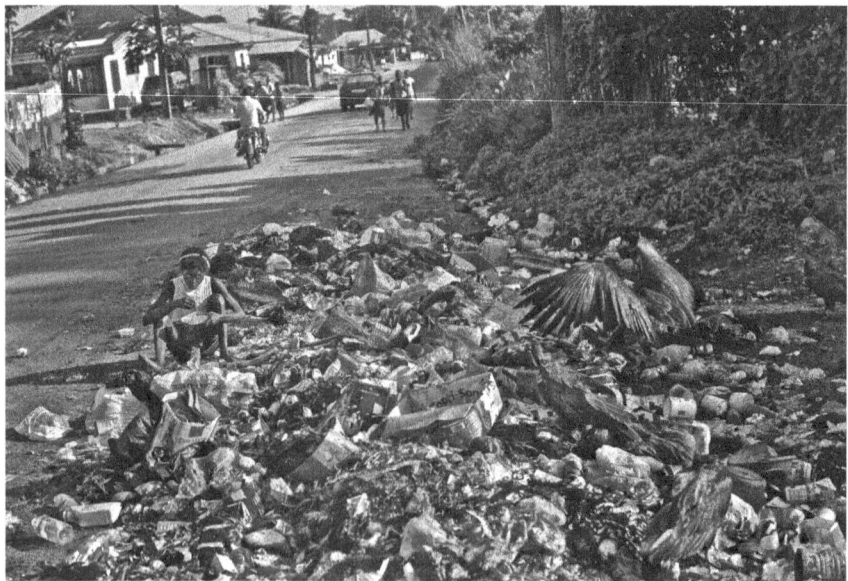

Figure 21.1 Mental health is not a priority to the state government of the Niger Delta. Many people with mental illness and/or intellectual disability are abandoned to the streets where they wander searching for food and shelter. The Niger Delta, Nigeria. October 2012. Photo Robin Hammond/Panos.

56 years) and nearly two-thirds of the continent's population live in slum-like conditions. Many countries have very small health budgets and large numbers of people die from infections and other preventable causes. Given this, it is perhaps no surprise that the care of people with long-term mental health problems is often a low priority. However, the lack of provision goes beyond simple poverty, and the financial allocation for mental health in many Sub-Saharan countries is proportionately much lower than one would expect.

A number of countries lack mental health legislation or policy, or have maintained woefully outdated versions. Attitudes are in some parts distressingly negative, for example a survey of Nigerian medical students 65% reported that mental illness was God's punishment (see Figure 21.2). The stigma of mental illness is a particularly persistent stain and affects help-seeking behaviour by individuals and families as well as working against the provision of adequate and humane treatment. This is undoubtedly implicated in the decision by many to turn to so-called traditional healers. Such practitioners vary enormously, and no doubt there are examples of humane and person-centred support. However, there are clear examples of neglect and abuse, highlighted in the literature and the photobook *Condemned* by Robin Hammond (2013). No cultural interpretation or adjustment is needed when discussing people being tied to trees, beaten, and inadequately fed.

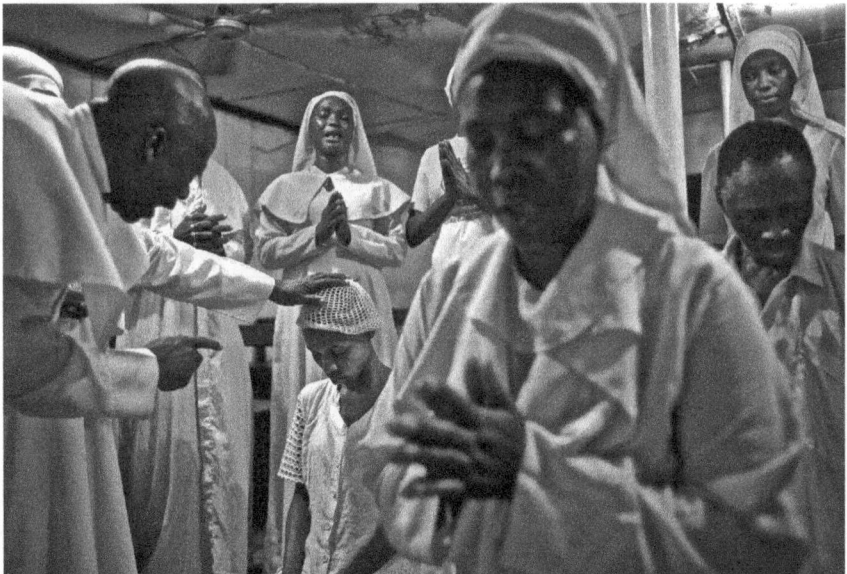

Figure 21.2 Christ's Universal Spiritual Hospital claims, through the power of prayer, to be able to heal mental illness. In a society that cannot trust government organizations, churches have become a sanctuary from the perceived wickedness and greed of the modern culture. In regions where both fortune and sickness are attributed to the spirit world, mental illness is considered a curse. Spiritual remedies are often sought. The Niger Delta, Nigeria. October 2012. Photo Robin Hammond/Panos.

Health centres provided by the state or non-governmental organizations often lack facilities for basic treatments. The absence of treatment is an under-recognized and under-discussed form of coercion. Inadequate treatment may result in more adverse effects and people may spend far longer in institutional settings, often with very limited comfort and freedom, than in wealthier countries. The impossibility of receiving evidence-based treatments for recognized health conditions is undoubtedly undermining of autonomy.

The Americas

Chapter 15 clearly articulates the striking differences between North and South America in terms of economy and culture. The USA and Canada both have highly funded and organized services with well-established and recently reviewed legislation. Countries further south do not have the same resources or (in general) organizational structures. The situation varies across countries, with an emphasis in North America on the state's response to illness while in the south the responsibility is often seen as shared with families, or even largely the family's domain.

Much of the research evidence and wider literature considered in this book originates in North America, especially the USA. It has come to dominate the field in both scope and amount. Perhaps the most influential of this research will, over time, come to be Monahan's seminal study on leverage in mental health care (Monahan 2005). This examines non-statutory pressures brought to bear upon individuals to encourage them to accept treatment.

Both the USA and Canada have adopted increasingly coercive mental health legislation over recent decades, with widespread coverage of laws to compel those in the community to accept treatment and support against their will. This is despite the lack of robust evidence for effectiveness as described in Chapters 4 and 5. Laws have often been introduced after high-profile tragedies, such as Kendra's Law in New York after the tragic murder of Kendra Webdale by a man with a psychotic illness who was off treatment (Sjöström et al. 2011). Both countries have complex federal legislatures, with states and provinces having different legal and practical arrangements for care, often very marked ones. This means that people living geographically close to each other or even in the same social network may be subject to strikingly different legislation when unwell, with no clear evidence or rationale for such differences. It is widely quoted that there are more mentally ill people in prison than in hospital in the USA (Fazel and Danesh 2002) and there have been a number of cases of shockingly degrading and coercive treatment in custody.

Countries in South America vary significantly in terms of economic resources, culture, and politics. Services are fairly rudimentary in many. Kohn (2005) reports that up to 75% of people do not get the care they need and Rondon (2009) states that in Peru 'the unavailability and inaccessibility of mental healthcare is the most important rights issue'. These echo some of the observed difficulties in Africa, and highlight the coerciveness inherent in the lack of necessary treatment. The situation in general, however, is less severe than in some parts of Africa, and most countries have some form of specific legislation with safeguards built in. Again, given the relative lack of statutory services, families are crucially important in the care of those with ongoing disability and this is poorly understood, little described, and hardly researched.

Asia

There are a bewildering variety of cultures and health-care systems in Asia, providing a major challenge to coverage in this volume. Themes of social inequality, stigma, and relative or absolute lack of health care are common. What care exists tends in countries, such as India and Pakistan, to be either institutional or provided by families. Extensive coercion can be a feature of both. In India the administration of covert medication is common. This usually involves placing medication surreptitiously in food or drink to achieve compliance without either the knowledge or the consent of the individual. There is little access to legislation with rights of appeal or other safeguards. At times covert medication may avoid damaging conflict but it is clearly coercive and denies individuals their right to make a key decision about their care. It appears to reflect the prevailing stigma in Indian society and elsewhere regarding the value of the mentally ill. The Erwadi tragedy, a dreadful incident in which more than 20 people died shackled as fire swept through the 'healing temple' where they were kept, demonstrated the damaging effects of stigma combined with an absence of modern, effective health care or a reluctance to accept it (Patel 2006). The use of ECT without an individual's consent also remains common, though reportedly less so than previously.

Other countries covered in Chapter 16 have health-care systems devastated by decades of conflict. Obvious examples are Iraq and Afghanistan. Both are rebuilding services significantly, and as is demonstrated by the developments in Aceh Province in Indonesia, terrible disaster (whether natural or human-made) can provoke positive change alongside investment.

Even wealthy countries such as Saudi Arabia have relatively poorly developed community services and most care is provided by families. Guilt and shame are important features of local culture and limit the autonomy of many mentally ill patients cared for in family homes.

The spread of legislation is increasing, as exemplified in Pakistan. As legislation is often modelled on Western legal frameworks, it generally promotes patients' rights and includes mechanisms for appeal. A pervasive issue, however, is an inability to fully and routinely implement legislation and thus protect rights because of inadequate resources and prevailing cultural assumptions.

Europe

One cannot discuss the care of the mentally ill in the community and human rights in Europe without acknowledging the grotesque abuses of the Nazi government in the late 1930s and 1940s, ably assisted by prominent psychiatrists (Strous 2007). The realization of the extent of these abuses has set the tone for much of what has happened since with the development of international legislation and safeguards. Despite these there have since been well-documented abuses of psychiatry in the Soviet Union (Bonnie 2002.). Developments in legislation and international agreements are outlined both in Chapter 18 on Europe and Chapter 13 on human rights. The majority of European countries have established mental health systems, recently updated specific legislation, and policies. There is significant variation in practice, however, with institutional care being the mainstay of treatment in a number of countries, especially those in the former Soviet Union (Knapp et al. 2006). The vast majority of European countries are high-income group countries, and they generally allocate significant resources to mental health care. All countries have mental health policy and legislation, though there are variations in content and approach. Many countries now have specific powers to compel acceptance of treatment in the community and well-resourced teams with 'no dropout' policies to provide intensive community service and enforce this. This combination of enabling legislation and available personnel is seen by some as unacceptably coercive; at the same time it may enable excellent care. The evidence does not support either position (Burns et al. 2013; Maughan 2013) and it is likely the reality is more nuanced, with variation between individuals and services. These variations are likely to be important but are poorly understood.

It is perhaps in Europe that those who use services have the loudest voice and are increasingly involved in designing and providing services. 'Co-production', the process by which patients and families are intrinsically involved in service design (Boyle and Harris 2009), is widely adopted in many states in western Europe across health and social care; mental health care is no exception. Quantitative and qualitative research on coercion is now being increasingly undertaken in Europe, an important recent example being the ambitious EUNOMIA study (Kallert et al. 2005).

Oceania

The majority of Oceania's population lives in its only two high-income group nations, Australia and New Zealand. Both countries have comprehensive mental health legislation with rights of appeal and independent scrutiny. They were also both early adopters of powers to compel in the community and, especially in some parts of Australia, are heavy users of community treatment orders (CTOs). Indeed, in one Australian state approximately 1 in every 1000 people is subject to community compulsion; this is the general population not specifically those with mental health problems! Elsewhere use is much lower in states with similar levels of education, health care, and funding and with similar civil societies. This variation, as with that in the USA, is disquieting and does not reflect an evidence-based approach to health care.

Elsewhere in Oceania, things are generally quite different. In Papua New Guinea (PNG), there are many challenges relating to lack of resources and structure. As has been described in other regions with very limited health care, other forms of healing are employed. Sorcery is a particular issue in PNG, both as a proposed treatment for mental illness and as a widely understood cause of it. Samoa has embraced 'family-focused mental health care' in which health staff and family work together on individualized care plans. It sounds a little like (but perhaps better than) what many wealthy countries aspire to in their highly funded specialized teams. The legislation in Samoa is based on an Australian model but CTOs are little used.

Southeast Asia

Several regional experts declined the opportunity to contribute to the chapter on Southeast Asia (Chapter 17), citing concerns regarding negative outcomes from describing the situation in China. We are immensely grateful to those who agreed. This serves to highlight wider concerns that will be no surprise to the reader. Our information regarding China is therefore 'external'. It is striking that in the world's most populous country the use of unarguably the 'world's best medication' for psychosis (clozapine) is so extensive. It undoubtedly leads to greater rates of symptomatic recovery and functioning. The evidence suggests, however, that it is used without the safeguards that are mandatory in other countries and this means that patients are not protected from the 1% risk of agranulocytosis. This is a condition where the medication destroys a person's resistance to infection and means that a common cold can kill (and frequently does). The authors suggest that this position may stem from the very strong collectivist culture in China particularly, with the overall 'good' for society weighing more heavily than the rights of an individual to protection from harm. Collectivism is a common theme in this chapter, as are shame and guilt, especially in a Japanese context. It appears that in Japan the stigma surrounding mental health problems in general and schizophrenia in particular is severe. A name change from 'Seishin Bunretsu Byo' or 'mind split disease' to 'Togo Shitcho Sho' or 'integration disorder' in 2002 has significantly improved the information given by psychiatrists to their patients, with an increase in diagnosis sharing from 36% to 70% (Sato 2006).

The positive developments in Aceh following the higher rates of mental illness after the devastating tsunami of 2004 gives hope that even relatively low-income countries can embrace principles of community care, fairness, and autonomy. Reportedly, this collaboration between the state, foreign non-governmental organizations, and the local population has led to significant increases in those receiving treatment and significant reductions in the use of shackling.

Emergent themes

Increasingly coercive legal regimes in high-income group countries

The developments in mental health laws in many countries over the last two decades has undoubtedly led to greater safeguards and certainty for many people with mental illness, both those in institutions and those in hospitals.

Across North America, Europe, and many countries in Asia, Africa, and the Americas rights of appeal and independent review of those in involuntary treatment have been introduced. However, at the same time, this process of updating has included the explicit provision of powers to compel acceptance of treatment for those not considered to require hospital admission. This includes people who are not in the acute phase of illness and who retain both insight and capacity. Such powers, as has been described previously, remain controversial and there is limited evidence to support their use. However, they are used. It is the variation in use that is perhaps most striking (Dawson 2007; HSCIC 2015), as illustrated in Table 21.2.

Table 21.2 Differing rates of use of community treatment orders (CTOs) between jurisdictions

Location	Rate of CTO use per 100,000 population
Victoria, Australia (2005)	60
District of Columbia, USA (2004)	54
New Zealand (2003)	44
Queensland, Australia (2004)	43
Maricopa County, Arizona, USA (2004)	31
England and Wales (2014)	15
Western Australia (2004)	10
Tennessee, USA (2004)	10
Ontario, Canada (2003)	2

Changes in mental health legislation in wealthy countries typically involve input from a wide variety of sources, including politicians, clinicians, lawyers, service user representatives, and the media and public. They are certainly not examples of a pure 'evidence-based' approach to health-care interventions, and probably rightly so. However, the competing demands of these groups can lead to the adoption of legislation in response to high-profile tragedies, such as Kendra's Law, or a general perception that community care is 'failing', as seems to have been at least partly the view in England and Wales. In other countries, such as some of the Scandinavian countries, the ideology behind introduction has been about treatment and integration. It may be that CTOs that are essentially a form of conditional discharge are less likely to be viewed as integrative than the more flexible 'community start' orders that can form an alternative to admission in countries such as New Zealand, Scotland, and Norway. Outreach services with 'no drop out' policies are seen by most stakeholders as a positive and empowering development, as their purpose is to maximize the delivery of treatment and thus promote social functioning and autonomy. However, when combined with a legal mandate they can undoubtedly be experienced as coercive.

The family as a source of support and control

All the regional chapters and Chapter 10 have highlighted the role of families in caring for the mentally ill. It is clear that the role of the family is of huge importance, even in countries with highly developed care systems and an individualistic orientation. The literature to date, with a few exceptions, fails to convey just how different and important the family is in middle- and low-income group countries across the world. In Africa, Asia, South America and the Caribbean, and Oceania the family may be the sole source of support with only rudimentary or even absent health service support. Families in these desperate situations clearly do what they can to care for their unwell relatives. This frequently involves coercion. The coercive use of covert medication is widespread, and is particularly well described in the Indian context. Undoubtedly it occurs elsewhere, including in wealthy countries where the issue is often 'skirted around' by professionals.

The use of domestic cells in Japan, strapping and tying in much of Africa and Asia, and the highly supportive but restrictive care by relatives in parts of the Middle East are all born out of a desire to help. They represent the same strategy of containment provided in other countries by statutory services with legal safeguards. Though international conventions have moved us forward enormously over recent decades, it is safe to assume that such conventions are irrelevant if you are caring for an acutely disturbed family member with no access to support or treatment. Not all the countries where these situations are described are poor, however. Japan and Saudi Arabia have highly developed economies, national mental health legislation, and well-funded health services. The issues of family containment here appear predominately related to shame and stigma.

The absence of care as coercion

The preceding chapters have eloquently and repeatedly reported on the absence of effective treatment for the mentally ill in many low- and middle-income group countries. For those with an illness it is a fundamental right to be able to access safe and effective care. Though most of this book and all of the preceding international literature focuses entirely on 'active coercion', this passive form of coercion is perhaps the most widespread, the most serious, and the most toxic of all. The situation where a person in distress does not have the ability to elect to receive treatment is undoubtedly one where they have diminished autonomy and are coerced to remain unwell. This often results in them then being subject to 'active coercion' such as shackling to prevent disturbed and/or damaging behaviour.

The lack of evidence outside a small number of countries

The overwhelming body of empirical evidence has been gathered in high-income group countries with developed services and a focus on the rights of the individual. For example research in Oceania is overwhelmingly from Australia and New Zealand, that in the Americas is from the USA and Canada, and that in Europe is from the UK, Scandinavia, and some other western European states. We tend to see this evidence as generalizable across cultures and it may well be—at least across high-income group countries with developed health-care systems and a high regard for individual rights. It is clear from the preceding chapters that it may not be generalizable to countries with fewer resources, less developed systems, and a collective culture. The evidence therefore does not serve the majority of the global population. The research funding structure perpetuates this inequality. One example is the expanding literature on CTOs and assertive community treatment. While this is undoubtedly important and affects the care of many thousands of people, the fact that many countries do not have any mental health laws or community services renders it irrelevant to them. Furthermore the concentration of resources and personnel on such questions is likely to reduce the focus on approaches to understanding and reducing the use of coercion elsewhere.

In the same way, most of the thought about ethical, legal, and human rights issues around coercion is heavily weighted towards Western societies. It also is irrelevant to many. Although there is some evidence of a new literature arriving from outside the traditional sources, particularly in India, there is a considerable way to go. A research agenda of coercion and global mental health is needed.

The limitations of legislation and international conventions

The United Nations Convention on Rights of Persons with Disabilities (UNCRPD) (United Nations 2006) has led to a significant shift in how we think about the care of the mentally ill, and in principle affords them much greater safeguards. However, it is presumably irrelevant to those families in most of the developing world striving to keep their relative alive without support or treatment. They will almost certainly not even have heard of it.

On a national level there are numerous examples in Sub-Saharan Africa and elsewhere of countries that have signed and ratified this convention and have their own national coverage of mental health legislation. An example could be somewhere such as Nigeria, mentioned in more detail in Chapter 19. However, resources in general and those allocated to mental health care in particular do not allow for the respect of either conventions or law. High levels of coercion thus persist in the vacuum left behind—a vacuum often filled, of necessity, by patients' families.

Stigma and shame

The examples of Japan and Saudi Arabia make it clear that the exclusion from society and coercion of the mentally ill is not just about finance. These two countries in particular have very serious difficulties with stigma, as described in the preceding chapters. There are active attempts in Japan to reduce this, including the radical step of changing the terminology used, but much work remains. The media play a significant role in stigma reduction (though in practice they often play a part in promoting stigma). This is the case across many countries (Thornicroft 2007; Wehring 2011), and there is evidence that it is not decreasing. Indeed it may become even more powerful in today's world where we are delivered news updates and information continuously. Stigma reduction programmes have had mixed success and it remains an issue everywhere, regardless of the availability of education, finance, or health care. It does appear to be a particularly damaging issue in some countries, however. In Indonesia, the story from Aceh is encouraging. Though it should not take one of the worst natural disasters of all time to improve mental health services it does appear that the combination of significant international resources and knowledge and a government willing to change things has led to a step change in provision, an increased focus on human rights, and the reduction of stigma. Perhaps most important was the experience of trauma. Following the severe trauma and dislocation experienced by nearly all the population, symptoms of mental illness became 'normal' and as a result perhaps something to be less ashamed and afraid of.

Conclusions

In the preceding chapters we have, probably for the first time, attempted to provide a global overview of coercion in community mental health care. The overview could never be comprehensive as there is simply too much to describe and a very limited literature on which to base such a description. However, a number of themes are clear and are described above.

The introduction of increasingly sophisticated mental health legislation in many countries with multiple layers of safeguards is undoubtedly a good thing. Legislative changes, however, have frequently ushered in increased powers to compel, particularly powers to compel outside institutions. This has made compulsion a reality to many more people and a possibility for even more. This shift has occurred in the absence of evidence for effectiveness.

International conventions to protect the rights of vulnerable people have increased in sophistication, scope, and ambition but are simply irrelevant for much of the world's population. Many are either unaware of them or do not have the luxury of living in a country that can attend to them, even if many have ratified them. Many of these places do not even have the ability to provide basic mental health care, and some do not seem to want to, as demonstrated by their very small allocations from overall health-care budgets. This combination of very limited resources, little legislation, and stigma is undoubtedly a toxic cocktail leading to the abuses of human rights described in some of the preceding chapters. Families are left alone to cope with burdens they should not have to carry and often feel themselves compelled to resort to mechanisms that severely limit freedom and autonomy. The resources invested internationally in medical and legal research in this field offer little for them or for policy makers in their countries as they draw too heavily on priorities and practices of wealthy countries with an alien societal structure.

It appears that coercion in wealthy countries may be an issue of 'too much' treatment and in poorer countries it is one of 'too little' treatment. While the richness of detail in the preceding chapters underlines the complexity beneath that bald distinction, perhaps there is something in it?

References

Bonnie RJ (2002). Political abuse of psychiatry in the Soviet Union and in China: complexities and controversies. *Journal of the American Academy of Psychiatry and the Law*, **30**:136–144.

Boyle D, Harris M (2009). *The challenge of co-production* [a discussion paper]. London: New Economics Foundation.

Burns T, Rugkåsa J, Molodynski A, et al. (2013). Community treatment orders for patients with psychosis (OCTET): a randomised controlled trial. *The Lancet*, **381**:1627–1633.

Dawson J (2007). Factors influencing the rate of use of community treatment orders. *Psychiatry*, **6**(2):42–44.

Fazel S, Danesh J (2002). Serious mental disorder in 23 000 prisoners: a systematic review of 62 surveys. *The Lancet*, **359**:545–550.

Hammond R (2013). Condemned. Mental health in African countries in crisis. Brooklyn, NY: FotoEvidence.

HSCIC (Health and Social Care Information Centre) (2015). Mental health. URL: http://www.hscic.gov.uk/mentalhealth

Kallert TW, Glöckner M, Onchev G, et al. (2005). The EUNOMIA project on coercion in psychiatry: study design and preliminary data. *World Psychiatry*, **4**:168–172.

Knapp M, McDaid D, Mossialos E, et al. (2006). *Mental health policy and practice across Europe*. London: McGraw-Hill International.

Kohn R, Levav I, de Almeida JM, et al. (2005). Mental disorders in Latin America and the Caribbean: a public health priority. *Revista Panamericana de Salud Pública*, **18**:229–240.

Maughan D, Molodynski A, Rugkåsa J, et al. (2013). A systematic review of the effect of community treatment orders on service use. *Social Psychiatry and Psychiatric Epidemiology*, **49**:651–663.

Monahan J, Redlich AD, Swanson J, et al. (2005). Use of leverage to improve adherence to psychiatric treatment in the community. *Psychiatric Services*, **56**:37–44.

Patel V, Saraceno B, Kleinman A (2006). Beyond evidence: the moral case for international mental health. *American Journal of Psychiatry*, **163**:1312–1315.

Rondon MB (2009). Peru: mental health in a complex country. *International Psychiatry*, **6**:12–14.

Sato M (2006). Renaming schizophrenia: a Japanese perspective. *World Psychiatry*, **5**:53–55.

Sjöström S, Zetterberg L, Markström U (2011). Why community compulsion became the solution—reforming mental health law in Sweden. *International Journal of Law and Psychiatry*, **34**:419–428.

Strous RD (2007). Psychiatry during the Nazi era: ethical lessons for the modern professional. *Annals of General Psychiatry*, **6**:8.

Thornicroft G, Rose D, Kassam A, et al. (2007). Stigma: ignorance, prejudice or discrimination? *British Journal of Psychiatry*, **190**:192–193.

United Nations (2006). *Convention on the Rights of Persons with Disabilities*. New York: United Nations. URL: http://www.un.org/disabilities/convention/conventionfull.shtml

United Nations (2010). Population Division: world population prospects. URL: http://esa.un.org/unpd/wpp/Excel-Data/population.htm

Wehring HJ, Carpenter WT (2011). Violence and schizophrenia. *Schizophrenia Bulletin*, **37**:877–878.

Wilkinson RG, Pickett K (2009). *The spirit level: why more equal societies almost always do better*. London: Allen Lane.

Chapter 22

Conclusions

Andrew Molodynski, Tom Burns,
and Jorun Rugkåsa

Introduction

In the preceding chapters, experts in the relevant fields have for the first time gathered clinical and research evidence from around the world and combined this with a focus on key aspects of coercion in the community. The task was not easy, as the lack of evidence and information from many countries was striking. The painstaking enquiries by the authors of a number of chapters, especially those recounting the issues from each geographical region, have allowed unprecedented exploration and documentation of the subject. The chapters have been wide ranging and embraced health-care provision, culture, legislation, stigma, societal structure, and (perhaps most crucially of all) economy. Also, at the heart of the care of the severely mentally ill everywhere is the interpersonal management of an individual in great distress and who may well be at risk; the vast majority of the time, regardless of location, a great proportion of care happens within families.

Much has been written previously about coercion within institutions. This has been for good reason: historically the majority of 'recognizable' mental health care occurred within institutions—examples of coercion have often been highlighted within them—and these aspects of coercion are more easily measured. Where records are kept, episodes of involuntary admission, restraint, and forced medication can be counted, logged, and compared. As will be obvious to the reader, such recording is more difficult with many of the coercive practices covered in this book. The use of legal compulsion in the community can be counted and comparisons made and we will shortly return to the striking results of such research efforts. What happens within relationships, whether they are with professionals, with family carers, or with others, is much harder to measure and document. These pressures, or informal coercion, are likely to be more important overall in community mental health care because relationships between people (whether they be professionals or family/community members) are ubiquitous whereas legislation permitting compulsion is not.

The changing face of mental health care provision

This book would have been strikingly different had it been written 50 years ago. The overwhelming majority of people treated for severe mental illness in high- and middle-income group countries at that time were managed in institutions with little (if any) provision for community care except within family networks or local communities. In low-income group countries the vast majority of care would also not have been provided by health services. The former situation has changed radically, the latter much less so. As outlined in the early chapters of this volume both the practice of community mental health care and the legal structures to support it have developed significantly in recent decades with deinstitutionalization and the 'move into the community'. The fact that many people with severe symptoms, poor psychosocial functioning, and risky behaviours were living outside hospital meant it was inevitable that powers to compel acceptance of treatment would be introduced.

Large asylums (the largest of which housed around 13,000 inhabitants) which were entirely self-contained societies with factories, farms, and social clubs, began shrinking from the 1950s and closing from the 1980s onwards. Admissions became shorter and more explicitly directed towards improving symptoms and functioning. While this was generally positive, concerns increased regarding the potential for many of those who were discharged to live lives of poverty and neglect and to have limited access to effective treatment. The phenomenon of the 'revolving-door patient' became prominent in psychiatric thought and writing. Such individuals would be admitted to hospital for treatment and support but then promptly disengage after discharge and deteriorate, requiring readmission. How would we manage these situations? The response was two-fold. First the provision of services to reach out to such people and second the introduction of powers to compel acceptance of medication and/or support. The provision of enhanced services has undoubtedly benefitted many, but at the same time (as described in Chapter 6) it can be perceived as pressurizing and coercive. The evidence regarding the effect of such services on patient outcomes is equivocal and contested but they are common in well-developed and adequately funded systems.

The deinstitutionalization movement did not occur to any significant extent outside North America, Europe, and Australasia. There were very many fewer institutions to begin with and many still provide the only meaningful psychiatric care available. This is described in the chapters covering Asia, Southeast Asia, and Africa in particular. Services to reach out to the mentally ill simply do not exist in these regions. Families are left with the very difficult alternatives of long journeys to distant facilities, seeking help from traditional or alternative healers, or of caring for their affected family member themselves as best they can.

The spread of legislation and the use of informal coercion

The early part of this book described the reasons for the spread of legislation permitting compulsion, its nature, and the justifications for it. Legislation has spread both geographically and in terms of the number of patients who are subject to it. In general, the increased adoption of legislation with safeguards of any type is positive. In many countries this has included powers to compel those outside hospital, and recent updates of legislation in different countries have broadened scope. There are now over 75 jurisdictions in over 30 countries with formal powers to compel in the community, as illustrated in the maps in Figures 3.1 and 3.2. International conventions have been developed by bodies such as the United Nations and adopted in many countries to support humane care and incentivize and/or enforce the introduction of safeguards. However, in many places the adoption of regulations on paper has not guaranteed adequate implementation of such safeguards.

The current state of the evidence, from rigorous randomized trials and systematic analyses to locally led descriptions, audits, and evaluations of services, does not support the effectiveness of such legislation, despite positive findings in some local studies. Even so, there is little doubt that such powers will continue to expand geographically, and possibly be enhanced where they already exist.

Informal coercion may be used alongside legal powers where they exist or instead of them. Pressures are ubiquitous in human relationships so their existence in health care is to be expected. Chapters 6–11 described in detail what these pressures might look like and how they might be experienced, and outlined the small but growing evidence base regarding their prevalence and associations. Again, this evidence is only from wealthy countries with established and relatively well-funded health-care systems. It seems reasonable to assume that similar pressures exist elsewhere but likely to be manifest in relationships with important members of the patient's social network. Statutory services that do not exist cannot be coercive, but the coercion will still be present and manifested in different forms and in different relationships.

The effect of society and stigma

Different societies perceive and manage those with mental illness differently. Several chapters in this book have suggested a particularly clear divide between those cultures that hold the rights of the individual and their autonomy paramount and those cultures that may be described as predominantly collectivist in outlook. It is important that we acknowledge cultural differences, as they affect both care and legislation. The chapters on Asia and Southeast Asia clearly describe the differences in approach in a number of countries that have led both to significant gains in autonomy and welfare but at times the continued use of very coercive treatment, such as beatings and the use of 'domestic cells' in Japan. It is perhaps too easy for those of us living in a very different cultural context to be critical of this. For example, the use of restraint and handcuffing by the authorities in many high-income group countries is an integral aspect of compulsion and in some sense analogous to the tying and restraint of individuals described in other regions of the world. How different in reality is the process of being handcuffed by law enforcement officers and transported to a hospital to being tied up by family members and driven to a traditional healing facility? Perhaps the former is more regulated and safer, with the training of staff and legislative safeguards, but the latter is done by people who are known to the affected person and is thus less impersonal.

The preceding chapters have repeatedly highlighted the negative role of stigma. No country can say it does not have problems with stigmatizing attitudes to the mentally ill, but the severity of their consequences varies. The evidence from medical students and health workers in Nigeria (Chapter 19) is striking, and it can be seen why alternative healers, with their frequent use of manifest coercion, may be turned to in such a culture. The pictures taken by Robin Hammond (Figures 19.1 and 19.2) require little explanation or interpretation. Similar situations appear to exist in countries where the protection of piety and honour are deemed particularly important, two highlighted examples being Japan and Saudi Arabia. Both are noteworthy as they are not countries with financial problems or limited health-care investment—quite the opposite. Stigmatizing media coverage of rare incidents of violence by the mentally ill has undoubtedly been important in the development of more coercive legislations. In the UK many more psychiatric patients are subject to legal compulsion now than at any other time in its history.

The effect of economic conditions

Health care for the mentally ill is limited or absent in many countries. Limited or absent treatment choices are a profoundly coercive force. People are simply unable to access evidence-based interventions for their illness and consequently remain unwell. The subsequent effect of this will often be significant coercion, whether from prolonged spells in institutional settings or periods of limited freedom of movement and autonomy in the family home. Practices such as chaining and tying are undoubtedly coercive and damaging and anything that can be done to reduce and stop such strategies must be pursued. However, it is important to recognize that such measures are generally born out of desperation. It is the absence of any other means to keep people alive and safe that is truly coercive. This is open to change; if countries investing only a tiny proportion of already meagre health resources would rethink their priorities then mental health care could be transformed.

In wealthier countries, community resources funded by the state or insurance systems can assertively follow up the severely mentally ill, supporting many who would previously have been held in institutions. However, seeing people frequently, 'no drop-out policies', and supervised medications may be experienced as coercive by patients. This is especially likely when interventions are backed up by compulsory powers and when pressures are felt in various domains of life, such as housing and finance. Rates of experienced coercion appear to be highest in the USA, perhaps reflecting different prevailing attitudes towards universal welfare benefits compared with more liberal societies in western Europe and Australasia with broadly similar services.

The inadequacy of the evidence

Evidence-based medicine and evidence-based justice are important. The evidence base that exists in regard to community compulsion and the use of 'informal coercion' is problematic. It originates almost exclusively from a small number of high-income countries with strong cultural traditions of promoting individual rights and with well-financed mental health services. There is little or nothing from whole continents or regions, particularly Asia and Africa. This renders the 'evidence' largely irrelevant to the majority of the world's population.

What evidence does exist tends to be contradictory and beset by methodological problems as this is a very difficult area, both ethically and practically, to research.

Randomized controlled trials (RCTs) are very hard to conduct and have been criticized on the grounds of representativeness. They do, however, report consistent results unlike the other sources of evidence and show no effects of community compulsion, positive or negative. So far no accurate and reliable measure of leverage or informal coercion has been developed. We are left, as a result, with instruments that have undeveloped psychometrics such as data on reliability and validity. The measurement of outcomes of coercion in community mental health care is in its infancy.

The future

Coercion is ubiquitous in human relationships and its impact most powerful in those that are imbalanced. Stigma, poverty, and the symptoms of illness combine to make the severely mentally ill amongst the most vulnerable in any society. It can be difficult to support the most unwell to access treatment where it exists, especially as the majority are now in the community rather than institutions. The widespread adoption of coercive practices is therefore understandable. Coercive practices of many sorts, whether the use of legal mechanisms, the employment of leverage, or the development of 'coercive contexts', are generally born out of a desire to help those who are suffering. The alternative of simply not intervening to help seems unthinkable.

However, little is known about these practices and we do not know whether they produce better or worse outcomes. The one area that does have a reasonably large evidence base is community treatment orders (CTOs). It provides a consistent picture of the kinds of people who are made subject to compulsion and the way in which it is deployed. The higher levels of evidence, RCTs, meta-analyses, and systematic reviews, uniformly conclude that the practice does not benefit patients. They also find no evidence of harm. Despite this lack of effectiveness, powers are being increasingly used where they exist and are increasingly adopted where they do not.

The first step in quantifying and understanding such complex phenomena as coercion in the community is to accurately define and measure them. We hope that this volume has helped with the former and identified ways in which we can do the latter and then put such knowledge to use. Identification and measurement are crucial, with a strong focus on research led by—or at the very least involving—those who have used services and been subject to compulsion. The issues are complex and may not be fully appreciated by those on the 'giving' as much as those on the 'receiving' end of coercive practices.

Mental health law with safeguards is being increasingly adopted around the world and most countries have ratified important human rights legislation over recent years. There is, however, a difference between ratification and real life adoption of the principles of such conventions, that renders them of limited (if any) use across large swathes of several continents. Where there are ineffective legal regimes and grossly inadequate health services how can we expect such safeguards to be upheld? The international literature and informed debate in this field tends to gloss over such inconvenient facts. In many countries in Africa, Asia, and South America the resources simply do not exist to provide even basic mental health care. Overall health budgets are small and competing demands are large. It is likely that this, combined with widespread stigma in some countries, leads to disproportionately small budgets. The real coercion here is the absence of services to treat people and support their families. This vacuum leads many to pursue what avenues they can to try to help and protect the affected individual. This may involve significant coercion with ongoing distress and psychiatric symptoms.

We hope this book has at least served to paint a global picture for the first time, shining a light on the plight of many. The issues are bewilderingly complex and surprisingly simple at the same time. There are many things we can do to move forwards and minimize the use of coercion, while allowing those who urgently need treatment and support to receive it, even if they are reluctant. The remedies differ in different places and are often primarily related to economic conditions. Even in impoverished conditions, education and support may lead to enhanced mental health budgets and thus less reliance on simple containment.

There is an urgent need to understand more about coercion, and this must start with identification and accurate measurement, before moving on to robust studies of outcome. If all such research is conducted in a small group of similar countries, as it has been so far, it will continue to serve us poorly. If research can be conducted more widely it will be enriched, be perceived to be more relevant, and as a result its findings much more likely to be applied.

Organizations such as the Mental Disability Advice Centre, service user groups, and some health professionals continue to advocate for refined and improved practice in line with international conventions, and robust enforcement of the latter. This is welcome and can be supported by the evidence gathering and material support of wealthier countries.

Campaigns against stigma are widespread but have had varying success. The need for them is obvious and ongoing and there are signs of change in many countries, as shown in Japan after the radical step of changing the name of schizophrenia. Some innovative projects supported by international organizations have enabled changes in societal attitudes and the availability of care. The example of Aceh, devastated by the 2004 tsunami, is described in Chapter 17 and may provide a model for other low-income countries to build on.

None of the things outlined above are easy, but all are possible. The first step, however, must be to acknowledge the central importance of the issue and talk openly and honestly about how we can improve the care of the most disadvantaged members of our societies.

Index